Advances in Management of Voice and Swallowing Disorders

Advances in Management of Voice and Swallowing Disorders

Editor

Renée Speyer

MDPI • Basel • Beijing • Wuhan • Barcelona • Belgrade • Manchester • Tokyo • Cluj • Tianjin

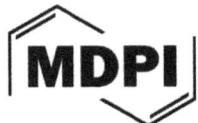

Editor
Renée Speyer
University of Oslo
Norway

Editorial Office
MDPI
St. Alban-Anlage 66
4052 Basel, Switzerland

This is a reprint of articles from the Special Issue published online in the open access journal *Journal of Clinical Medicine* (ISSN 2077-0383) (available at: https://www.mdpi.com/journal/jcm/special_issues/Voice_Swallowing_Disorders).

For citation purposes, cite each article independently as indicated on the article page online and as indicated below:

LastName, A.A.; LastName, B.B.; LastName, C.C. Article Title. *Journal Name* **Year**, *Volume Number*, Page Range.

ISBN 978-3-0365-4083-2 (Hbk)
ISBN 978-3-0365-4084-9 (PDF)

© 2022 by the authors. Articles in this book are Open Access and distributed under the Creative Commons Attribution (CC BY) license, which allows users to download, copy and build upon published articles, as long as the author and publisher are properly credited, which ensures maximum dissemination and a wider impact of our publications.

The book as a whole is distributed by MDPI under the terms and conditions of the Creative Commons license CC BY-NC-ND.

Contents

Renée Speyer
Advances in Management of Voice and Swallowing Disorders
Reprinted from: *J. Clin. Med.* **2022**, *11*, 2308, doi:10.3390jcm1109230 1

Katina Swan, Renée Speyer, Martina Scharitzer, Daniele Farneti, Ted Brown and Reinie Cordier
A Visuoperceptual Measure for Videofluoroscopic Swallow Studies (VMV): A Pilot Study of Validity and Reliability in Adults with Dysphagia
Reprinted from: *J. Clin. Med.* **2022**, *11*, 724, doi:10.3390/jcm11030724 5

Duy Duong Nguyen, Antonia M. Chacon, Daniel Novakovic, Nicola J. Hodges, Paul N. Carding and Catherine Madill
Pitch Discrimination Testing in Patients with a Voice Disorder
Reprinted from: *J. Clin. Med.* **2022**, *11*, 584, doi:10.3390/jcm11030584 21

Daniel Novakovic, Meet Sheth, Thomas Stewart, Katrina Sandham, Catherine Madill, Antonia Chacon and Duy Duong Nguyen
Supraglottic Botulinum Toxin Improves Symptoms in Patients with Laryngeal Sensory Dysfunction Manifesting as Abnormal Throat Sensation and/or Chronic Refractory Cough
Reprinted from: *J. Clin. Med.* **2021**, *10*, 5486, doi:10.3390/jcm10235486 35

Catherine Madill, Antonia Chacon, Evan Kirby, Daniel Novakovic and Duy Duong Nguyen
Active Ingredients of Voice Therapy for Muscle Tension Voice Disorders: A Retrospective Data Audit
Reprinted from: *J. Clin. Med.* **2021**, *10*, 4135, doi:10.3390/jcm10184135 57

Jin-Woo Park, Chi-Hoon Oh, Bo-Un Choi, Ho-Jin Hong, Joong-Hee Park, Tae-Yeon Kim and Yong-Jin Cho
Effect of Progressive Head Extension Swallowing Exercise on Lingual Strength in the Elderly: A Randomized Controlled Trial
Reprinted from: *J. Clin. Med.* **2021**, *10*, 3419, doi:10.3390/jcm10153419 87

Felix Caffier, Tadeus Nawka, Konrad Neumann, Matthias Seipelt and Philipp P. Caffier
Validation and Classification of the 9-Item Voice Handicap Index (VHI-9i)
Reprinted from: *J. Clin. Med.* **2021**, *10*, 3325, doi:10.3390/jcm10153325 95

Yuna Kim, Hyun-Il Kim, Geun-Seok Park, Seo-Young Kim, Sang-Il Choi and Seong Jae Lee
Reliability of Machine and Human Examiners for Detection of Laryngeal Penetration or Aspiration in Videofluoroscopic Swallowing Studies
Reprinted from: *J. Clin. Med.* **2021**, *10*, 2681, doi:10.3390/jcm10122681 111

Anna Sinkiewicz, Agnieszka Garstecka, Hanna Mackiewicz-Nartowicz, Lidia Nawrocka, Wioletta Wojciechowska and Agata Szkiełkowska
The Effectiveness of Rehabilitation of Occupational Voice Disorders in a Health Resort Hospital Environment
Reprinted from: *J. Clin. Med.* **2021**, *10*, 2581, doi:10.3390/jcm10122581 121

Wen Song, Felix Caffier, Tadeus Nawka, Tatiana Ermakova, Alexios Martin, Dirk Mürbe and Philipp P. Caffier
T1a Glottic Cancer: Advances in Vocal Outcome Assessment after Transoral CO_2-Laser Microsurgery Using the VEM
Reprinted from: *J. Clin. Med.* **2021**, *10*, 1250, doi:10.3390/jcm10061250 131

Renée Speyer, Anna-Liisa Sutt, Liza Bergström, Shaheen Hamdy, Bas Joris Heijnen, Lianne Remijn, Sarah Wilkes-Gillan and Reinie Cordier
Neurostimulation in People with Oropharyngeal Dysphagia: A Systematic Review and Meta-Analyses of Randomised Controlled Trials—Part I: Pharyngeal and Neuromuscular Electrical Stimulation
Reprinted from: *J. Clin. Med.* **2022**, *11*, 776, doi:10.3390/jcm11030776 . . . . **149**

Renée Speyer, Anna-Liisa Sutt, Liza Bergström, Shaheen Hamdy, Timothy Pommée, Mathieu Balaguer, Anett Kaale and Reinie Cordier
Neurostimulation in People with Oropharyngeal Dysphagia: A Systematic Review and Meta-Analysis of Randomised Controlled Trials—Part II: Brain Neurostimulation
Reprinted from: *J. Clin. Med.* **2022**, *11*, 993, doi:10.3390/jcm11040993 . . . . **201**

Renée Speyer, Reinie Cordier, Anna-Liisa Sutt, Lianne Remijn, Bas Joris Heijnen, Mathieu Balaguer, Timothy Pommée, Michelle McInerney and Liza Bergström
Behavioural Interventions in People with Oropharyngeal Dysphagia: A Systematic Review and Meta-Analysis of Randomised Clinical Trials
Reprinted from: *J. Clin. Med.* **2022**, *11*, 685, doi:10.3390/jcm11030685 . . . . **243**

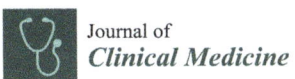

Editorial

Advances in Management of Voice and Swallowing Disorders

Renée Speyer [1,2,3]

1. Department Special Needs Education, Faculty of Educational Sciences, University of Oslo, 0318 Oslo, Norway; renee.speijer@isp.uio.no
2. Curtin School of Allied Health, Faculty of Health Sciences, Curtin University, Perth, WA 6102, Australia
3. Department of Otorhinolaryngology and Head and Neck Surgery, Leiden University Medical Centre, 2333 ZA Leiden, The Netherlands

Dysphagia (swallowing disorders) and dysphonia (voice disorders) are both common disorders within the area of laryngology. Recent research has focused on instrument development and psychometrics, and the development of methods with robust measurement properties (i.e., validity, reliability and responsiveness). In addition, newly developed interventions are waiting to be evaluated to objectify treatment effects. The outcomes of both instrument development and intervention studies will support evidence-based clinical practice and research [1]. This current Special Issue of the *Journal of Clinical Medicine* (*JCM*) describes both ongoing instrument development and intervention studies targeting people with dysphagia and dysphonia.

A reliability study by Kim et al. [2] confirmed that computer analysis using a deep learning model could detect laryngeal penetration or aspiration in recordings of videofluoroscopic swallowing studies (VFSS) as reliably as human examiners. These results provide further evidence to support the clinical application of deep learning technology in addition to the visuoperceptual evaluation of videofluoroscopic and possibly endoscopic recordings of swallowing. A second study on VFSS by Swan et al. [3] reported on the development of the Visuoperceptual Measure for Videofluoroscopic swallow studies (VMV). The authors piloted their newly developed measure to determine its validity and reliability using classical test theory analysis, informed by the consensus-based standards for the selection of health measurement instruments (COSMIN) guidelines [4]. The results are promising and validation will be continued using larger sample sizes and an item response theory paradigm approach.

Two studies refer to assessment in dysphonia. The study by Caffier et al. [5] determined the test–retest reliability of the nine-item Voice Handicap Index (VHI-9i), a self-reported questionnaire on the subjective impact of voice disorders on patients' daily lives. The authors found high reliability and, as presented here, revised the VHI-9i severity levels based on receiver operating characteristic (ROC) curve analysis. The second study, by Nguyen et al. [6], used pitch discrimination as a key index of auditory perception, to discriminate between people with and without a voice disorder. The authors advocate the use of pitch discrimination testing during comprehensive voice assessment.

Three studies report on behavioural interventions in people with voice and swallowing problems. Madill et al. [7] describe the efficacy of active ingredients in the treatment of muscle-tension voice disorders, whereas Sinkiewicz et al. [8] present the results of a rehabilitation program for occupational voice disorders in teachers. A third study by Park et al. [9] on lingual strengthening training in older adults compares a new progressive resistance exercise with a conventional isometric tongue strengthening exercise. Two other intervention studies by Song et al. [10] and Novakovic et al. [11] report on CO_2 laser microsurgery in patients with unilateral vocal fold cancer [10] and supraglottic botulinum toxin injection in laryngeal sensory dysfunction [11], respectively. All five of these intervention studies contribute to evidence-based clinical practice by objectifying the effects of distinct interventions in laryngology.

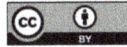

This Special Issue includes three more studies by Speyer et al. [12–14]: three systematic reviews and meta-analyses of interventions in people with oropharyngeal dysphagia. All three reviews use the same study methods. The reviews follow the PRISMA guidelines [15,16], and include the highest level of evidence only, thus excluding any other study designs except for randomised controlled trials. Two reviews report on neurostimulation: (1) pharyngeal and neuromuscular electrical stimulation; and (2) brain neurostimulation. Although describing promising results, protocol heterogeneity, potential moderators and inconsistent reporting of the methodology resulted in conservative generalisations and interpretations of the meta-analyses. Both reviews confirmed the need for further randomised controlled trials with larger population sizes using standard protocols and reporting guidelines as achieved by international consensus. The third review reports on behavioural interventions. Again, although behavioural interventions show promising effects in people with oropharyngeal dysphagia, due to high heterogeneity between studies, generalisations of meta-analyses must be interpreted with care.

In summary, the studies included in this Special Issue contribute to instrument development and psychometrics, and to objectifying the effects of interventions in the area of laryngology. Future studies will continue to contribute to evidence-based clinical practice and research.

Funding: This research received no external funding.

Institutional Review Board Statement: Not applicable.

Informed Consent Statement: Not applicable.

Data Availability Statement: Not applicable.

Conflicts of Interest: The author declares no conflict of interest.

References

1. Speyer, R.; Cordier, R.; Farneti, D.; Nascimento, W.; Pilz, W.; Verin, E.; Walshe, M.; Woisard, V. White Paper by the European Society for Swallowing Disorders: Screening and Non-instrumental Assessment for Dysphagia in Adults. *Dysphagia* **2022**, *37*, 333–349. [CrossRef] [PubMed]
2. Kim, Y.; Kim, H.-I.; Park, G.; Kim, S.; Choi, S.-I.; Lee, S. Reliability of Machine and Human Examiners for Detection of Laryngeal Penetration or Aspiration in Videofluoroscopic Swallowing Studies. *Clin. Med.* **2021**, *10*, 2681. [CrossRef] [PubMed]
3. Swan, K.; Speyer, R.; Scharitzer, M.; Farneti, D.; Brown, T.; Cordier, R. A Visuoperceptual Measure for Videofluoroscopic Swallow Studies (VMV): A Pilot Study of Validity and Reliability in Adults with Dysphagia. *J. Clin. Med.* **2022**, *11*, 724. [CrossRef] [PubMed]
4. Mokkink, L.B.; Prinsen, C.A.; Bouter, L.M.; de Vet, H.C.; Terwee, C.B. The COnsensus-based Standards for the selection of health Measurement INstruments (COSMIN) and how to select an outcome measurement instrument. *Braz. J. Phys. Ther.* **2016**, *20*, 105–113. [CrossRef] [PubMed]
5. Caffier, F.; Nawka, T.; Neumann, K.; Seipelt, M.; Caffier, P.P. Validation and Classification of the 9-Item Voice Handicap Index (VHI-9i). *J. Clin. Med.* **2021**, *10*, 3325. [CrossRef] [PubMed]
6. Nguyen, D.D.; Chacon, A.M.; Novakovic, D.; Hodges, N.J.; Carding, P.N.; Madill, C. Pitch Discrimination Testing in Patients with a Voice Disorder. *J. Clin. Med.* **2022**, *11*, 584. [CrossRef]
7. Madill, C.; Chacon, A.; Kirby, E.; Novakovic, D.; Nguyen, D.D. Active Ingredients of Voice Therapy for Muscle Tension Voice Disorders: A Retrospective Data Audit. *J. Clin. Med.* **2021**, *10*, 4135. [CrossRef] [PubMed]
8. Sinkiewicz, A.; Garstecka, A.; Mackiewicz-Nartowicz, H.; Nawrocka, L.; Wojciechowska, W.; Szkiełkowska, A. The Effectiveness of Rehabilitation of Occupational Voice Disorders in a Health Resort Hospital Environment. *J. Clin. Med.* **2021**, *10*, 2581. [CrossRef] [PubMed]
9. Park, J.W.; Oh, C.H.; Choi, B.U.; Hong, H.J.; Park, J.H.; Kim, T.Y.; Cho, Y.J. Effect of Progressive Head Extension Swallowing Exercise on Lingual Strength in the Elderly: A Randomized Controlled Trial. *J. Clin. Med.* **2021**, *10*, 3419. [CrossRef] [PubMed]
10. Song, W.; Caffier, F.; Nawka, T.; Ermakova, T.; Martin, A.; Mürbe, D.; Caffier, P.P. T1a Glottic Cancer: Advances in Vocal Outcome Assessment after Transoral CO_2-Laser Microsurgery Using the VEM. *J. Clin. Med.* **2021**, *10*, 1250. [CrossRef] [PubMed]
11. Novakovic, D.; Sheth, M.; Stewart, T.; Sandham, K.; Madill, C.; Chacon, A.; Nguyen, D.D. Supraglottic Botulinum Toxin Improves Symptoms in Patients with Laryngeal Sensory Dysfunction Manifesting as Abnormal Throat Sensation and/or Chronic Refractory Cough. *J. Clin. Med.* **2021**, *10*, 5486. [CrossRef] [PubMed]

12. Speyer, R.; Sutt, A.L.; Bergström, L.; Hamdy, S.; Heijnen, B.J.; Remijn, L.; Wilkes-Gillan, S.; Cordier, R. Neurostimulation in People with Oropharyngeal Dysphagia: A Systematic Review and Meta-Analyses of Randomised Controlled Trials—Part I: Pharyngeal and Neuromuscular Electrical Stimulation. *J. Clin. Med.* **2022**, *11*, 776. [CrossRef] [PubMed]
13. Speyer, R.; Sutt, A.L.; Bergström, L.; Hamdy, S.; Pommée, T.; Balaguer, M.; Kaale, A.; Cordier, R. Neurostimulation in People with Oropharyngeal Dysphagia: A Systematic Review and Meta-Analysis of Randomised Controlled Trials—Part II: Brain Neurostimulation. *J. Clin. Med.* **2022**, *11*, 993. [CrossRef] [PubMed]
14. Speyer, R.; Cordier, R.; Sutt, A.L.; Remijn, L.; Heijnen, B.J.; Balaguer, M.; Pommée, T.; McInerney, M.; Bergström, L. Behavioural Interventions in People with Oropharyngeal Dysphagia: A Systematic Review and Meta-Analysis of Randomised Clinical Trials. *J. Clin. Med.* **2022**, *11*, 685. [CrossRef] [PubMed]
15. Page, M.J.; McKenzie, J.E.; Bossuyt, P.M.; Boutron, I.; Hoffmann, T.C.; Mulrow, C.D.; Shamseer, L.; Tetzlaff, J.M.; Akl, E.A.; Moher, D.; et al. The PRISMA 2020 statement: An updated guideline for reporting systematic reviews. *Int. J. Surg.* **2021**, *88*, 105906. [CrossRef] [PubMed]
16. Page, M.J.; Moher, D.; Bossuyt, P.M.; Boutron, I.; Hoffmann, T.C.; Mulrow, C.D.; Shamseer, L.; Tetzlaff, J.M.; Akl, E.A.; McKenzie, J.E.; et al. PRISMA 2020 explanation and elaboration: Updated guidance and exemplars for reporting systematic reviews. *BMJ* **2021**, *372*, n160. [CrossRef] [PubMed]

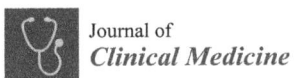

Article

A Visuoperceptual Measure for Videofluoroscopic Swallow Studies (VMV): A Pilot Study of Validity and Reliability in Adults with Dysphagia

Katina Swan [1], Renée Speyer [1,2,3], Martina Scharitzer [4], Daniele Farneti [5], Ted Brown [6] and Reinie Cordier [1,7,*]

1 Curtin School of Allied Health, Faculty of Health Sciences, Curtin University, Bentley, WA 6102, Australia; katina.swan@postgrad.curtin.edu.au (K.S.); renee.speijer@isp.uio.no (R.S.)
2 Department Special Needs Education, University of Oslo, 0315 Oslo, Norway
3 Department of Otorhinolaryngology and Head and Neck Surgery, Leiden University Medical Centre, 2333 ZA Leiden, The Netherlands
4 Department of Biomedical Imaging and Image-Guided Therapy, Medical University of Vienna, Waehringer Guertel 18-20, 1090 Vienna, Austria; martina.scharitzer@meduniwien.ac.at
5 Audiologic Phoniatric Service, Infermi Hospital Rimni, 47900 Rimini, Italy; lele.doc@libero.it
6 Department of Occupational Therapy, Faculty of Medicine, Nursing and Health Sciences, Monash University—Peninsula Campus, Frankston, VIC 3199, Australia; ted.brown@monash.edu
7 Department of Social Work, Education and Community Wellbeing, Northumbria University, Newcastle upon Tyne NE7 7YT, UK
* Correspondence: reinie.cordier@northumbria.ac.uk

Abstract: The visuoperceptual measure for videofluoroscopic swallow studies (VMV) is a new measure for analysing the recordings from videofluoroscopic swallow studies (VFSS). This study evaluated the reliability and validity of the pilot version of the VMV using classical test theory (CTT) analysis, informed by the consensus-based standards for the selection of health measurement instruments (COSMIN) guidelines. Forty participants, diagnosed with oropharyngeal dysphagia by fibreoptic endoscopic evaluation of swallowing, were recruited. The VFSS and administration of bolus textures and volumes were conducted according to a standardised protocol. Recordings of the VFSS were rated by three blinded raters: a speech-language pathologist, a radiologist and a phoniatrician. Inter- and intra-rater reliability was assessed with a weighted kappa and resulted in 0.889 and 0.944 overall, respectively. Structural validity was determined using exploratory factor analyses, which found four and five factor solutions. Internal consistency was evaluated with Cronbach's alpha coefficients, which found all but one factor scoring within an acceptable range (>0.70 and <0.95). Hypothesis testing for construct validity found the expected correlations between the severity of dysphagia and the VMV's performance, and found no impact of gender on measure performance. These results suggest that the VMV has potential as a reliable and valid measure for VFSS. Further validation with a larger sample is required, and validation using an item response theory paradigm approach is recommended.

Keywords: classic test theory; dysphagia; measure; psychometrics; videofluoroscopic swallow studies; VMV

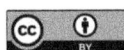

1. Introduction

Oropharyngeal dysphagia (OD) is a disorder that disturbs the sensory and physical processes of swallowing [1]. As not all aspects of OD can be observed externally, investigation of OD often necessitates the use of specialised instrumental examination procedures. The videofluoroscopic swallow study (VFSS) is an instrumental exam that uses recordings of dynamic fluoroscopies in an assessment of swallowing physiology and kinematics. VFSS is recognised as a gold-standard instrumental swallowing assessment and is widely used in clinical and research settings around the world [2]. However, the video recordings require skilled analysis for meaningful interpretation. Clinicians typically examine the videos by visuoperceptual means to make judgments about impairments and to plan and trial interventions [3]. Measures suitable for visuoperceptual analysis of dynamic images with robust psychometric properties are therefore essential for the assessment and treatment of OD.

Several visuoperceptual analysis measures have been developed for VFSS. Some target a single construct, such as aspiration, while others attempt to measure multiple constructs, such as lingual and pharyngeal movement, residue, cough and upper oesophageal sphincter (UES) function [4]. The constructs included in measures are just one facet the clinician must consider when choosing an appropriate tool for OD analysis. Measures must be reliable, valid and responsive, with key psychometric properties that describe whether a measure evaluates what it claims to assess and whether it does so in a consistent, repeatable manner [5].

Understanding the psychometric properties of OD measures is important given the complexity of OD as a clinical and diagnostic construct, where a phenomenon viewed on VFSS may be interpreted in multiple ways. For example, the presence of pharyngeal residue may be explained by any of the following: the contrast material preparation in the oral phase (weak tongue squeeze), poor pharyngeal constriction, anatomical abnormalities, surgeries obstructing bolus flow, impaired upper oesophageal sphincter functioning, and other dysfunctions [6]. Analysis of psychometric properties provides statistical evidence about the relationships between the items in the measure, the precision of the scale, and the association between the measure and the construct(s) of interest [7].

In recent years, the science of psychometric analyses applied to outcome measures has been scrutinised through the consensus-based standards for the selection of health measurement instruments (COSMIN) initiative [8]. The COSMIN initiative applied international multi-disciplinary expertise in psychometrics, research and measure development to formulate a methodology for evaluating outcome measures [5]. In a series of Delphi studies, consensus was reached on standardised definitions of psychometric properties, quality criteria for which properties should be reported, and recommended statistical methods to be used to investigate them. The COSMIN taxonomy encompasses nine psychometric properties, divided into three domains: reliability, validity and responsiveness [9–13]. The COSMIN checklist is an inventory of recommended criteria and statistical methods for studies on measurement properties [8].

The checklist was applied to VFSS visuoperceptual measures in a 2018 study, where psychometric properties were assessed in a combination of COSMIN ratings and quality criteria [4]. The authors found that visuoperceptual VFSS measures had overall indeterminate, limited or conflicting evidence of psychometric quality and concluded that there was insufficient evidence to recommend any of the VFSS measures reviewed [4]. Unclear or inadequate psychometric properties risk misapplication of the measure, while inaccurate measurement wastes resources and undermines the evidence base for clinical practice [14]. Thus, there is an urgent need for studies that focus on the development of VFSS measures that utilise sound statistical methods.

A new measure, the visuoperceptual measure for videofluoroscopic swallow studies (VMV) was created to address this gap. The process of developing a measure involves conceptualisation of the construct of interest, item/response scale generation (content validity), piloting the measure, preliminary evaluation, item refinement and reduction, and finally a large trial [15]. The VMV's content validity was established in an international Delphi study involving more than 50 experts in OD and VFSS from 27 countries. The constructs to be included in the VFSS analysis, the conversion of these constructs to items, and the operationalisation of these items were established via consensus across three Delphi rounds. The Delphi identified 32 constructs recommended for analysis, and between one and four items per construct [16]. These findings were used to create the pilot version of the VMV, which comprised 97 items. As a new measure, its psychometric properties are not established. Therefore, the aim of this study is to conduct a pilot evaluation of the VMV's

psychometric quality. Specifically, the objectives are to evaluate the following psychometric properties:
- inter- and intra-rater reliability
- structural validity
- internal consistency
- hypothesis testing for construct validity

2. Methods

2.1. Participants

This study was granted ethical approval by the Human Research Ethics Committees of The Medical University of Vienna And Curtin University (HRE2018-0151, April 2018 and March 2019). Adults with OD, diagnosed by fibreoptic endoscopic evaluation of swallowing (FEES) and referred for VFSS as part of their assessment plan, were recruited from the Medical University of Vienna between July 2019 and March 2020. As FEES and VFSS are complementary instrumental assessments, diagnosis of OD by FEES supported appropriate participant selection [17]. Informed consent was obtained from all participants.

In- and out-patients accessing services for OD were eligible if they satisfied the following inclusion criteria: (1) adults (>18yo) with a diagnosis of OD, (2) had been deemed by their treating clinician to be medically and cognitively appropriate for VFSS, and (3) to require VFSS to assess or manage their OD. Participants who had radical surgery of the head and/or neck were excluded.

A total of 40 participants were recruited. One patient was excluded due to data loss on the medical archive imaging system. Of the 39 remaining, 64% (n = 25) of participants were men and 36% (n = 14) were women. Participants ranged in age from 21 to 91 years (mean = 63.0 years, SD ± 17.0 years). The onset of OD (defined as the date of first symptoms) ranged from six days to five years prior to the VFSS, with onset less than 1 month prior to VFSS for 33% (n = 13), 1–6 months prior for 36% (n = 14), 7–12 months prior for 13% (n = 5), and more than 13 months prior for 18% (n = 7). Medical diagnoses in the participant group, while heterogeneous, can be grouped into four categories: cancer (primarily of head and neck), neurological disorder, surgery, and anatomical abnormality (Table S1—Aetiology of Oropharyngeal Dysphagia). Participants were assigned to groups based on the diagnosis which appeared most strongly associated with their OD diagnosis, based on consensus of the three authors (KS, RS, RC). For example, a participant with a history of lung cancer 20 years prior to VFSS who had a stroke the month before the VFSS was classified as 'Neurological disorder'. The anatomical abnormality group was comprised of conditions in which physical changes to bodily structures adjacent to and involved in the process of swallowing were the most likely cause of the OD (e.g., cervical spine abnormalities).

2.2. Equipment and Materials

The VFSS were performed by a radiologist on a fluoroscopy unit (Axiom Sireskop S3 fluoroscopy system, Siemens Healthineers; Siemens AG, Erlangen, Germany) with a Siricon high-dynamic-range image intensifier, spot film device and analog/digital acquisition at an image rate of 30 pulses/s. Patients were placed upright in a sitting position. The oropharynx and the proximal oesophagus were viewed in lateral projection and anterior-posterior positions. Boluses consumed was comprised of a non-ionic low-osmolar contrast (Omnipaque™), thickener (Nutilis Clear®), water and a cracker (Mini Toast, Delhaize®; Delhaize Group SA, Brussels, Belgium).

2.3. Protocol

Participants had part of their VFSS conducted according to a standardised protocol (Supplementary Materials, Figure S1). The protocol was designed to ensure participant safety by starting with small volumes of each texture (5 mL) and including cessation points if severe aspiration or residue was observed by the radiologist. As swallowing is affected by volume, texture and verbal instructions [18,19], the protocol included four different textures. These were administered using a standardised order, method and set of verbal instructions to maximise the variety of swallowing behaviours related to textures/volumes elicited, while controlling for the influence of the administrator. Textures/volumes were as follows: three trials of Thick (L3 International Dysphagia Diet Standardisation Initiative (IDDSI)), three trials of Thin (L0 IDDSI), four trials of pudding (L4 IDDSI), and one cracker (L7 IDDSI) [20] in four different volumes (5 mL, 10 mL, 20 mL, bite sized cracker). The average number of trials completed by the participants was seven (range 1–11), with the most common trial completed being 5 mL thick (completed by all 39 participants; however, data were lost from one due to technical issues, resulting in data from 38 participants for this trial). The VFSS was conducted by an experienced radiologist (>10 years' experience). The non-ionic low-osmolality contrast was mixed with food and fluids according to a standard recipe (Supplementary Materials, Table S2: Administration protocol [21]) and each was kept at room temperature prior to the procedure.

In addition to the VFSS, assessment of the participants' self-reported and observed functional health status (FHS) and clinician-perceived symptoms on VFSS were completed. Measures of FHS assess severity of OD symptoms from the perspective of daily functioning and impacts on participation in daily activities [22]. Participants who were referred for VFSS completed the Deglutition Handicap Index, Symptom subscale (DHI-S) [23] (a self-report FHS measure), and clinicians scored the Functional Oral Intake Scale (FOIS) [24] (an observational FHS measure) along with a 5-point ordinal scale to indicate the radiologist's overall impression of OD severity based on viewing VFSS. To overcome the pragmatic limitation of having a single rater scoring OD severity, data were triangulated by using two separate measures of OD severity. (Supplementary Materials, Table S3. Functional Health Status and Severity measures and Table S4. Functional Health Status and Severity measures scoring.).

2.4. Manual

A manual was constructed based on Delphi study results. This manual includes: detailed instructions on contrast preparation, administration, patient positioning, items with descriptions, response scales, instructions for rating items, and anchor images [16].

2.5. Raters, Consensus Meetings, Training and Rating

Three raters used the draft VMV, informed by the Delphi results [16]. One rater had qualifications in speech-language pathology, the others were physicians with qualifications in radiology and phoniatrics, respectively. All three raters had over 10 years of experience with OD and VFSS. In a consensus meeting, the raters scored one patient through a full protocol, including all 11 trials, working item by item as a group. Each draft VMV item was discussed, and the manual regularly referenced by the raters on the first trial (5 mL Thick). As the raters progressed through the trials in the protocol, only new items were discussed in detail unless there was disagreement in scoring. Adjustments were made to items and the manual based on this feedback. These adjustments included removing ambiguous language, adding additional anchor images and expanding response options. After six hours, a 100% group consensus was reached for each item. The raters then scored three VFSS recordings independently and convened for an additional two-hour consensus meeting to discuss questions about measure use and resolve any differences in ratings. This consensus process led to the development of the pilot version of the VMV. An overview of measure development and versions of the VMV is depicted in Figure 1.

All of the VFSS recordings were deidentified. Ratings were completed on 100% of recordings using the pilot VMV on Qualtrics (www.qualtrics.com accessed on 3 July 2020). The raters referred to the manual as needed. At least two weeks after initial rating, repeated ratings were completed on an additional six (15%) randomly selected participants' recordings by all three raters.

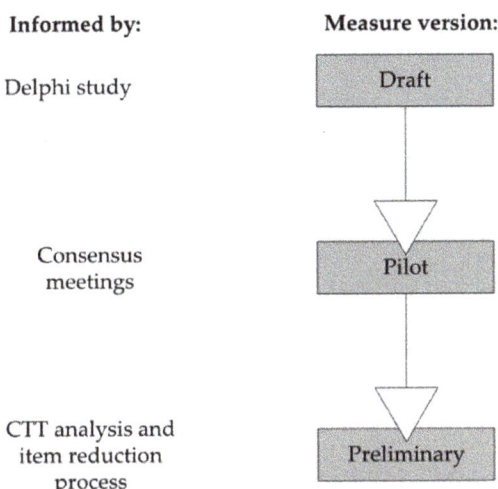

Figure 1. Overview of measure development and versions of the VMV.

2.6. Item Reduction

The pilot version of the VMV included 97 items, derived from results of the international Delphi study on visuoperceptual analysis of VFSS [16] and informed by the results of the consensus meetings regarding the draft version. After completing the ratings, the raters and the authors met to review the pilot version of the VMV item by item and reach consensus on whether each item should be kept, modified or rejected in the next iteration of the measure.

Decisions to retain or remove items were first made based on the clinical relevance of the item, where items considered less clinically important by a two-thirds majority of authors were removed. Consideration was then given to feasibility (e.g., items that are excessively time-consuming or difficult to view), redundancy between items, and the potential for multiple items to be consolidated into one (e.g., posterior movement of base of tongue and posterior pharyngeal wall contact with base of tongue). Lastly, all items which existed solely for the purposes of skip logic within the Qualtrics version (i.e., items which directed raters to a point further in the VMV based on their response) were removed and that item's response options consolidated to a related scale (Figure 2—skip logic—original question structure vs. skip logic removed with retained concept.). Skip logic questions contribute to survey structure by allowing only relevant questions to be shown to participants, but their content overlaps with constructs assessed by other items. Removal prevents this overlap from causing issues in statistical analysis. Reducing these items prior to statistical analysis simplified this analysis and allowed analysis to meet statistical assumptions. For example, factor analysis has minimum sample size requirements (100 observations and 5 times the number of cases per items) [25], meaning that factor analysis of 97 items would require a minimum of 485 cases, which was beyond the scope of the current pilot study.

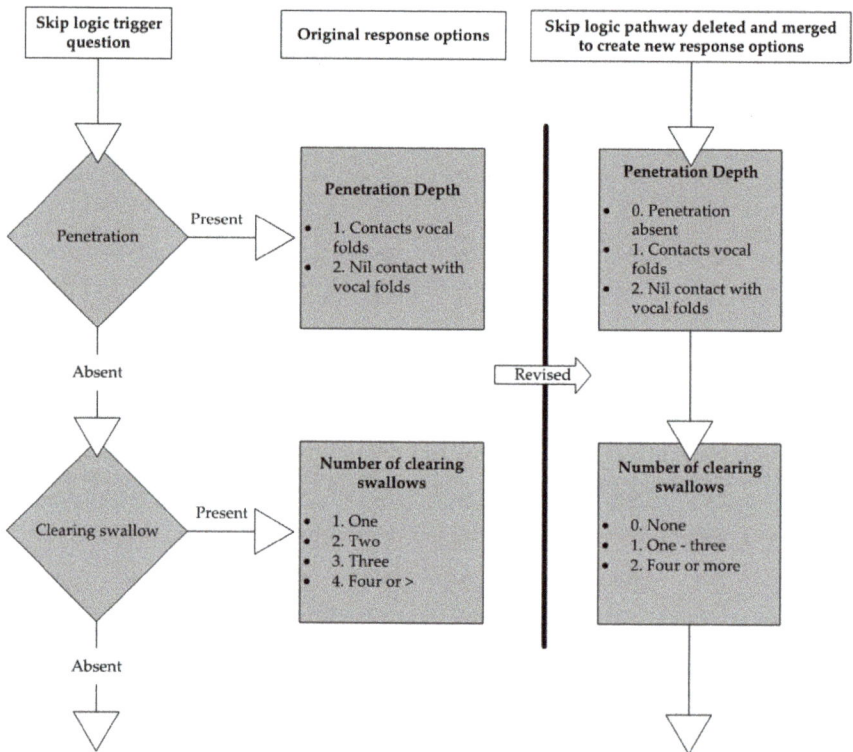

Figure 2. Skip logic—original question structure vs. removed skip logic with retained concept.

Item reduction following rater feedback is summarized in Figure 3, Item reduction from rater feedback. Details of items removed and rationales behind these decisions are described in Supplementary Materials, Table S5: Items removed or altered following rater consensus.

Item reduction resulted in the retention of 56 items. One new item, 'clearing swallow efficacy', was created with data derived from items rating the volume residue that remained after clearing swallow/s. An overview of items retained per domain is displayed in Supplementary Materials, Table S6: Included items per domain. The researchers then evaluated whether each of the items was clear (i.e., whether it was evident what the item was assessing, whether the manual clearly described what to examine and when to assess) and whether the response scale was adequate (i.e., whether there were too many/too few options in the response scale or ambiguous wording). Of the 57 items evaluated, one was considered unclear and 30 required revisions to their respective response scales.

2.7. Psychometric Properties

An analysis of psychometric properties was conducted using the COSMIN taxonomy guidelines [5]. The COSMIN initiative, formulated as a response to the differing terminology found in the literature, developed a unified taxonomy to describe the different measurement properties of instruments [8]. The COSMIN taxonomy was used within this study to define the properties from the domains of reliability and validity, and COSMIN recommendations for the statistical analysis of their quality were also applied [5,11–13].

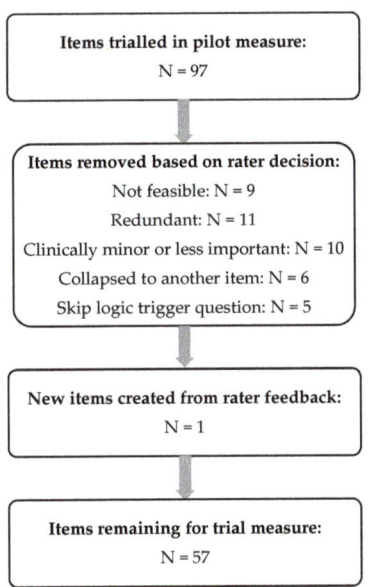

Figure 3. Item reduction from rater feedback.

Psychometric properties were determined if the characteristics of the data were appropriate for the intended statistical analysis (i.e., if the assumptions for statistical processing could be met) or if the analyses were feasible for the scope of a pilot study. Psychometric properties included in these analyses were:

- Reliability: The amount of variance in scores which are reflective of true differences in participant function rather than errors in the measure or process of rating [8]. This study included analysis of inter-rater (differences in scores between raters) and intra-rater (differences within a single rater's scores applied to repeated measures of the same participant).
- Structural Validity: The degree to which the scores adequately reflect the dimensionality of the construct of interest [8]. For example, the VFSS is expected to be multidimensional due to the complexity of the analysis, illustrated by the number of different constructs being assessed (e.g., movement of the bolus, actions of the anatomical structures) and distinct ways constructs are operationalised (i.e., spatial, volume, temporal).
- Internal consistency: The degree of interrelatedness among the VFSS items. Items which measure the same construct should demonstrate a relationship [8]. For example, the items 'lip seal', 'lingual movement', 'glossopalatal seal' and 'bolus control' are likely to show a close relationship and score highly on analysis of inter-relatedness as a group.
- Hypotheses testing for construct validity: The extent to which the scores on the measure agree with hypotheses which are theoretically consistent with the condition and the construct being measured [8]. In the case of the VFSS, for example, it is expected that lingual movement correlates strongly with oral residue, with a weaker correlation between lingual movement and parameters of the UES.

Psychometric properties omitted from this analysis were excluded if analysis was not possible, relevant or appropriate for the scope of a pilot. Criterion validity (Diagnostic performance) refers to the degree to which scores adequately reflect a gold-standard measure [8]. This measure for assessment of OD is generally considered to be instrumental assessment [2,26]; however, both FEES and VFSS require the use of visuoperceptual measures to analyse them. There is currently no measure with sufficient evidence of psychometric quality for it to be recommended as a gold-standard for VFSS or FEES [4]. Therefore, criterion validity could not be determined. Cross-cultural validity describes how well a translation of a culturally adapted measure replicates the original [8]. As this is a novel measure, developed only in English and tested in a single geographical location and cultural group, this property was irrelevant. Content validity is the degree to which the content of a measure is an accurate reflection of the construct of interest based on cognate literature and expert opinion [8]. Although not examined in this study, the VMV's content validity was developed via a Delphi study that is reported in a separate manuscript [16].

Responsiveness refers to a measure's ability to detect clinically important change over time [8]. Repeated VFSS procedures and assessment pre-post intervention were beyond the scope of the current pilot study. Systematic and random errors in scores that are due to rater or measure errors rather than a true representation of patient change are classed as measurement errors [8]. Statistical analysis requires a total score (summed score) to examine this property, which the pilot measure did not include. Finally, interpretability, the degree to which clinically meaningful connotations can be assigned to the numerical scores or to changes in scores [8], was excluded. Although this is not a psychometric property, its importance is recognised in the COSMIN taxonomy due to the clinical relevance of applying qualitative meaning to quantitative data [5]. This property was not included in this analysis due to the relatively small sample size and the preliminary form of the VMV.

2.8. Statistical Analysis

Reliability was analysed using quadratic weighted kappa. The quadratic weighted kappa assesses the degree of disagreement between raters (scale of difference between ordered scorings). Kappa was computed for each rater pair, then averaged to provide a single index of inter-rater reliability [27]. Cronbach's alpha coefficients were calculated to assess internal consistency for each factor individually as well as for the whole measure. A low Cronbach's alpha value (alpha < 0.70) indicates inadequate internal consistency, whereas a very high Cronbach's alpha value (alpha > 0.95) suggests redundancy of items in the factor, which could mean that there are too many items to assess the target construct [28].

With the exception of the inter- and intra-rater reliability analyses, scores from all three raters for 5 mL Thick were used for all analyses as this volume/texture had the largest case numbers available, allowing for statistical assumptions to be met. In the case of inter- and intra-rater reliability, analyses were performed between and within all raters, but were grouped by texture group (i.e., all volumes of Thick were grouped together for analysis). The grouping allowed for comparison of reliability between textures, as swallow behaviours and kinematics may be altered by texture differences [18].

The normality of the dataset will inform the use of parametric or nonparametric statistics. Structural validity was analysed via exploratory factor analysis (EFA) using principal component analysis. Factor analysis is a multivariate technique which identifies the strength of the relationships between items and the underlying latent constructs in the dataset [25]. These latent constructs are referred to as factors, or dimensions. For example, some items in the measure may demonstrate strong relationships with 'severity' while others appear related to 'aetiology'. In EFA, all items are tested for a relationship to every latent construct. A second analysis, known as confirmatory factor analysis (CFA), may be performed to assess whether the model's factor structure can be replicated. A CFA is only performed if a model of factors is an adequate representation of the theoretical constructs of interest. A CFA was not performed in this study due to the small sample size, which meant that statistical assumptions were not met [25].

Hypothesis testing for construct validity was conducted using Spearman rho correlations and Mann–Whitney U to test the following hypotheses, respectively:

Hypothesis 1 (H1). *70% of factors will be significantly positively correlated with the FOIS and 5-point ordinal scale.*

Hypothesis 2 (H2). *No significant differences between genders are expected on any of the item scores.*

3. Results

3.1. Functional Health Status and Severity Scores

DHI-S scores describe patient severity from self-rating of physical symptoms. Scores ranged from 13–43, with a median of 28.0 (SD ± 7.9, Q1 = 20.0, Q3 = 32.0). Five-point ordinal scale scores ranged from 1–5, with a median of 3.0 (SD ± 1.2, Q1 = 2.0, Q3 = 4.0). FOIS (reversed) scores ranges from 1–7, with a median of 3.0 (SD ± 1.9, Q1 = 2.0, Q3 = 5.0).

3.2. Reliability (Intra- and Inter-Rater Reliability)

A quadratic weighted Kappa assessed the degree to which raters produced consistency in the scores they applied between participants, and agreement within scores given to participants on repeated measures [29]. Weighted Kappas between pairs of raters ranged from 0.842 to 0.939, with minor differences between consistencies or views (Table 1. Inter-rater reliability—Weighted Kappa per Texture). The resulting overall average inter-rater weighted Kappa was in the 'strong' range, with an average weighted Kappa of 0.889 [27]. This indicates that raters had a high degree of agreement and suggests that the function or impairment of swallowing as measured by VMV items was coded similarly and consistently across the three raters.

Table 1. Interrater reliability—Weighted Kappa per Texture.

	Rater One vs. Two	Rater One vs. Three	Rater Two vs. Three	Average
Thick (L3)	0.932	0.886	0.882	0.900
Thin (L0)	0.930	0.866	0.860	0.885
Pudding (L4)	0.939	0.874	0.868	0.894
Solids (L7)	0.934	0.892	0.852	0.893
Anterior-Posterior view	0.868	0.910	0.842	0.873
Total (Average)	0.921	0.886	0.861	0.889

Total intra-rater weighted Kappa on repeated measures of six participants showed excellent intra-rater reliability, resulting in a Kappa of 0.944 (Rater One Mean = 0.948, Rater Two Mean = 0.962, Rater Three Mean = 0.921). Agreement was not calculated between textures due to small data sets. Overall, these results suggest that there is a high level of consistency between raters and that a minimal amount of error was introduced by the independent raters. Ratings were therefore deemed to be suitable to conduct hypothesis testing as outlined before.

3.3. Structural Validity

Exploratory Factor Analysis

Fifteen items of the 57 retained for the trial measure were excluded from the EFA, as they pertained solely to textures or views (e.g., solids or anterior/posterior) other than 5 mL Thick (lateral view). This resulted in 42 items being assessed in the EFA. The trial using 5 mL Thick was selected for EFA due to this being the trial with the highest number of cases (n = 114), being the first trial in the protocol, and thus being best suited to meeting statistical assumptions for EFA. EFA requires a minimum of fives times the number of cases per item [25], and given 114 cases for 5 mL Thick, the maximum number of items permitted for EFA was 22 (22 × 5 = 110). Therefore, the 42 items were divided into two groups.

Item groupings were initially constructed based on theory and clinical reasoning, with items pertaining to anatomically close regions (e.g., oral and oropharyngeal) and/or impairments or events which are closely related (e.g., aspiration and penetration) being grouped. Initial analysis revealed eight factors in both groups. New groupings were created by moving a single item at a time between groups. This process was informed by clinical reasoning, empirical literature and factor loadings (i.e., if a single item was creating a factor by itself, it was moved to another group to attempt to eliminate a one-item factor). The impact of moving single items was evaluated by examining changes in factor loading and total variance, and allowing the items to demonstrate relationships to other items. For example, items related to aspiration or penetration loaded on different factors when items related to the UES functioning were included in the factor analysis, whereas if UES items were excluded from the analyses, both aspiration and penetration items loaded on the same factor.

After the total number of factors was reduced as much as possible, clinical reasoning was used to allocate ambiguous items (i.e., those which loaded approximately equally on more than one factor) to a factor. During this process, three items, 'Piecemeal Deglutition', 'Volume Tracheal residue' and 'Coordination of the upper oesophageal sphincter' were removed due to erratic behaviour (creating weak, theoretically inconsistent single or two-item factors). Finally, the groupings with the combination of items which best represented the most concise and theoretically coherent factors of item loadings were retained.

This process resulted in two EFA models consisting of five and four factors, respectively (Tables 2 and 3, Exploratory Factor Analysis). In Group One, five factors explained 71.8% of the total variance, with most items loading on Factors One and Two. Factor One explained 18.6% of the variance, indicating multidimensionality, as Factor One accounted for <20% of the variability and the ratio of the variance from Factor One to Two is less than four [30]. The Group Two factor loadings reflected similar findings. A four-factor solution explained 77.4% of the total variance, with most items loading on Factors 6 and 7 (factors are named with sequential numbers continuing from group One to Two), and a ratio of less than four in variance between the two factors. These findings also suggest multidimensionality.

Table 2. Exploratory factor analysis—factor loadings of model one.

Item No.	Item Descriptor	Factor 1	Factor 2	Factor 3	Factor 4	Factor 5	Communalities
1.1	Number of swallows	0.120	**0.867**	0.126	−0.060	−0.105	0.797
1.2	Lingual motion (liquids)	**0.748**	0.091	0.349	0.088	−0.053	0.701
1.3	Bolus formation (liquids)	**0.777**	0.019	0.112	−0.156	0.132	0.659
1.4	Bolus transport (liquids)	**0.728**	0.194	0.069	0.138	−0.236	0.647
1.5	Base of tongue retraction	**0.620**	0.086	0.090	0.412	−0.071	0.574
1.6	Velum elevation	**0.530**	−0.052	0.413	0.120	−0.099	0.478
1.7	Premature Spillage location	0.239	0.056	0.169	**0.781**	0.145	0.719
1.8	Location material at swallow initiation	−0.037	−0.067	0.057	**0.820**	0.002	0.681
1.9	Hyoid excursio—superior movement	0.245	0.079	**0.827**	0.081	−0.162	0.783
1.10	Hyoid excursion—anterior movement	0.233	0.286	**0.793**	0.023	0.094	0.774
1.11	Laryngeal excursion	0.104	0.071	**0.898**	0.170	−0.136	0.870
1.12	Pharyngeal constriction pharyngeal obliterated space	0.225	**0.571**	0.297	0.279	0.001	0.543
1.13	Clearing Swallow—Location of residue when swallow triggered	−0.047	**0.904**	0.088	−0.021	0.102	0.837
1.14	Clearing swallows (number)	−0.155	**0.927**	0.115	−0.109	0.097	0.917
1.15	Width of UES opening	−0.032	0.124	−0.072	−0.015	**0.922**	0.872
1.16	UES closure impedes flow	−0.185	0.037	−0.113	0.110	**0.909**	0.886
1.17	Oral residue volume	**0.629**	−0.063	0.262	0.350	−0.276	0.666
1.18	Oropharynx residue volume	**0.559**	0.008	0.054	0.593	−0.050	0.670
1.19	Valleculae residue volume	0.383	**0.592**	−0.148	0.078	0.196	0.564
	Eigenvalue	3.525	3.282	2.704	2.139	1.989	
	% of Total Variance	18.55	17.27	14.23	11.26	10.47	
	Total variance			71.78%			

The bold represent the proposed models for the loading on these factors.

3.4. Internal Consistency

Cronbach's alpha was calculated per factor and for the whole measure for 5 mL Thick data on the 39 items retained from the EFA results, following the removal of three items creating erratic behaviour (Table 4. Internal Consistency). Scores for all factors and overall were adequate (Cronbach's alpha >0.70 and <0.95), except for Factor Four (0.698) [28].

Table 3. Exploratory factor analysis—factor loadings model two.

Item No.	Item Descriptor	Factor 6	Factor 7	Factor 8	Factor 9	Communalities
2.1	Laryngeal vestibule closure (LVC)—base to arytenoids	0.248	**0.754**	0.160	0.191	0.691
2.2	Epiglottic tilting	0.148	**0.716**	0.036	0.259	0.604
2.3	Laryngeal vestibule closure—base to arytenoids contact relative to UES opening	0.136	**0.722**	−0.102	0.212	0.595
2.4	Pharyngeal wall movement	−0.051	0.361	−0.307	**0.400**	0.387
2.5	Aspiration present on x number of swallows	0.233	**0.835**	0.012	−0.003	0.751
2.6	Response to aspiration	**0.978**	0.171	0.086	0.052	0.995
2.7	Cough ability to eject material	**0.952**	0.166	0.066	0.097	0.948
2.8	Cough latency (ordinal)	**0.962**	0.167	0.070	0.088	0.966
2.9	Aspiration occurrence timing	**0.955**	0.168	0.098	0.013	0.950
2.10	Aspiration volume	**0.978**	0.171	0.086	0.052	0.995
2.11	Penetration present on x number of swallows	0.160	−0.065	**0.839**	0.179	0.765
2.12	Penetration occurrence timing	0.147	0.026	**0.907**	0.053	0.848
2.13	Penetration depth	0.018	0.478	**0.757**	0.217	0.849
2.14	Response to penetration	0.167	**0.772**	0.485	0.143	0.881
2.15	Permanence of penetration	0.132	**0.723**	0.523	0.164	0.841
2.16	Post. pharyngeal wall of hypopharynx residue volume	0.138	0.161	0.089	**0.674**	0.507
2.17	Pyriform sinus residue volume	0.052	0.088	0.153	**0.872**	0.794
2.18	Laryngeal surface epiglottis residue volume	**0.582**	0.369	0.350	0.032	0.598
2.19	Laryngeal vestibule residue volume	0.164	**0.799**	−0.010	0.043	0.667
2.20	Clearing Swallow Efficacy	0.018	0.212	0.214	**0.869**	0.845
	Eigenvalue	5.300	4.777	2.971	2.432	
	% of Total Variance	26.48	23.89	14.86	12.16	
	Total variance	77.38%				

The bold represent the proposed models for the loading on these factors.

Table 4. Internal Consistency.

Factors and Description of Items within the Factor	Cronbach's Alpha
Factor 1. Lingual control and motion, velum motion, oral and oropharynx residue	0.810
Factor 2. Number of swallows, clearing swallows and pharyngeal contraction	0.861
Factor 3. Hyoid and larynx movement	0.876
Factor 4. Premature spillage and swallow initiation	0.698
Factor 5. Upper oesophageal sphincter function	0.836
Factor 6. Aspiration and underside epiglottis residue	0.934
Factor 7. Epiglottis movement, aspiration, penetration permanence and response and laryngeal vestibule closure	0.873
Factor 8. Penetration	0.853
Factor 9. Pharyngeal wall movement, pharyngeal residue and clearing swallows	0.714
Total Measure	0.902

3.5. Hypothesis Testing for Construct Validity

The data were not normally distributed, therefore nonparametric correlations were calculated.

Hypothesis One, which stated that factor scores will be significantly positively correlated with FOIS and 5-point ordinal scale scores in 70% of factors, was partially supported (Table 5. Factors' correlation with FOIS and 5-point ordinal scale). The hypothesis was partially supported with a weak to moderate positive correlation (FOIS mean: 0.171, range = −0.157–0.415; 5-point ordinal scale mean: 0.199, range −0.055–0.432) that was statistically significant in seven of nine (77%) factors, and positive but non-significant in one (Factor 8: Penetration) [31,32]. The factor containing UES Function items generated weak inverse correlations (−0.157 and −0.055).

Table 5. Factors' correlation with FOIS and 5-point ordinal scale.

Factor		FOIS	5-Point Scale
		Correlation coefficient	Correlation coefficient
1	Lingual control and motion, velum motion, oral and oropharynx residue	0.228 **	0.226 **
2	Number of swallows, clearing swallows and pharyngeal contraction	0.289 **	0.324 **
3	Hyoid and larynx movement	0.415 **	0.432 **
4	Premature spillage and swallow initiation	0.185 **	0.264 **
5	Upper oesophageal sphincter function	−0.157 *	−0.055
6	Aspiration and underside epiglottis residue	0.199 **	0.225 **
7	Epiglottis movement, aspiration, penetration permanence and response and Laryngeal Vestibule closure	0.231 **	0.234 **
8	penetration	0.063	0.058
9	Pharyngeal wall movement, pharyngeal residue and clearing swallows	0.086 **	0.086 **

* Correlation is significant at the 0.05 level (2-tailed). ** Correlation is significant at the 0.01 level (2-tailed).

Hypothesis 2, which stated that there will be no significant difference on item scores between genders, was supported. The hypothesis was supported by a Mann–Whitney U test, which found no significant difference between the scores of male and female patients: Mean Rank$_{Male}$ = 2393.28 (Sum of Ranks = 7,237,279.00); Mean Rank$_{Female}$ = 2396.59 (Sum of Ranks = 4,227,587.00); U = 2,663,479.00; p = 0.932, two-tailed.

4. Discussion

The psychometric properties of the pilot VMV were evaluated in this study. The analysis was conducted with reference to a classical test theory (CTT) psychometric paradigm and the COSMIN framework [9–13]. CTT is well-suited for initial investigations of psychometric properties [33] and is useful in measure development, as many constructs of interest are not directly observable in health practice. For example, laryngeal vestibule closure may be purported to be assessed by VFSS analysis; however, 'closure' is not directly measured. The clinician's perception of the proximity of pixels produced by digitisation of fluoroscopy is the observable data. Clinicians assign meaning to this 'proxy indicator' to measure the unobserved construct of 'closure'. CTT-informed analysis determines the success of the proxy indicator in measuring the unobservable phenomenon [34]. A key tenet of CTT is that the scores of each item are produced by a combination of the unobservable 'true' score, summed with the unavoidable errors and biases introduced by the use of a proxy indicator. Errors in CTT are assumed to be random and unique to each item [34]. The COSMIN framework was used to define the psychometric terms applied and to guide the statistical methodology used [11–13].

Statistical analysis found that the inter-rater reliability coefficients of the VMV were in the 'strong' range overall and included scores in the excellent range between Raters One and Two. This indicated that the target concepts were clearly and consistently understood between the three raters from different professions—speech-language pathology (SLP), radiology and phoniatrics. This was reflected in the item reduction process, where the majority of items selected for the next version of the measure were considered 'clear/unambiguous' by all raters. Intra-rater reliability was excellent, indicating that the pilot VMV supports a consistent internal schema within raters that is stable across time [27].

Structural validity analysis via EFA produced a 5-factor and 4-factor solution. Group One contained variables primarily relating to swallowing events and kinematics occurring superiorly in the oropharyngeal tract and early in the swallowing process (e.g., hyoid movement). Group Two resulted in items pertaining to laryngeal, hypopharyngeal and late-stage events (e.g., residue post swallow). However, some items behaved erratically (i.e., 'piecemeal deglutition' caused a factor with a single item loading on it) and some items had ambiguous loadings (e.g., 'Oropharynx residue volume' loaded similarly on two factors). This is likely related to sample size. Items with ambiguous loadings were allocated to a group and factor based on theoretical consistency of the grouping (e.g., oropharynx residue volume was grouped with the factor containing 'oral residue volume' as opposed to the factor containing 'location of material at swallow initiation', as the pairing with another item measuring residue, rather than a temporal event, is more logically consistent). Three items, 'Piecemeal deglutition', 'Volume tracheal residue' and 'Coordination of the upper oesophageal sphincter' were removed as they created single item factors or groupings which were illogical. Therefore, the groups represent preliminary proposals at this time; conclusive evidence of factor structure will require greater numbers of participants.

EFA indicated that the measure is multidimensional, meaning that the construct under assessment has two or more dimensions. In VFSS, a simple construct such as velum movement may be unidimensional (i.e., the underlying dimension of the construct is velum elevation). A multidimensional construct might be aspiration, where the dimensions contributing to the construct include volume of aspirate, time when aspiration occurs, and the patient's awareness of the event. In the context of the pilot VMV, this finding means that visuoperceptual examination of VFSS likely involves multiple underlying dimensions. However, this needs to be confirmed in a larger sample with an EFA that includes all items in a single analysis (as opposed to split into two groups) followed by a confirmatory factor analysis. Total percentage of variance explained was >70% for both models, indicating that random error was not excessive [35].

Internal consistency was good (alpha > 0.7 but < 0.95) for 8 of the 9 factors and overall, with only one factor (Factor Four, which contained items pertaining to premature spillage and swallow initiation) not reaching this zone alpha by only 0.002 [28]. This indicates good content coverage, but item reduction may be possible to streamline the measure. Further analysis of the preliminary measure using the Rasch measurement model (RMM), a type of item response theory, would provide additional information about the dimensionality, differential item functioning, person-ability scores, and item difficulty scores. This would assist in identifying items that do not meet RMM person and item fit criteria and could subsequently be discarded [33].

Hypothesis testing for convergent validity tested two hypotheses. The first, an expected positive relationship between VMV and both FOIS and 5-point ordinal scale scores was partially supported. All but one factor had a weak, positive statistically significant correlation. That is, as the degree of impairment increased (as measured by texture prescription) and the radiologist's perception of overall severity of OD increased, so did scores on the VMV. The factor containing the UES items was negatively correlated with both FOIS and the 5-point ordinal scale. It might be expected that the UES, as the terminal part of the pharynx, would reflect dysfunction from superior abnormalities of the oral cavity, pharyngeal shortening and constriction, cervical spine and hyolaryngeal function [36]. However, the inverse correlation indicates that this was not the case in this pilot. This finding may be a related to the small sample size or the texture/volume analysed; 5 mL Thick may not be ideal to reveal UES deficits because the small volume is less likely to be problematic for passage through the UES, given that larger thick volumes produce greater durations of opening, amplitudes of relaxation and earlier opening onset (i.e., thick volumes induce greater challenges to the swallow system) [37]. The inverse correlation result may also be related to the construct itself. For instance, the UES items were the only items where 'opening' was measured, while other items assess contact with other structures, volumes of material and timing of kinematics. As this was a pilot study, explanation of this finding cannot be conclusive. Further analysis in a larger sample is required.

The second hypothesis, a lack of association between scores on VMV and gender, was supported. This result was expected given that OD severity as perceptually analysed on VFSS should have no association with gender [38]. These two findings indicate that it is likely that the VMV is measuring the target construct. Finally, a review by the authors of the feasibility, clinical relevance and redundancy of the items found that approximately half of the items could be removed. This is expected in measure construction, where multiple items may assess the same construct in the pilot and then the most suitable are retained following initial testing. Removal of items also assists in developing a measure's suitability for clinical use; the pilot iteration of the measure was excessively time consuming, taking over 40 min for analysis. A measure useful for practice must balance adequate content coverage with feasible administration time.

The pilot VMV exhibits evidence of content validity [16], intra- and inter-reliability, structural validity, internal consistency and hypothesis testing. In a psychometric review of current visuoperceptual VFSS measures, only nine measures were found where evidence of the scale's validity and reliability were reported. The quality of the reported psychometric properties was limited, primarily due to unclear reporting and methodological flaws. [4]. The VMV represents the first visuoperceptual measure for VFSS that has been constructed with reference to the international best practice guidelines of the COSMIN initiative [10,39]. The VMV has evidence of its robust content validity, established through an extensive international Delphi process involving 50 experts from 27 countries [16]. In addition, this measure was piloted using raters from three different disciplines (SLP, radiology and phoniatrics) and their expertise informed measure refinement and item reduction. No other measure has utilised such comprehensive and robust methodology [4]. Similarly, initial evidence of the VMV's structural validity and dimensionality was provided through the EFA results.

Limitations and Future Research

Limitations of this study are the small sample size, which resulted in the reliability and EFA analyses being limited to 5 mL Thick to meet statistical assumptions. The study was conducted at a single site, and while the population was reasonably heterogenous, the sample does not comprehensively reflect all possible aetiologies and comorbidities of the OD population. The analysis was conducted using only a CTT framework, which is known to have a number of limitations. For example, each item's score is comprised of its 'true' score and random error in CTT, and as the distribution of the error is random around a mean of zero, errors from different items will generally negate each other. This means that scales which include many items may yield disproportionately strong reliability [34]. However, the application of CTT represents a first step in the psychometric evaluation of the VMV. The combination of CTT with another theoretical framework, such as the RMM, would yield further valuable insights about the measurement properties of the VMV [12,40]. In addition, some psychometric properties (e.g., test re-test, measurement error) and interpretability were out of the scope of this study. Finally, this study reports on a pilot version of the VMV that is not yet ready for formal clinical use. It is anticipated that future studies involving larger patient populations will allow additional statistical analysis (e.g., EFA and RMM analysis including all items), investigation of additional psychometric properties, and investigation using psychometric paradigms that complement each other (i.e., CTT and IRT). Together, these will help create a refined version of the preliminary VMV which is suitable for clinical use.

5. Conclusions

The CTT analysis indicates that the initial psychometric properties of a pilot version of the VMV may be adequate for analysing VFSS in a valid and reliable manner. The VMV appears to have good inter and intra rater reliability. The VMV is multidimensional, based on EFA results, and exhibits good internal consistency. Hypothesis testing for construct validity indicates that the relationship between OD severity and population characteristics is as expected, with VMV severity scores increasing as functional severity on other measures increase. Future studies of the preliminary VMV with larger samples and additional statistical analysis using the RMM is recommended as this will add to the psychometric evidence of the VMV. The VMV pilot study represents the first step in developing a robustly validated measure for visuoperceptual analysis of VFSS which is intended to be suitable for research and clinical purposes in its final version.

Supplementary Materials: The following supporting information can be downloaded at: https://www.mdpi.com/article/10.3390/jcm11030724/s1, Table S1: Aetiology of Oropharyngeal Dysphagia; Figure S1: VFSS protocol; Table S2: Administration protocol; Table S3: Functional Health Status and Severity measures; Table S4: Functional Health Status and Severity measures scoring; Table S5: Items removed or altered following rater consensus; Table S6: Included items per domain.

Author Contributions: Conceptualization, R.S. and R.C.; methodology, R.S., R.C.; formal analysis, K.S., R.S.; investigation, K.S., M.S., D.F.; resources, M.S.; data curation, K.S.; writing—original draft preparation, K.S.; writing—review and editing, K.S., R.S., T.B., R.C.; supervision, R.S., T.B., R.C.; project administration, K.S. All authors have read and agreed to the published version of the manuscript.

Funding: The authors wish to acknowledge Curtin University and the Australian Federal Government for the Curtin University Postgraduate Scholarship (CUPS) and the Australian Postgraduate Award (APA).

Institutional Review Board Statement: The study was conducted in accordance with the Declaration of Helsinki, and approved by the Human Research Ethics Committees of The Medical University of Vienna And Curtin University (HRE2018-0151, 11/04/2018 and March 2019).

Informed Consent Statement: Informed consent was obtained from all subjects involved in the study.

Data Availability Statement: The data presented in this study are available on request from the first author. The data are not publicly available due to conditions of approval from the governing Human Research Ethics Committee.

Conflicts of Interest: The authors declare no conflict of interest.

References

1. Philpott, H.; Garg, M.; Tomic, D.; Balasubramanian, S.; Sweis, R. Dysphagia: Thinking outside the box. *World J. Gastroenterol.* **2017**, *23*, 6942. [CrossRef] [PubMed]
2. Langmore, S.E. History of fiberoptic endoscopic evaluation of swallowing for evaluation and management of pharyngeal dysphagia: Changes over the years. *Dysphagia* **2017**, *32*, 27–38. [CrossRef] [PubMed]
3. Lee, J.W.; Randall, D.R.; Evangelista, L.M.; Kuhn, M.A.; Belafsky, P.C. Subjective assessment of videofluoroscopic swallow studies. *Otolaryngol.-Head Neck Surg.* **2017**, *156*, 901–905. [CrossRef] [PubMed]
4. Swan, K.; Cordier, R.; Brown, T.; Speyer, R. Psychometric properties of visuoperceptual measures of videofluoroscopic and fibre-endoscopic evaluations of swallowing: A systematic review. *Dysphagia* **2019**, *34*, 2–33. [CrossRef]
5. Mokkink, L.B.; Prinsen, C.A.; Bouter, L.M.; de Vet, H.C.; Terwee, C.B. The COnsensus-based Standards for the selection of health Measurement INstruments (COSMIN) and how to select an outcome measurement instrument. *Braz. J. Phys. Ther.* **2016**, *20*, 105–113. [CrossRef]
6. Clavé, P.; Rofes, L.; Carrión, S.; Ortega, O.; Cabré, M.; Serra-Prat, M.; Arreola, V. Pathophysiology, relevance and natural history of oropharyngeal dysphagia among older people. In *Stepping Stones to Living Well with Dysphagia*; Karger Publishers: Basel, Switzerland, 2012; pp. 57–66.
7. Anunciacao, L. An overview of the history and methodological aspects of psychometrics-history and methodological aspects of psychometrics. *J. ReAttach Ther. Dev. Divers.* **2018**, *1*, 44–58. [CrossRef]
8. Mokkink, L.B.; Terwee, C.B.; Knol, D.L.; Stratford, P.W.; Alonso, J.; Patrick, D.L.; Bouter, L.M.; De Vet, H.C. The COSMIN checklist for evaluating the methodological quality of studies on measurement properties: A clarification of its content. *BMC Med. Res. Methodol.* **2010**, *10*, 22. [CrossRef]
9. Mokkink, L.B.; Boers, M.; van der Vleuten, C.P.M.; Bouter, L.M.; Alonso, J.; Patrick, D.L.; De Vet, H.C.; Terwee, C.B. COSMIN Risk of Bias tool to assess the quality of studies on reliability or measurement error of outcome measurement instruments: A Delphi study. *BMC Med. Res. Methodol.* **2020**, *20*, 293. [CrossRef]
10. Mokkink, L.B.; Prinsen, C.A.; Patrick, D.L.; Alonso, J.; Bouter, L.M.; de Vet, H.C.; Terwee, C.B. *COSMIN Study Design Checklist for Patient-Reported Outcome Measurement Instruments*; Amsterdam Public Health Research Institute: Amsterdam, The Netherlands, 2019.
11. Terwee, C.B.; Prinsen, C.A.; Chiarotto, A.; Westerman, M.J.; Patrick, D.L.; Alonso, J.; Bouter, L.M.; De Vet, H.C.; Mokkink, L.B. COSMIN methodology for evaluating the content validity of patient-reported outcome measures: A Delphi study. *Qual. Life Res.* **2018**, *27*, 1159–1170. [CrossRef]
12. Mokkink, L.B.; De Vet, H.C.; Prinsen, C.A.; Patrick, D.L.; Alonso, J.; Bouter, L.M.; Terwee, C.B. COSMIN risk of bias checklist for systematic reviews of patient-reported outcome measures. *Qual. Life Res.* **2018**, *27*, 1171–1179. [CrossRef]

13. Prinsen, C.A.; Mokkink, L.B.; Bouter, L.M.; Alonso, J.; Patrick, D.L.; De Vet, H.C.; Terwee, C.B. COSMIN guideline for systematic reviews of patient-reported outcome measures. *Qual. Life Res.* **2018**, *27*, 1147–1157. [CrossRef]
14. Ioannidis, J.P. How to make more published research true. *Rev. Cuba. De Inf. En Cienc. De La Salud (ACIMED)* **2015**, *26*, 187–200. [CrossRef]
15. El-Den, S.; Schneider, C.; Mirzaei, A.; Carter, S. How to measure a latent construct: Psychometric principles for the development and validation of measurement instruments. *Int. J. Pharm. Pract.* **2020**, *28*, 326–336. [CrossRef]
16. Swan, K.; Cordier, R.; Brown, T.; Speyer, R. Visuoperceptual Analysis of the Videofluoroscopic Study of Swallowing: An International Delphi Study. *Dysphagia* **2021**, *36*, 595–613. [CrossRef]
17. Giraldo-Cadavid, L.F.; Leal-Leaño, L.R.; Leon-Basantes, G.A.; Bastidas, A.R.; Garcia, R.; Ovalle, S.; Abondano-Garavito, J.E. Accuracy of endoscopic and videofluoroscopic evaluations of swallowing for oropharyngeal dysphagia. *Laryngoscope* **2017**, *127*, 2002–2010. [CrossRef]
18. Steele, C.M.; Alsanei, W.A.; Ayanikalath, S.; Barbon, C.E.; Chen, J.; Cichero, J.A.; Coutts, K.; Dantas, R.O.; Duivestein, J.; Giosa, L.; et al. The influence of food texture and liquid consistency modification on swallowing physiology and function: A systematic review. *Dysphagia* **2015**, *30*, 2–26. [CrossRef]
19. Curtis, J.A.; Troche, M.S. Effects of Verbal Cueing on Respiratory-Swallow Patterning, Lung Volume Initiation, and Swallow Apnea Duration in Parkinson's Disease. *Dysphagia* **2020**, *35*, 460–470. [CrossRef]
20. Steele, C.M.; Namasivayam-MacDonald, A.M.; Guida, B.T.; Cichero, J.A.; Duivestein, J.; Hanson, B.; Lam, P.; Riquelme, L.F. Creation and initial validation of the international dysphagia diet standardisation initiative functional diet scale. *Arch. Phys. Med. Rehabil.* **2018**, *99*, 934–944. [CrossRef]
21. Bonilha, H.S.; Blair, J.; Carnes, B.; Huda, W.; Humphries, K.; McGrattan, K.; Michel, Y.; Martin-Harris, B. Preliminary investigation of the effect of pulse rate on judgments of swallowing impairment and treatment recommendations. *Dysphagia* **2013**, *28*, 528–538. [CrossRef]
22. Speyer, R.; Kertscher, B.; Cordier, R. Functional health status in oropharyngeal dysphagia. *J. Gastroenterol. Hepatol. Res.* **2014**, *3*, 1043–1048.
23. Woisard, V.; Andrieux, M.; Puech, M. Validation of a self-assessment questionnaire for swallowing disorders (Deglutition Handicap Index). *Rev. De Laryngol.-Otol.-Rhinol.* **2006**, *127*, 315–325.
24. Crary, M.A.; Mann, G.D.C.; Groher, M.E. Initial psychometric assessment of a functional oral intake scale for dysphagia in stroke patients. *Arch. Phys. Med. Rehabil.* **2005**, *86*, 1516–1520. [CrossRef]
25. Suhr, D.D. Exploratory or confirmatory factor analysis? In Proceedings of the SAS SUGI Proceedings: Statistics, Data Analysis and Data Mining (SUGI 31), San Francisco, CA, USA, 26–29 March 2006. Paper 200-31.
26. Brady, S.; Donzelli, J. The modified barium swallow and the functional endoscopic evaluation of swallowing. *Otolaryngol. Clin. N. Am.* **2013**, *46*, 1009–1022. [CrossRef]
27. McHugh, M.L. Interrater reliability: The kappa statistic. *Biochem. Med.* **2012**, *22*, 276–282. [CrossRef]
28. Terwee, C.B.; Bot, S.D.; de Boer, M.R.; van der Windt, D.A.; Knol, D.L.; Dekker, J.; Bouter, L.M.; de Vet, H.C. Quality criteria were proposed for measurement properties of health status questionnaires. *J. Clin. Epidemiol.* **2007**, *60*, 34–42. [CrossRef]
29. Cohen, J. Weighted kappa: Nominal scale agreement provision for scaled disagreement or partial credit. *Psychol. Bull.* **1968**, *70*, 213. [CrossRef]
30. Prinsen, C.A.; Vohra, S.; Rose, M.R.; Boers, M.; Tugwell, P.; Clarke, M.; Williamson, P.R.; Terwee, C.B. How to select outcome measurement instruments for outcomes included in a "Core Outcome Set"—A practical guideline. *Trials* **2016**, *17*, 449. [CrossRef]
31. Dancey, C.P.; Reidy, J. *Statistics without Maths for Psychology*; Pearson Education: New York, NY, USA, 2007.
32. Akoglu, H. User's guide to correlation coefficients. *Turk. J. Emerg. Med.* **2018**, *18*, 91–93. [CrossRef]
33. Petrillo, J.; Cano, S.J.; McLeod, L.D.; Coon, C.D. Using classical test theory, item response theory, and Rasch measurement theory to evaluate patient-reported outcome measures: A comparison of worked examples. *Value Health* **2015**, *18*, 25–34. [CrossRef]
34. DeVellis, R.F. Classical test theory. *Med. Care* **2006**, *11*, S50–S59. [CrossRef]
35. Hinkin, T.R. A brief tutorial on the development of measures for use in survey questionnaires. *Organ. Res. Methods* **1998**, *1*, 104–121. [CrossRef]
36. Belafsky, P.C.; Kuhn, M.A. *The Clinician's Guide to Swallowing Fluoroscopy*; Springer: Berlin/Heidelberg, Germany, 2014.
37. Butler, S.G.; Stuart, A.; Castell, D.; Russell, G.B.; Koch, K.; Kemp, S. Effects of age, gender, bolus condition, viscosity, and volume on pharyngeal and upper esophageal sphincter pressure and temporal measurements during swallowing. *J. Speech Lang. Hear. Res.* **2009**, *52*, 240–253. [CrossRef]
38. Nabieh, A.A.; Emam, A.M.; Mostafa, E.M.; Hashem, R.M. Gender Differences in Normal Swallow. *Egypt. J. Neck Surg. Otorhinolaryngol.* **2018**, *4*, 1–7. [CrossRef]
39. Terwee, C.B.; Prinsen, C.A.C.; Garotti, M.R.; Suman, A.; De Vet, H.C.W.; Mokkink, L.B. The quality of systematic reviews of health-related outcome measurement instruments. *Qual. Life Res.* **2016**, *25*, 767–779. [CrossRef] [PubMed]
40. Edelen, M.O.; Reeve, B.B. Applying item response theory (IRT) modeling to questionnaire development, evaluation, and refinement. *Qual. Life Res.* **2007**, *16*, 5–18. [CrossRef]

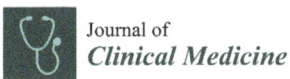

Article

Pitch Discrimination Testing in Patients with a Voice Disorder

Duy Duong Nguyen [1,2,*], Antonia M. Chacon [1], Daniel Novakovic [1,3], Nicola J. Hodges [4], Paul N. Carding [5] and Catherine Madill [1]

1. Voice Research Laboratory, Discipline of Speech Pathology, Faculty of Medicine and Health, The University of Sydney, Sydney, NSW 2006, Australia; antonia.chacon@sydney.edu.au (A.M.C.); daniel.novakovic@sydney.edu.au (D.N.); cate.madill@sydney.edu.au (C.M.)
2. National Hospital of Otorhinolaryngology, Hanoi 11519, Vietnam
3. The Canterbury Hospital, Campsie, NSW 2194, Australia
4. School of Kinesiology, University of British Columbia, Vancouver, BC V6T 1Z1, Canada; nicola.hodges@ubc.ca
5. Faculty of Health and Life Sciences, Oxford Institute of Nursing, Midwifery and Allied Health Research, Oxford OX3 0BP, UK; pcarding@brookes.ac.uk
* Correspondence: duong.nguyen@sydney.edu.au

Abstract: Auditory perception plays an important role in voice control. Pitch discrimination (PD) is a key index of auditory perception and is influenced by a variety of factors. Little is known about the potential effects of voice disorders on PD and whether PD testing can differentiate people with and without a voice disorder. We thus evaluated PD in a voice-disordered group (n = 71) and a non-voice-disordered control group (n = 80). The voice disorders included muscle tension dysphonia and neurological voice disorders and all participants underwent PD testing as part of a comprehensive voice assessment. Percentage of accurate responses and PD threshold were compared across groups. The PD percentage accuracy was significantly lower in the voice-disordered group than the control group, irrespective of musical background. Participants with voice disorders also required a larger PD threshold to correctly discriminate pitch differences. The mean PD threshold significantly discriminated the voice-disordered groups from the control group. These results have implications for the voice control and pathogenesis of voice disorders. They support the inclusion of PD testing during comprehensive voice assessment and throughout the treatment process for patients with voice disorders.

Keywords: auditory discrimination; voice control; voice assessment; voice disorders

1. Introduction

Laryngeal muscle control in voice production is affected by auditory feedback and sensorimotor reflexes [1]. There are overlapping anatomical pathways in the brain that encode similar acoustic information presented in both music and voice, such as waveform periodicity and amplitude envelope [2]. Coordination of laryngeal muscles in phonation depends upon motor planning, muscle activation, and feedback provided by auditory systems [1,3]. It has been demonstrated that disturbances in auditory perception/discrimination are related to problems within auditory motor reflexes governing effective laryngeal control. These perception problems lead to abnormal motor control patterns as observed in people with hyperfunctional dysphonia [4,5]. The impairment of temporal auditory function in patients with behavioral dysphonia may affect the success of voice therapy, suggesting the need for auditory processing assessment [6].

A disordered voice is defined as a voice that does not meet the occupational or social needs of the speaker and is inappropriate given the speaker's age, gender, or situation [7]. Voice disorders can be classified according to the aetiology of the voice dysfunction [8]. Functional voice disorders include muscle tension voice disorder (MTVD) and psychogenic voice disorders [9]. Functional voice disorders may result from poor detection of pitch, volume, and voice quality dimensions in the absence of any neurological motor and sensory deficit [8,10]. In contrast, in neurological voice disorders, there is damage to the motor and/or sensory pathways. Distinguishing between different types of voice disorders requires not only voice quality assessment but also perception assessment, which allows conclusions to be made about the dependence of patient's perception and vocal production upon specific sensory and motor pathways.

Auditory perception function can be evaluated using pitch discrimination (PD) testing. Pitch is a perceptual attribute of sound that has important roles in the human voice and PD is the ability to correctly detect intervals/differences between pitches of pure or complex tones. This ability to perceive different pitches is reflected in the experience of both perceiving and producing sound. PD also reflects auditory discrimination function. Tonal language speakers show greater pitch perception accuracy than non-tonal language speakers [11] and people with a musical background discriminate pitches more accurately than those with a non-musical background [12,13].

The neural processing of pitch is complicated. It involves hierarchical responses and mainly occurs in the right hemisphere of the brain; including the superior temporal gyrus, lateral Heschl's gyrus, inferior frontal gyrus, insular cortex, and the inferior colliculus [14,15]. People possess variable pitch perception ability with some apparently having more difficulties in PD than others, probably due to their use of sub-optimal brain regions (e.g., left hemisphere) for pitch processing [16]. It was also found that there is differential neural pitch processing in the left and right hemispheres that allows the auditory system to detect temporal and spectral changes in the auditory feedback necessary for voice control [17]. PD is impaired in some congenital and acquired neurological conditions that involve organic neurological dysfunction. Congenital amusia (prevalence of 1.5%) [18] results in impaired pitch processing due to abnormal deactivation of the right inferior frontal gyrus [19]. Given that the auditory cortex shows normal responses to pitch in this condition, the suggestion has been made that the impairments are due to reduced white matter functional connections between the auditory and inferior frontal cortices [19]. Traumatic brain injury is also known to affect pitch perception ability due to damages of the underlying pitch processing regions [20].

Auditory discrimination problems have been shown in people with functional voice disorders. Abur et al. [4] showed that patients with hyperfunctional voice disorders had poorer auditory discrimination and more atypical adaptive responses to fundamental frequency (F0) shifts than those without the condition. Stepp et al. [5] showed that patients with hyperfunctional voice disorders demonstrated different patterns of adaptive responses in pitch perturbation tasks compared with controls. They suggested a disruption between auditory processing and laryngeal motor control. The pitch-shift reflex shows how well individuals can adapt their own pitch according to auditory feedback and has been examined in patients with muscle tension dysphonia (MTD) [21]. Compared with a control group without dysphonia, MTD patients had a significantly larger magnitude adaptive response to changes in auditory feedback, suggesting some type of dysfunction or dysregulation between pitch perception and voice production [21]. There were signs of deficits in temporal auditory processing, auditory discrimination, and adaptive responses in those with voice disorders, compared with those without [6].

Despite some evidence that voice disorders are associated with auditory processing problems, there are several studies which show discrepant results. Davis and Boone [22] compared PD and tonal memory between 30 adult patients with hyperfunctional voice disorders and 30 control participants and showed no significant differences between the two groups. However, there were participants who demonstrated difficulties in PD or remembering a tonal sequence [22]. Another study showed no relationship between PD and voice production in children with and without vocal nodules [23]. The above-mentioned literature has therefore shown conflicting findings related to the association between PD and voice disorders.

In patients with neurological voice disorders, some studies have also reported dysfunctional auditory perception. In spasmodic dysphonia, a neurological voice dystonia of cortical origin, dysfunctional sensory-motor processing was shown when these patients were presented with altered pitch feedback [24]. Patients with unilateral vocal fold paralysis had reduced auditory-processing ability and vocal motor function compared with healthy controls after surgical vocal fold augmentation procedures, as well as differences in the neural areas associated with vocal motor function [25,26]. These studies provide evidence for the impact of damage to the lower motor neuron pathways, involved in production impacting the upper motor neuron pathways (i.e., cortical) involved in perception. Given that vocal production ability shares some neurological pathways in tasks such as speech and musical processing [27,28], it is reasonable to hypothesize that dysfunction in voice production might have effects on PD. Clarifying whether there is such a link between voice quality and pitch perception would be the basis to deliver relevant/specific perception training in parallel to voice restoration/treatment.

We used the Newcastle Assessment of Pitch Discrimination (NeAP) [29] as part of a routine comprehensive assessment of voice function and auditory discrimination. In a previous study, this tool was shown to be reliable and clinically applicable [30]. The aims of the present study were to (1) examine PD characteristics in patients with voice disorders in comparison with non-voice-disordered speakers; and (2) evaluate the value of PD testing in differentiating voice-disordered patients from non-disordered speakers. The overall purpose was to provide clinical data on the use of PD testing in voice-disordered patients to determine the need to pay attention to patient's auditory perception function for successful voice treatment and provide insight into voice control mechanisms and pathogenesis of voice disorders.

2. Materials and Methods

2.1. Study Design

This was a cross-sectional study where both voice and auditory discrimination data were collected at a teaching voice clinic at The University of XX. The clinic performed comprehensive standardized voice assessment, including PD testing.

2.2. Participants

2.2.1. Voice-Disordered Groups

There were 71 patients (54 females and 17 males) with a confirmed diagnosis of primary or secondary MTVD or a neurological voice disorder. The mean age was 38.5 years (standard deviation, SD = 15.5 years, range = 18–82). Five (7.0%) were vocal performers, 29 (40.8%) were professional voice users, and 37 (52.1%) worked in other occupations. All patients were diagnosed by a laryngologist following conduction of standardized multidimensional voice assessment protocols in the University of XX's voice clinic. Diagnosis was based on patient-reported outcome measures, such as the Voice Handicap Index (VHI-10) [31], speech language pathologist's (SLP) voice assessment, voice recordings for acoustic analysis, and videostrobolaryngoscopy. There were no patients with hearing impairments as confirmed through audiometric screening (i.e., passing 20-decibel threshold in a pure-tone at 500 Hz, 1 kHz, 2 kHz, and 4 kHz). Participants were excluded if there were self-reported symptoms or clinical signs of speech disorders, cognitive impairments, neurodegenerative conditions, or hearing loss.

In the voice-disordered group there were two sub-groups: MTVD and neurological voice disorder. Table 1 shows patient numbers in each group. In the MTVD group, 26 were diagnosed as primary MTVD and 24 had secondary MTVD with lesions deemed related to phonotrauma such as vocal nodules, pre-nodular swellings, and mucosal thickening. There were 21 patients with neurological voice disorders including vocal fold paresis ($n = 11$), vocal fold paralysis ($n = 4$), tremor ($n = 3$), and laryngeal dystonia ($n = 3$). No patient in the neurological disorder group had Parkinson's disease, other neurodegenerative, or neuro-cognitive problems. There was a total of 45 voice-disordered patients with a musical training background and 26 without a musical training background.

Table 1. Number of participants by groups. MTVD: muscle tension voice disorder.

Groups	Musical Background		Total
	No	Yes	
Control	40	40	80
MTVD no lesions	7	19	26
MTVD with lesions	11	13	24
Neurological dysphonia	8	13	21
Total	66	85	151

2.2.2. Control Group

There were 80 participants, all female, with a mean age of 23.5 years (SD = 4.3 years, range = 18–40). All were speech language pathology students. They self-reported as having no voice problems at the time of the study and underwent voice screening using a case history questionnaire and the VHI-10 [31]. Inclusion criteria included no current voice symptoms, VHI-10 < 7.5 [32], normal hearing, and no current upper respiratory problems. Two certified practicing speech language pathologists perceptually assessed their voices using a standardized protocol and confirmed that their voices were non-dysphonic.

Participants in both groups completed a case history questionnaire to determine history of voice disorders, current voice problems, language backgrounds, musical background, and voice/musical training. Musical background was defined as having formally practiced a musical instrument for at least a year past the 5 years of age.

2.3. Voice Assessment

Mean VHI-10 score for the voice-disordered group was 20.48 (SD = 10.34, 95% confidence interval, CI = 18.03–22.93), which was above the cut-off score for a voice disorder (>7.5) [32]. Mean VHI-10 score for the control group was 2.28 (SD = 2.03, 95% CI = 1.82–2.73) which fell within the non-disordered range [32].

Acoustic analyses were performed as part of the voice assessment protocols on standardized vocal tasks (middle three seconds of sustained vowel /a/, the third CAPEV phrase [33], and the 2nd and 3rd sentences of the Rainbow Passage [34]). Acoustic measures analyzed for each participant included the harmonics-to-noise ratio (HNR), and cepstral/spectral index of dysphonia (CSID) [35,36]. Acoustic voice data for the groups are presented in Table 2.

Table 2. Mean (SD) and 95% confidence intervals for the mean of voice data for voice-disordered and control groups. The p value indicates significance level of independent t-test comparisons of the voice-disordered group (n = 71) and control group (n = 80) for each measure. HNR: harmonics-to-noise ration; CSID: cepstral/spectral index of dysphonia.

Measures (Normative Values)	Voice-Disordered Group			Control (n = 80)	p
	MTVD (n = 50)	Neurological Voice Disorders (n = 21)	All (n = 71)		
HNR (dB) (20 dB) [37]	23.90 (4.16) 22.71–25.10	21.36 (7.80) 17.81–24.91	23.14 (5.57) 21.81–24.47	24.90 (2.46) 24.35–25.45	0.016
CSID of vowel (NA)	9.03 (18.17) 3.81–14.25	25.43 (31.79) 10.96–39.90	13.95 (24.08) 8.21–19.69	−10.81 (7.38) (−12.45)–(−9.17)	<0.001
CSID of CAPEV-3 (NA)	−10.18 (20.78) (−16.15)–(−4.21)	1.42 (30.05) (−12.26)–15.10	−6.70 (24.31) (−12.49)–(−0.90)	−16.36 (9.48) (−18.47)–(−14.25)	<0.001
CSID Rainbow Passage (24.27) [36]	17.49 (14.05) 13.45–21.52	21.13 (17.84) 13.01–29.25	18.58 (15.24) 14.95–22.21	−3.16 (19.19) (−7.43)–1.12	<0.001

2.4. Pitch Discrimination Testing

2.4.1. Pitch Discrimination Testing Tool

We used the NeAP [29], which is a two-tone computer-based PD task, where listeners are required to stipulate which tone of a given pair is higher in pitch, or whether they are the same. One study reported on the use of this tool in assessing PD [30], showing it to be reliable, with a moderate to good prediction value in ascertaining one's musical background.

2.4.2. Protocols

All PD tasks were performed in a sound-protected room with ambient noise measured between 50 and 55 dB sound pressure level (SPL) to avoid effects of noise on auditory discrimination. The NeAP program included 20 tone pairs of sine waves. Each tone pair had a lower frequency tone and a higher frequency tone, with a range of pitch differences between the lower tone and higher tone (Appendix A). The lowest and highest frequency of the lower tones was 123.47 Hz and 293.66 Hz, respectively. The lowest and highest frequency of the higher tones was 130.81 Hz and 311.13 Hz, respectively. The pitch differences between tone pairs ranged from 2.29 Hz to 32.03 Hz (29.98 to 200.01 cents). One semitone is equal to 100 cents.

The tone pairs were played on a Dell computer (Latitude 7280) via two speakers (Harman/Kardon HK645) calibrated to 65.0–65.2 dBA hearing level (HL). Hearing level was measured at 5 cm lateral to the external ear meatus using a lingWAVES sound pressure level meter II model IEC 651. The participant was seated 1 m away equidistantly from the speakers. Participants completed the default protocol of the NeAP program. No training or trial was provided apart from instructions to listen to the tone pairs and to indicate which tone was higher in pitch or if the pitch sounded the same. Participants provided their responses by clicking on one of three buttons on the computer screen. Each button represented 'tone 1 was higher', 'tone 2 was higher' or 'both tones were the same'. The 20 tone pairs were presented a second time in a new random order in the same session for reliability analysis. The duration of each tone was 300 milliseconds (ms) and the pause between any two tones was 500 ms. The procedure lasted on average 6 min. The percentage of accurate responses was calculated for each tone pair by dividing the number of accurate responses by the total responses for that tone pair. Outcome measures included the percentage of accurate responses (%) and the mean PD threshold (cent) of correct responses.

2.5. Statistical Analysis

Statistical analyses were completed using SPSS 28.0 [38] and MedCalc 20.014 [39]. Data were checked for normal distribution. Intraclass correlation coefficients (ICC) [40] were used to determine the level of agreement between the first and second (repeated) PD responses. ICC was calculated using a two-way mixed model consistency type and single measure analysis [ICC (3,1)]. To help interpret reliability, ICC < 0.5 indicates poor correlation, 0.5–0.75 moderate, 0.75–0.9 good, and >0.9 indicates excellent correlation [41]. Box-Cox transformation was implemented in SPSS for variables with non-normal distribution to obtain a near-normal distribution for parametric tests. A two-way analysis of variance (ANOVA) was used to compare PD scores between groups with a musical background as a fixed factor. Effect sizes are reported as partial Eta squared (η_p^2). Effect size of 0.01, 0.1, and 0.25 indicated small, medium, and large statistical effects, respectively [42].

A Receiver Operating Characteristic (ROC) Curve Analysis was calculated to evaluate the value of PD testing in differentiating the voice-disordered groups from the control group. Where there were multiple tests, we used Sidak's adjustment to the observed p values to minimize Type I error. In all calculations, statistical significance testing was two-tailed, $p < 0.05$.

3. Results

3.1. Reliability of PD Testing

Table 3 shows reliability results for PD testing for all groups. There was good to excellent agreement in PD responses between the first and second trials within all groups.

Table 3. Reliability of PD testing. ICC: intraclass correlation coefficient; CI: confidence interval, MTVD: muscle tension voice disorders.

Groups	Single Measures (ICC, 95% CI)	Average Measures (ICC, 95% CI)	p
Whole cohort	0.899 (0.863–0.926)	0.947 (0.927–0.961)	<0.001
Control (n = 80)	0.880 (0.819–0.921)	0.936 (0.901–0.959)	<0.001
MTVD (n = 50)	0.847 (0.746–0.910)	0.917 (0.854–0.953)	<0.001
Neuro (n = 21)	0.972 (0.933–0.989)	0.986 (0.965–0.994)	<0.0001

3.2. Percentage of Accurate Responses

3.2.1. Voice-Disordered vs. Non-Voice-Disordered Groups

The percentage of correct responses for the PD test is shown in Figure 1. A two-way ANOVA was calculated to compare the correct scores between the voice-disordered group (n = 71) and the control group (n = 80). Musical background was included as a factor given previous findings of better PD in people with a musical background than those without [12,13]. There were significant effects of group, (F(1, 147) = 9.97, p = 0.002, η_p^2 = 0.064), and musical background, (F(1, 147) = 57.94, p < 0.001, η_p^2 = 0.28), but there was no significant interaction (p = 0.31). The mean (95% CI) of the percentage of accurate responses was lower by 10.32% (3.86–16.78) in the voice-disordered group compared with the control group (p = 0.002).

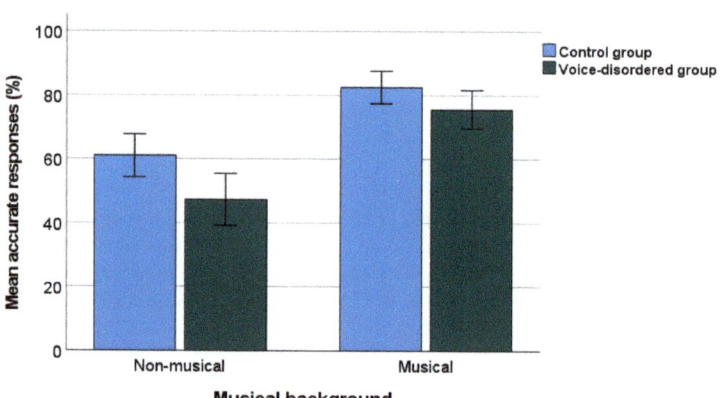

Figure 1. Percentage of PD accuracy in voice-disordered and control groups. Error bars indicate standard errors.

3.2.2. Sub-Group Comparisons

Figure 2 shows the percentage of correct PD responses for sub-groups. Sub-group comparisons were calculated using a two-way ANOVA, comparing across three groups (control, MTVD, neurological) and the two backgrounds (musical, non-musical). Again there was a significant effect of group (F(2, 145) = 7.632, p < 0.001, η_p^2 = 0.095) and musical background (F(1, 145) = 52.130, p < 0.001, η_p^2 = 0.264) but no significant interaction (p = 0.376).

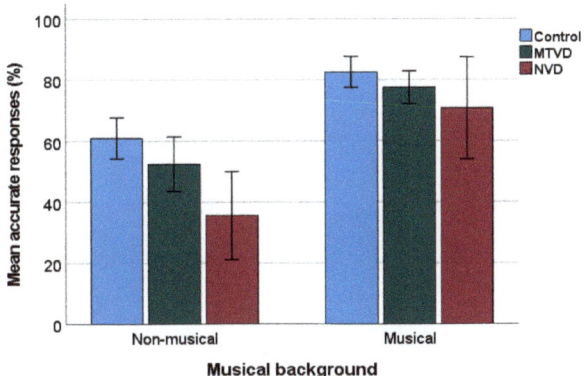

Figure 2. Percentage of PD accuracy in sub-groups. Error bars indicate standard errors. MTVD: muscle tension voice disorder; NVD: neurological voice disorder.

Post-hoc test using Sidak's adjustment to the p values showed that compared with the control group, the mean of percentage of accurate response was significantly lower by 18.55% (95% CI = 6.77–30.33%) in the neurological group ($p < 0.001$), but not in the MTVD group (mean difference = 6.75%, 95% CI = −1.93–15.43%, $p = 0.176$). The two voice-disordered groups were not significantly different (Mean difference = 11.8%, 95% CI = −0.81–24.41%, $p = 0.074$).

There was no statistical difference (t = 0.153, $p = 0.879$) in the percentage of correct responses (%) between the primary MTVD (n = 26; mean = 68.08, SD = 23.24) and secondary MTVD groups ($n = 24$, mean = 68.96, SD = 17.38).

3.3. Pitch Discrimination Threshold

3.3.1. Voice-Disordered vs. Non-Voice-Disordered Groups

Figure 3 shows the PD threshold data for the voice-disordered (Mean = 108.08 cents) and control groups (Mean = 98.65 cents) by musical background. For statistical analysis, the mean PD threshold for each participant were Box-Cox transformed due to non-normal distribution. A two-way ANOVAs as reported for PD, showed significant effects of group (F(1, 147) = 16.704, $p < 0.001$, $\eta_p^2 = 0.102$) and musical background (F(1, 147) = 17.212, $p < 0.001$, $\eta_p^2 = 0.105$), but no interaction ($p = 0.122$). Overall, the PD threshold in voice-disordered patients was 9.43 cents higher than that in the control group.

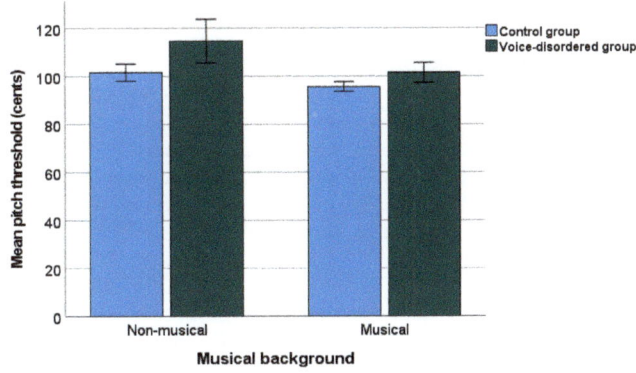

Figure 3. Pitch discrimination threshold in voice-disordered group and control group. Error bars indicate standard errors.

3.3.2. Sub-Group Comparisons

Figure 4 shows the data of the mean PD threshold by sub-groups. Descriptively, mean PD threshold (cents) was higher in each voice-disordered group (MTVD = 105.12; neurological voice disorder = 109.18) than in the control group (Mean = 98.65).

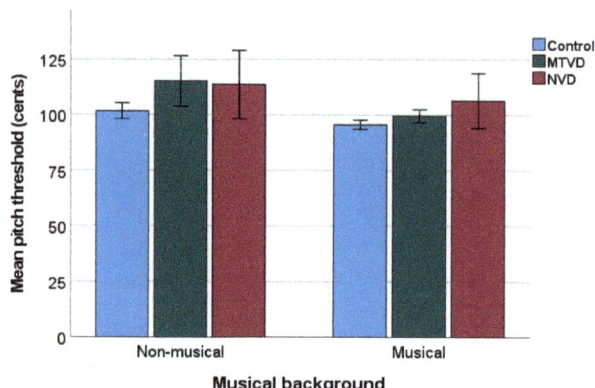

Figure 4. Mean pitch discrimination threshold of sub-groups. The lower pitch threshold, the better discrimination ability. Error bars indicate standard errors. MTVD: muscle tension voice disorder; NVD: neurological voice disorder.

A two-way ANOVA showed significant sub-group ($F_{(2, 145)}$ = 8.723, p < 0.001, η_p^2 = 0.107) and musical background ($F_{(1, 145)}$ = 12.735, p < 0.001, η_p^2 = 0.081) effects, but there was no interaction (p = 0.163). Post hoc comparisons showed that the PD threshold was significantly higher in both the MTVD group (by 8.66 cents, p = 0.003) and neurological voice disorder group (by 11.38 cents, p = 0.004), than in the control group. The two voice-disordered groups did not differ (p = 0.848).

Pair-wise comparison across sub-groups of the same musical background showed that in the non-musical background group, the mean PD threshold was significantly higher for the MTVD group than for the control group (by 13.49 cents, p = 0.002), but there were no differences between the neurological voice disorder group and control group (p = 0.080). In the musical background group, the mean PD threshold in the neurological voice disorder group was 10.806 cents higher than that in the control group (p = 0.047) whilst this measure was not statistically different between MTVD and controls (p = 0.570).

The mean (SD) of the PD threshold (cents) of the primary MTVD and secondary MTVD groups was 105.66 (22.59) and 104.53 (9.54). An independent samples t-test showed no statistically significant difference in the PD threshold between primary and secondary MTVD groups (t = 0.235, p = 0.816).

The Pearson's correlation coefficients calculated using the combined sample size of both voice-disordered and control groups (n = 151) showed significant correlations between the percentage of correct responses and mean PD threshold (r = −0.695, p < 0.001), median pitch threshold (r = −0.483, p < 0.001), and minimal pitch threshold (r = −0.488, p < 0.001). These implied that the accuracy of responses was associated with the size of the pitch intervals of tone pairs.

3.4. Predictive Value of PD Testing in Differentiating Voice-Disordered from Control Groups

An ROC curve (as shown in Figure 5) was analyzed to evaluate the predictive value of PD testing in differentiating the voice-disordered group from the control group. This measure significantly differentiated the two groups (area under the ROC curve, AUC = 0.630, 95% CI = 0.547–0.707, Z-statistic = 2.828, p = 0.005). With a Youden index (J) of 0.243 and the associated cut-off value >106.28 cents, this measure differentiated the two groups at a specificity of 86.25% and a sensitivity of 38.03%. At a cut-off of >85.02 cents, sensitivity was

98.59% but specificity was low (2.5%). The cut-off value of >97.45 cents had a balance of both sensitivity (64.79%) and specificity (53.75%).

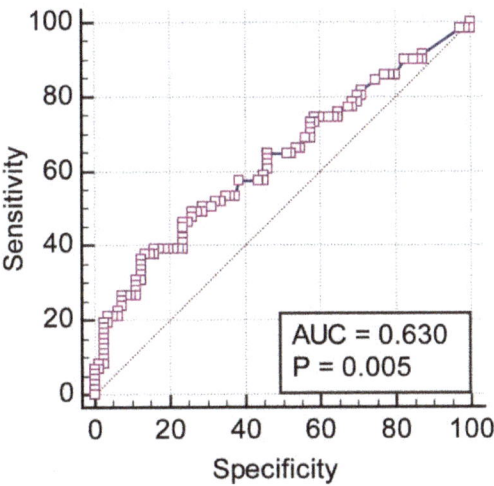

Figure 5. ROC curve for mean pitch discrimination threshold (cents).

4. Discussion

4.1. Pitch Discrimination in Voice-Disordered Patients

As predicted, pitch discrimination accuracy was significantly lower in the voice-disordered group than in the non-voice-disordered group. Based on effect size calculations, the size of this effect was medium. However, with respect to the units of measurement, the difference might be considered small (i.e., 9.43 cents). These differences in pitch discrimination support a previous study [6] showing that patients with behavioral dysphonia had worse pitch perception ability than non-dysphonic speakers. The patients with either MTVD or neurological voice disorder required a larger pitch threshold (above 100 cents) to correctly discriminate the pitch differences compared with the healthy speaker control group (again yielding a medium effect size). Patients with a neurological disorder needed a slightly larger threshold (109.18 cents) than those with a functional voice disorder (105.12 cents), although this difference was not statistically significant.

These results are suggestive of an impairment in auditory discrimination in both functional (MTVD) and neurological voice-disordered individuals. These data are also congruent with work by Abur et al. [4] who showed that the auditory discrimination threshold was significantly larger in patients with hyperfunctional voice disorders (mean = 47 cents, SD = 32 cents) than in control participants (mean = 35 cents, SD = 20 cents). The differences in the auditory discrimination thresholds between our current data and their study likely stemmed from the study design and type of test stimuli. Here, we did not test the just-noticeable-difference (JND) in pitch, but rather used pure tones. In summary, reliable group differences were noted in pitch perception between voice and non-voice-disordered samples, although the clinical relevance of the difference remains to be studied.

In the voice-disordered group, patients with a neurological voice disorder did not show statistically significantly poorer PD than those with MTVD. This suggests voice disorder types and/or dysphonic severity may not be linked to the auditory perception function. This finding appeared to agree with observations by Abur et al. [4] who found no relationship between the overall severity of dysphonia and auditory discrimination threshold. It is important to note that their study [4] only included patients with hyperfunction voice disorders, which might have had smaller range of vocal dysfunction than in our study.

The pitch interval of the pure tones used in the PD testing tool (NeAP) ranged between 29.98 and 200.01 cents. At the smallest pitch interval, the accurate responses for control, MTVD, and neurological group were 29 (19.2%), 18 (11.9%), and 9 (6.0%), respectively. This suggests that the voice-disordered group, particularly the neurological group, had more difficulties discriminating small pitch intervals than controls. We recommend that in future work the JND for different types of voice disorders with different severity should be investigated. This would help to further understand the impact of voice disorders on the minimum pitch difference that a patient can detect, and explore the relationship between voice perception and production.

It is believed that aberrant auditory discrimination plays a role in the pathogenesis of hyperfunctional voice disorder [4]. Current neural models of voice/speech production can be used to explain the poorer PD in those with a voice disorder. In the first place, auditory dysfunction may occur first. The DIVA neural model of phonation [3] states that the control of voice production includes two components: feedforward control (motor components) and feedback control (auditory and somatosensory targets). When the auditory discrimination system is dysfunctional, the ability to detect the mismatch between the expected and real feedback would be decreased. Consequently, this would lead to suboptimal use of the laryngeal motor system in phonation due to the feedforward system failing to update the corrective motor plan provided by the auditory feedback system [4]. This explanation appears to be applicable to MTVD and is supported by previous findings on the mismatch between the auditory-motor control system in patients with hyperfunctional voice disorders [4,5].

In patients with a neurological voice disorder, the model of neural plasticity [43] might explain the poorer PD compared with the non-voice-disordered controls. In patients with neurological voice disorders, neural plasticity may explain the adjustment (increase) in the auditory response threshold to allow for the variability in motor response. Neuroplastic models are well-known when explaining voice and laryngeal syndromes that involve a sensory pathway dysfunction such as the irritable larynx syndrome [44] or the laryngeal hypersensitivity syndromes [45]. A similar neuroplastic process may exist in those with a neurological voice disorder. Increasing the auditory discrimination threshold would benefit the auditory-motor control system in that auditory feedback would be less sensitive to feedback errors and the feedforward system would be less likely to provide motor commands that exceed the capability of the neurologically impaired laryngeal motor system. This model provides an explanation for shifting internal PD thresholds, or other auditory discrimination/perception thresholds to adapt to a worsening voice quality. Over time, if laryngeal coordination is worsened, further feedback would be added to the system, exacerbating the threshold sensitivity. Eventually, there may be more adaptive adjustments in auditory-motor control system, leading to compensatory/suboptimal laryngeal muscle use, or compensatory hyperfunction.

Musical background was factored in the between-subjects analysis due to its known impact on pitch perception. Despite overall differences between individuals in terms of musical background improving pitch discrimination, supporting previous research [12], there were no interactions involving the voice group. Group effects related to musical training background were descriptively similar to those due to voice for pitch accuracy, but for pitch threshold, musical background appeared to have larger and more reliable impacts on pitch perception than voice disorder.

The non-significant interaction effect between groups and musical background in this study was surprising given previous research indicating that both musicians and singers have a greater ability to compensate for pitch disturbances [46,47]. The above-mentioned mechanisms explaining the reasons for poor pitch discrimination in voice-disordered individuals might bypass or over-ride the well-established reflexes or processes formed in those with musical and/or singing training. This non-interaction between voice groups and musical background also implied that training does allow individuals, regardless of pathology, to improve pitch discrimination.

4.2. Predictive Value of PD Testing

Results of the ROC curve analyses showed that the PD threshold had a predictive ability to discriminate between voice-disordered and control groups. This suggests that it is possible to use PD testing as a method to differentiate a voice-disordered group from non-disordered speakers. It is necessary to develop/revise the PD testing tool to include a wider range of pitch intervals/differences and test its sensitivity and specificity in different levels of dysphonic severity and different voice disorder types. This development will allow validation of its applicability in clinical settings. In the present study, the sensitivity and specificity of this measure were relatively low if a balance between them is used in determining a cut-off value.

Previous research showed that people without musical training required thresholds between 1 and 3 semitones (100–300 cents) to be able to discriminate pitch intervals [48]. In the present study we found that a cut-off of >97.45 cents had a reasonable balance between sensitivity and specificity of testing. However, the relatively low sensitivity and specificity probably resulted from heterogeneity within the voice-disordered groups (i.e., including both functional and neurological voice disorders). We did not perform the ROC analyses separately for the MTVD and neurological voice disorder groups and for the two musical background due to the small sample size of each subgroup. It may also be the case that the current NeAP protocol was not associated with optimal prediction ability given the number of tone pairs used (20) and the range of PD threshold. Smaller thresholds would probably be more likely to differentiate the groups with better sensitivity and/or specificity.

This study had several limitations that should be addressed in future research to help with internal and external validity. Firstly, this was a cross-sectional observational study and not a prospective cohort study. Consequently, this design did not allow the determination of PD of the dysphonic speaker prior to having a voice disorder. Therefore, we cannot state that PD deteriorated in these patients when they acquired a voice disorder. A second issue related to validity, was that the control group comprised all females at a younger age range than the dysphonic group. As auditory perception may vary as a function of age, better matched comparison groups will be needed to determine the size and reliability of any effects due to voice pathology. Lastly, despite its utility and functionality, there is a lack of literature exploring the sensitivity and specificity of the NeAP testing tool in differentiating those with and without voice disorders according to their PD abilities. Further studies are needed to validate this tool for clinical application.

5. Conclusions

Here we showed that patients with a voice disorder had poorer PD than non-voice-disordered controls. Patients with MTVD and neurological voice disorders had a lower percentage of accurate PD responses and required larger pitch discrimination thresholds to correctly identify pitch differences between tone pairs. These findings provided more evidence for a possible dysfunction or dysregulation of both auditory discrimination pathways and laryngeal motor control in these voice-disordered groups. The mechanisms for poorer PD might be different between functional/MTVD voice disorders and neurological voice disorders given the differences in the pathogenesis of each disorder type.

PD testing significantly differentiated voice-disordered patients (MTVD and neurological voice disorders) from non-disordered speakers. This finding is important as PD testing can serve as not only a diagnostic tool but also a follow-up tool during the treatment process. Moreover, the fact that musical background significantly distinguished PD ability irrespective of voice disorder, suggests that problems in perception can be overcome with training. These data highlight the need to evaluate both auditory discrimination function and voice quality across the diagnosis, treatment, and follow-up stages for voice disorders. It would be necessary to clarify whether PD changes reflect treatment outcome.

Author Contributions: Conceptualization, D.D.N. and C.M.; methodology, C.M. and D.D.N.; formal analysis, D.D.N.; investigation, C.M. and D.D.N.; data curation, A.M.C. and D.D.N.; writing—original draft preparation, D.D.N. and C.M.; writing—review and editing, C.M., D.D.N. A.M.C., N.J.H., P.N.C. and D.N.; project administration, C.M.; visualization, D.N.; funding acquisition, C.M. and D.N. All authors have read and agreed to the published version of the manuscript.

Funding: This research was funded by The Dr Liang Voice Program at The University of Sydney.

Institutional Review Board Statement: This project was approved by Human Research Ethics Committee of the University of Sydney (protocol number: 2020/027). All participants read a participant information sheet and signed a consent form prior to participating in the study.

Informed Consent Statement: All participants signed a written consent form prior to taking part in the present study.

Data Availability Statement: Data supporting reported results is retained by The University of Sydney in a de-identified form and is confidential under the conditions of the Human Research Ethics Committee of The University of Sydney approval.

Acknowledgments: We would like to thank the participants for participating in the study.

Conflicts of Interest: A.M.C., C.M., D.D.N. and D.N. are employees of The University of Sydney and are part or fully funded by the Dr Liang Voice Program, a philanthropically funded program of research and post-graduate education in laryngology. The funders had no role in the design of the study; in the collection, analyses, or interpretation of data; in the writing of the manuscript, or in the decision to publish the results.

Appendix A

Table A1. Frequency of tone pairs of the NeAP.

Tone Pairs		Frequency 1 (Hz)	Frequency 2 (Hz)	Hz Difference	Cent Difference
C3 (130.81)	D3 (146.83)	130.81	146.83	16.02	200.01
A3 (220.00)	B3 (246.94)	220	246.94	26.94	199.99
C4 (261.63)	D4 (293.66)	261.63	293.66	32.03	199.94
B2 (123.47)	C3 (130.81)	123.47	130.81	7.34	99.97
E3 (164.81)	F3 (174.61)	164.81	174.61	9.8	100.00
F3 (174.61)	F#3 (185.00)	174.61	185	10.39	100.07
C3 (130.81)	C#3 (138.59)	130.81	138.59	7.78	100.02
G3 (196.00)	G#3 (207.65)	196	207.65	11.65	99.96
D4 (293.66)	D#4 (311.13)	293.66	311.13	17.47	100.04
A3 (220.00)	A#3 (233.08)	220	233.08	13.08	99.99
D4 (293.66)	D4.5 (302.26)	293.66	302.26	8.6	49.97
F3 (174.61)	F3.5 (179.73)	174.61	179.73	5.12	50.03
C3 (130.31)	C3.5 (134.64)	130.31	134.64	4.33	56.59
A3 (220.00)	A3.5 (226.45)	220	226.46	6.46	50.10
E3 (164.81)	E3.5 (169.64)	164.81	169.64	4.83	50.01
D3 (146.83)	D3.5 (151.13)	146.83	151.13	4.3	49.97
B3 (246.94)	B3.5 (254.18)	246.94	254.18	7.24	50.03
G3 (196.00)	G3.5 (201.74)	196	201.74	5.74	49.97
C3 (130.81)	C3.3 (133.1)	130.81	133.1	2.29	30.05
F3 (174.61)	F3.3 (177.66)	174.61	177.66	3.05	29.98

References

1. Ludlow, C.L. Central nervous system control of the laryngeal muscles in humans. *Respir. Physiol. Neurobiol.* **2005**, *147*, 205–222. [CrossRef]
2. Patel, A.D. Why would Musical Training Benefit the Neural Encoding of Speech? The OPERA Hypothesis. *Front. Psychol.* **2011**, *2*, 142. [CrossRef]
3. Tourville, J.A.; Guenther, F.H. The DIVA model: A neural theory of speech acquisition and production. *Lang. Cogn. Process.* **2011**, *26*, 952–981. [CrossRef]
4. Abur, D.; Subaciute, A.; Kapsner-Smith, M.; Segina, R.K.; Tracy, L.F.; Noordzij, J.P.; Stepp, C.E. Impaired auditory discrimination and auditory-motor integration in hyperfunctional voice disorders. *Sci. Rep.* **2021**, *11*, 13123. [CrossRef]
5. Stepp, C.E.; Lester-Smith, R.A.; Abur, D.; Daliri, A.; Pieter Noordzij, J.; Lupiani, A.A. Evidence for Auditory-Motor Impairment in Individuals with Hyperfunctional Voice Disorders. *J. Speech Lang. Hear. Res.* **2017**, *60*, 1545–1550. [CrossRef]
6. Ramos, J.S.; Feniman, M.R.; Gielow, I.; Silverio, K.C.A. Correlation between Voice and Auditory Processing. *J. Voice* **2018**, *32*, 771.e725–771.e736. [CrossRef]
7. Aronson, A.E.; Bless, D.M. *Clinical Voice Disorders*, 4th ed.; Thieme: New York, NY, USA, 2009.
8. Mathieson, L. *The Voice and Its Disorders*, 6th ed.; Whurr Publishers Ltd.: London, UK, 2001.
9. Payten, C.; Madill, C. Frameworks, Terminology and Definitions used for the Classification of Voice Disorders: A scoping review. *J. Voice*, 2021; in press.
10. Verdolini, K.; Rosen, C.; Branski, R. *Classification Manual for Voice Disorders-I*; Lawrence Erlbaum Associates, Inc.: Mahwah, NJ, USA, 2006.
11. Bidelman, G.M.; Hutka, S.; Moreno, S. Tone language speakers and musicians share enhanced perceptual and cognitive abilities for musical pitch: Evidence for bidirectionality between the domains of language and music. *PLoS ONE* **2013**, *8*, e60676. [CrossRef]
12. Micheyl, C.; Delhommeau, K.; Perrot, X.; Oxenham, A.J. Influence of musical and psychoacoustical training on pitch discrimination. *Hear. Res.* **2006**, *219*, 36–47. [CrossRef]
13. Mary Zarate, J.; Ritson, C.R.; Poeppel, D. Pitch-interval discrimination and musical expertise: Is the semitone a perceptual boundary? *J. Acoust. Soc. Am.* **2012**, *132*, 984–993. [CrossRef]
14. Bianchi, F.; Hjortkjaer, J.; Santurette, S.; Zatorre, R.J.; Siebner, H.R.; Dau, T. Subcortical and cortical correlates of pitch discrimination: Evidence for two levels of neuroplasticity in musicians. *Neuroimage* **2017**, *163*, 398–412. [CrossRef] [PubMed]
15. Hall, D.A.; Plack, C.J. Pitch processing sites in the human auditory brain. *Cereb. Cortex* **2009**, *19*, 576–585. [CrossRef] [PubMed]
16. Foxton, J.M.; Weisz, N.; Bauchet-Lecaignard, F.; Delpuech, C.; Bertrand, O. The neural bases underlying pitch processing difficulties. *Neuroimage* **2009**, *45*, 1305–1313. [CrossRef]
17. Behroozmand, R.; Korzyukov, O.; Larson, C.R. ERP correlates of pitch error detection in complex tone and voice auditory feedback with missing fundamental. *Brain Res.* **2012**, *1448*, 89–100. [CrossRef]
18. Peretz, I.; Vuvan, D.T. Prevalence of congenital amusia. *Eur. J. Hum. Genet.* **2017**, *25*, 625–630. [CrossRef]
19. Hyde, K.L.; Zatorre, R.J.; Peretz, I. Functional MRI evidence of an abnormal neural network for pitch processing in congenital amusia. *Cereb. Cortex* **2011**, *21*, 292–299. [CrossRef] [PubMed]
20. Anderson, K.S.; Gosselin, N.; Sadikot, A.F.; Lague-Beauvais, M.; Kang, E.S.H.; Fogarty, A.E.; Marcoux, J.; Dagher, J.; de Guise, E. Pitch and Rhythm Perception and Verbal Short-Term Memory in Acute Traumatic Brain Injury. *Brain Sci.* **2021**, *11*, 1173. [CrossRef]
21. Ziethe, A.; Petermann, S.; Hoppe, U.; Greiner, N.; Bruning, M.; Bohr, C.; Dollinger, M. Control of Fundamental Frequency in Dysphonic Patients During Phonation and Speech. *J. Voice* **2019**, *33*, 851–859. [CrossRef]
22. Davis, D.S.; Boone, D.R. Pitch discrimination and tonal memory abilities in adult voice patients. *J. Speech Hear. Res.* **1967**, *10*, 811–815. [CrossRef]
23. Murray, E.S.H.; Hseu, A.F.; Nuss, R.C.; Woodnorth, G.H.; Stepp, C.E. Vocal Pitch Discrimination in Children with and without Vocal Fold Nodules. *Appl. Sci.* **2019**, *9*, 3042. [CrossRef]
24. Thomas, A.; Mirza, N.; Eliades, S.J. Auditory Feedback Control of Vocal Pitch in Spasmodic Dysphonia. *Laryngoscope* **2021**, *131*, 2070–2075. [CrossRef]
25. Naunheim, M.L.; Yung, K.C.; Schneider, S.L.; Henderson-Sabes, J.; Kothare, H.; Hinkley, L.B.; Mizuiri, D.; Klein, D.J.; Houde, J.F.; Nagarajan, S.S.; et al. Cortical networks for speech motor control in unilateral vocal fold paralysis. *Laryngoscope* **2019**, *129*, 2125–2130. [CrossRef] [PubMed]
26. Naunheim, M.L.; Yung, K.C.; Schneider, S.L.; Henderson-Sabes, J.; Kothare, H.; Mizuiri, D.; Klein, D.J.; Houde, J.F.; Nagarajan, S.S.; Cheung, S.W. Vocal motor control and central auditory impairments in unilateral vocal fold paralysis. *Laryngoscope* **2019**, *129*, 2112–2117. [CrossRef]
27. Peretz, I.; Vuvan, D.; Lagrois, M.E.; Armony, J.L. Neural overlap in processing music and speech. *Philos. Trans. R. Soc. B Biol. Sci.* **2015**, *370*, 20140090. [CrossRef]
28. Angulo-Perkins, A.; Concha, L. Discerning the functional networks behind processing of music and speech through human vocalizations. *PLoS ONE* **2019**, *14*, e0222796. [CrossRef]
29. Drinnan, M. *Newcastle Assessment of Pitch Discrimination*; Newcastle University: Newcastle, UK, 2012.
30. Yun, E.W.-T.; Nguyen, D.D.; Carding, P.; Hodges, N.J.; Chacon, A.M.; Madill, C. The relationship between pitch discrimination and acoustic voice measures in a cohort of female speakers. *J. Voice* **2021**, in press.

31. Rosen, C.A.; Lee, A.S.; Osborne, J.; Zullo, T.; Murry, T. Development and validation of the Voice Handicap Index-10. *Laryngoscope* **2004**, *114*, 1549–1556. [CrossRef]
32. Behlau, M.; Madazio, G.; Moreti, F.; Oliveira, G.; Dos Santos Lde, M.; Paulinelli, B.R.; Couto Junior Ede, B. Efficiency and Cutoff Values of Self-Assessment Instruments on the Impact of a Voice Problem. *J. Voice* **2016**, *30*, 506.e509–506.e518. [CrossRef]
33. Kempster, G.B.; Gerratt, B.R.; Verdolini Abbott, K.; Barkmeier-Kraemer, J.; Hillman, R.E. Consensus auditory-perceptual evaluation of voice: Development of a standardized clinical protocol. *Am. J. Speech Lang. Pathol.* **2009**, *18*, 124–132. [CrossRef]
34. Fairbanks, G. *Voice and Articulation Drillbook*, 2nd ed.; Harper & Row: New York, NY, USA, 1960.
35. Awan, S.N.; Roy, N.; Jette, M.E.; Meltzner, G.S.; Hillman, R.E. Quantifying dysphonia severity using a spectral/cepstral-based acoustic index: Comparisons with auditory-perceptual judgements from the CAPE-V. *Clin. Linguist. Phon.* **2010**, *24*, 742–758. [CrossRef]
36. Awan, S.N.; Roy, N.; Zhang, D.; Cohen, S.M. Validation of the Cepstral Spectral Index of Dysphonia (CSID) as a Screening Tool for Voice Disorders: Development of Clinical Cutoff Scores. *J. Voice* **2016**, *30*, 130–144. [CrossRef] [PubMed]
37. Boersma, P.; Weenink, D. Praat: Doing Phonetics by Computer. Available online: http://www.fon.hum.uva.nl/praat/ (accessed on 26 January 2018).
38. IBM Corp. IBM SPSS Software. Available online: https://www.ibm.com/analytics/data-science/predictive-analytics/spss-statistical-software (accessed on 8 February 2018).
39. MedCalc Software. MedCalc—User-Friendly Statistical Software. Available online: https://www.medcalc.org/ (accessed on 15 September 2021).
40. Shrout, P.E.; Fleiss, J.L. Intraclass correlations: Uses in assessing rater reliability. *Psychol. Bull.* **1979**, *86*, 420–428. [CrossRef] [PubMed]
41. Koo, T.K.; Li, M.Y. A Guideline of Selecting and Reporting Intraclass Correlation Coefficients for Reliability Research. *J. Chiropr. Med.* **2016**, *15*, 155–163. [CrossRef] [PubMed]
42. Murphy, K.R. *Statistical Power Analysis: A Simple and General Model for Traditional and Modern Hypothesis Tests*, 4th ed.; Routledge: New York, NY, USA, 2014.
43. Zarate, J.M.; Delhommeau, K.; Wood, S.; Zatorre, R.J. Vocal accuracy and neural plasticity following micromelody-discrimination training. *PLoS ONE* **2010**, *5*, e11181. [CrossRef]
44. Morrison, M.; Rammage, L.; Emami, A.J. The irritable larynx syndrome. *J. Voice* **1999**, *13*, 447–455. [CrossRef]
45. Vertigan, A.E.; Bone, S.L.; Gibson, P.G. Laryngeal sensory dysfunction in laryngeal hypersensitivity syndrome. *Respirology* **2013**, *18*, 948–956. [CrossRef]
46. Patel, S.; Gao, L.; Wang, S.; Gou, C.; Manes, J.; Robin, D.A.; Larson, C.R. Comparison of volitional opposing and following responses across speakers with different vocal histories. *J. Acoust. Soc. Am.* **2019**, *146*, 4244. [CrossRef]
47. Kim, J.H.; Larson, C.R. Modulation of auditory-vocal feedback control due to planned changes in voice f_o. *J. Acoust. Soc. Am.* **2019**, *145*, 1482. [CrossRef]
48. McDermott, J.H.; Keebler, M.V.; Micheyl, C.; Oxenham, A.J. Musical intervals and relative pitch: Frequency resolution, not interval resolution, is special. *J. Acoust. Soc. Am.* **2010**, *128*, 1943–1951. [CrossRef]

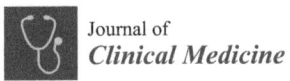

Article

Supraglottic Botulinum Toxin Improves Symptoms in Patients with Laryngeal Sensory Dysfunction Manifesting as Abnormal Throat Sensation and/or Chronic Refractory Cough

Daniel Novakovic [1,2,3,*], Meet Sheth [1,4], Thomas Stewart [1,3], Katrina Sandham [3], Catherine Madill [1], Antonia Chacon [1] and Duy Duong Nguyen [1,5]

[1] Voice Research Laboratory, Discipline of Speech Pathology, Faculty of Medicine and Health, The University of Sydney, Sydney, NSW 2006, Australia; meet.c.sheth@gmail.com (M.S.); thomas.e.stewart@sydney.edu.au (T.S.); cate.madill@sydney.edu.au (C.M.); antonia.chacon@sydney.edu.au (A.C.); duong.nguyen@sydney.edu.au (D.D.N.)
[2] The Canterbury Hospital, Campsie, NSW 2194, Australia
[3] Sydney Voice and Swallowing, St. Leonards, NSW 2065, Australia; kate.sandham@gmail.com
[4] Department of Otolaryngology, Christian Medical College, Vellore 632004, India
[5] National Hospital of Otorhinolaryngology, Hanoi 11519, Vietnam
* Correspondence: daniel.novakovic@sydney.edu.au

Citation: Novakovic, D.; Sheth, M.; Stewart, T.; Sandham, K.; Madill, C.; Chacon, A.; Nguyen, D.D. Supraglottic Botulinum Toxin Improves Symptoms in Patients with Laryngeal Sensory Dysfunction Manifesting as Abnormal Throat Sensation and/or Chronic Refractory Cough. *J. Clin. Med.* **2021**, *10*, 5486. https://doi.org/10.3390/jcm10235486

Academic Editor: Renee Speyer

Received: 2 November 2021
Accepted: 19 November 2021
Published: 23 November 2021

Publisher's Note: MDPI stays neutral with regard to jurisdictional claims in published maps and institutional affiliations.

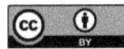

Copyright: © 2021 by the authors. Licensee MDPI, Basel, Switzerland. This article is an open access article distributed under the terms and conditions of the Creative Commons Attribution (CC BY) license (https://creativecommons.org/licenses/by/4.0/).

Abstract: Laryngeal sensory dysfunction (LSD) encompasses disorders of the vagal sensory pathways. Common manifestations include chronic refractory cough (CRC) and abnormal throat sensation (ATS). This study examined clinical characteristics and treatment outcomes of LSD using a novel approach of laryngeal supraglottic Onabotulinum toxin Type A injection (BTX). This was a retrospective review of clinical data and treatment outcomes of supraglottic BTX in patients with LSD. Between November 2019 and May 2021, 14 patients underwent 25 injection cycles of supraglottic BTX for treatment of symptoms related to LSD, including ATS and CRC. Primary outcome measures included the Newcastle Laryngeal Hypersensitivity Questionnaire (LHQ), Cough Severity Index (CSI), Reflux Symptom Index (RSI), and Voice Handicap Index-10 (VHI-10) at baseline and within three months of treatment. Pre- and post-treatment data were compared using a linear mixed model. After supraglottic BTX, LHQ scores improved by 2.6. RSI and CSI improved by 8.0 and 5.0, respectively. VHI-10 did not change as a result of treatment. Short-term response to SLN block was significantly associated with longer term response to BTX treatment. These findings suggest that LSD presents clinically as ATS and CRC along with other upper airway symptoms. Supraglottic BTX injection is a safe and effective technique in the treatment of symptoms of LSD.

Keywords: laryngeal sensory dysfunction; chronic refractory cough; botulinum toxin; larynx; laryngeal hypersensitivity; cough hypersensitivity syndrome; globus pharyngeus; laryngopharyngeal reflux; neuropathic cough; throat irritation

1. Introduction

The larynx is innervated by branches of the vagus nerve with complex coordination of afferent (sensory) and efferent (motor) pathways in the brainstem required for optimal physiological functioning [1,2]. Neurological dysfunction can occur secondary to central or peripheral pathology affecting the vagal pathways. Depending upon the level and nature of injury, vagal dysfunction can have either or both sensory and motor effects manifesting within and outside the larynx. Motor manifestations of vagal dysfunction involving the larynx can be broadly classified into hypofunctional (e.g., vocal fold paralysis or paresis) or hyperfunctional (e.g., inducible laryngeal obstruction) with laryngeal movement disorders affecting higher centers. Sensory manifestations of vagal dysfunction are less well understood but can present independently or in conjunction with apparent motor effects.

Laryngeal sensory dysfunction (LSD) represents disorders of laryngeal afferent sensory pathways presenting with abnormal laryngeal sensation. Several phenotypes related to hyperfunctional vagal sensation have been described manifesting in the larynx sharing similar features [3]. These include chronic refractory cough (CRC) [4], various forms of inducible laryngeal obstruction including recurrent laryngospasm, paradoxical vocal fold movement [5,6] and irritable larynx syndrome [7], globus pharyngeus [3] and laryngeal sensory neuropathy [8] with various proposed etiologies. We prefer to use the umbrella term laryngeal sensory dysfunction [3] which recognizes the role of abnormal laryngeal afferent sensory pathways in these conditions which may be affected at one or more levels (peripheral receptors, afferent vagal fibers, central pathways), and which present with abnormal/altered laryngeal sensation, without attribution to a specific underlying pathological process or cause. Accurate evaluation of laryngeal dysfunction and hypersensitivity would allow for accurate diagnosis and effective treatment [9].

Laryngeal hypersensitivity has been best described in the context of CRC [10], which is defined as a cough persisting beyond 8 weeks despite guideline-based treatment. Other terms for CRC include neurogenic cough, idiopathic cough, psychogenic cough, habitual cough and (laryngeal) cough hypersensitivity syndrome [11]. Increased sensitivity of the afferent limb of the cough reflex has been demonstrated in CRC [4], with those affected exhibiting a lower cough threshold in the capsaicin challenge test [12,13]. Furthermore, Vertigan and Gibson observed abnormal laryngeal sensation (laryngeal paresthesia) in 94% of patients with CRC [4], consistent with a sensory neuropathic disorder.

The concept of sensory neuropathy causing laryngeal symptoms was first proposed by Morrison et al. using the term irritable larynx syndrome [7]. They described laryngospasm, dysphonia, globus pharyngeus, pain and/or chronic cough as potential symptoms arising from a hyperexcitable state of the laryngeal neuronal sensory network. Laryngeal sensory neuropathy has also been described in the context of hypofunctional laryngeal sensation associated with a high risk of dysphagia in head and neck cancer patients [14]. Neuropathy represents a disturbance of function or pathological change in one or more nerves which can change the normal sensitivity or thresholds of afferent nerves causing neuropathic symptoms. Neuropathic pain is characterized by the clinical features of paresthesia, hyperalgesia and allodynia [15] with equivalent laryngeal features manifesting as abnormal throat sensation, hypertussia and allotussia (Table 1) [4].

Table 1. Equivalent laryngeal features of neuropathic pain.

Features of Neuropathic Pain	Explanation	Laryngeal Equivalents
Paresthesia	Abnormal sensation in the absence of a stimulus	Abnormal throat sensation—tickle, lump, globus pharyngeus
Hyperalgesia	Pain triggered at an abnormally low level by a noxious or painful stimulus	Hypertussia—cough triggered at an abnormally low threshold by a recognized cough stimulus
Allodynia	pain triggered by a non-noxious stimulus	Allotussia—cough triggered by non-cough stimuli, e.g., talking (mechanical) or cold air (thermal)

Laryngeal sensory receptors project centrally towards the nucleus tractus solitarius, primarily via the internal branch of the superior laryngeal nerve (iSLN), where activation can lead to a variety of reflexive responses including cough, swallow and laryngospasm [16]. The laryngeal adductor reflex (LAR) is one such robust and well-studied response which causes bilateral involuntary airway protective closure in response to supraglottic stimuli [17]. Topographic mapping of sensory receptors related to the LAR has recently been achieved. The highest density of LAR sensory receptors and afferent nerve fibers are found in the posterior supraglottis followed by the false vocal folds and epiglottic tip with no LAR activation with stimulation of the membranous vocal folds [18].

Peripheral and central sensitization are features of neuropathy. Peripheral sensitization describes both nociceptive and non-nociceptive sensory afferents becoming sensitized [15,19], with a lowered threshold for signaling, and/or an increase in the magnitude of responsiveness at the peripheral ends of sensory nerve fibers. A wide range of signaling molecules are involved in mediating peripheral sensitization including such neuropeptides as calcitonin gene-related peptide (CGRP) and substance P (SP). Laryngeal sensory dysfunction may occur at the periphery when laryngeal sensory receptors and nociceptive fibers become dysfunctional and undergo peripheral sensitization. The prolonged process of peripheral sensitization can lead to sensitization of the central sensory pathways, where potentiation by neurotransmitter signaling results in a net increase in neuronal spinal output [15,19].

1.1. Etiology of LSD/Mechanisms of Injury

The etiologies of LSD are yet to be fully elucidated, although numerous causes have been proposed in the literature. Morrison et al. [7] suggested viral infection, emotional distress, chronic reflux and habitual muscle misuse as potential contributing factors amongst other more common organic causes of nerve injuries [7].

Amin and Koufman [8] reported cases with laryngeal electromyographic evidence of lesions to both superior and recurrent laryngeal nerves. They maintained that damage to the vagal nerves was linked to a preceding viral upper respiratory tract infection as a one-off phenomenon rather than an ongoing/progressive degeneration or regeneration process [8]. Rees, Henderson and Belafsky [20] proposed Post-Viral Vagal Neuropathy as a clinical entity resulting from upper respiratory tract infection presenting with chronic cough, excessive throat clearing, dysphonia, and vocal fatigue with laryngoscopic signs of laryngeal motor weakness.

Honey et al. proposed neurovascular compression of the vagus nerve rootlets identified on magnetic resonance imaging [21] as a potential cause of vagal dysfunction presenting in the larynx with sensory symptoms of abnormal throat sensations [22] associated with motor symptoms of laryngospasm/choking, neurogenic cough or intermittent stridor [23].

Altman et al. suggested various factors (including topical airway infectious agents, inflammatory cytokines, viscosity of the airway mucus, gene regulation producing altered mucus in disease, the temperature and pH of the airway surface) may act synchronously to sensitize the larynx [24]. They activate and upregulate multiple upper airway receptors, including TRPV1 (transient receptor potential vanilloid 1, stimulated by acids, protons, and capsaicin). There is evidence that sensitization of the TRPV1 channel underlies hypersensitivity in neuropathic pain [25].

1.2. Assessment and Diagnosis of LSD

To date, no diagnostic criteria have been established for LSD. Consequently, the assessment of abnormal laryngeal sensation is based largely on patient history, clinical evaluation, appropriate questionnaires/patient-reported outcome measures (PROMs) and laryngeal investigations [9], along with limited response to treatment of other conditions which can present with similar symptomatology.

Several PROMs can be used for assessment of LSD (see methods). These questionnaires provide easily obtainable subjective baseline data which can then be used to monitor patient progress and treatment outcomes [26].

1.3. Superior Laryngeal Nerve Block

Local anesthetics are used extensively during endotracheal intubation and other procedures requiring upper airway manipulation to suppress normal physiological responses including cough and laryngospasm. Topical lidocaine (lignocaine) applied to the larynx has been shown to suppress laryngeal reflexes activated by mechanoreceptor and chemoceptor stimulation [27]. Superior laryngeal nerve block is another way to suppress these reflexes whereby the supraglottic larynx can be anesthetized in an awake patient by delivering local anesthesia around the internal branch of the superior laryngeal nerve at the thyro-hyoid membrane as it enters the larynx [28]. Lidocaine blockade of the SLN has been shown to temporarily relieve symptoms of laryngospasm due to known SLN injuries [29]. This opens the potential therapeutic pathway of modulating laryngeal sensation to treat conditions such as chronic refractory cough where LSD is a contributing factor. The temporary duration of this proposed modality as well as ease of administration makes this an excellent initial test to potentially predict response to treatments which can modulate sensation in the distribution of the SLN.

1.4. Treatment of LSD

Treatment of potential coexisting medical conditions that can present with similar symptoms is crucial in the management of LSD. A limited response will help support the diagnosis, but it is also important to control pathologies which can alter laryngeal sensitivity (including LPR, OSAS and chronic inflammation). Furthermore, any pathological process which can stimulate or irritate the laryngeal mucosa can act as a trigger of hypersensitized laryngeal sensory pathways and reflexes and reducing this sensory input can help with control of symptoms.

Centrally acting neuromodulators including amitriptyline, gabapentin, pregabalin and tramadol have some effectiveness in reducing symptoms linked to vagal neuropathy and have acceptance in the treatment of CRC [30,31]. There is evidence that gabapentin, which is effective mostly in pain due to nerve damage in postherpetic neuralgia and peripheral diabetic neuropathy [32], is also effective in treatment of odynophonia [8], neck pain [8], chronic cough and laryngospasm due to suspected sensory neuropathy of the SLN [33].

Behavioral treatment provided by a speech language pathologist (SLP) or physiotherapist has been found effective in management of CRC by reducing cough frequency [34] and cough reflex sensitivity [35]. Treatment typically includes some or all of the four elements described in the John Hunter Hospital Chronic Refractory Cough (JHCRC) Program: patient education regarding nature of cough, exercises to improve voluntary control over cough and/or suppression of the cough, reduction of behaviors that cause laryngeal irritation and psycho-educational counselling [36]. Improving voluntary control over one's cough and reducing the sources of irritation that trigger coughing are complementary approaches that are of equal importance in alleviating this behavior [37]. The treating clinician must emphasize the commitment required for behavioral change to occur and provide additional supports as necessary to facilitate the patient's independent management and control over their presenting symptoms.

1.5. Botulinum Toxin in the Larynx, and Its Potential Role as a Sensory Neural Modulator

Onabotulinum toxin Type A (BTX) is a proteolytic enzyme that cleaves neuronal SNARE proteins which play a crucial role in the mediation of neurotransmitter release. The primary studied effect of BTX is in motor nerves, where neuromuscular conduction is inhibited by the toxin, resulting in a localized but reversible chemical denervation of the associated muscle fibers.

The putative mechanism by which BTX may modulate laryngeal sensation can be best understood in the context of chronic refractory cough (CRC) and its correlation with neuropathic pain [30]. The therapeutic effects of BTX in CRC are thought to be due to its effects on sensory transmission and peripheral sensitization. Transient receptor potential (TRP) channels are a group of ion channels present on the plasma membrane of multiple mammalian cell types. In airway physiology, they play an important protective role in pathways inducing inflammation, mucus secretion, airway constriction, and reflexes such as cough and sneezing [38]. The reduced cough threshold in CRC is associated with increased expression of TRPV1 receptors on airway nerves [39,40]. Changes in these, and associated channels, along with the development of sensitization is the understood mechanism by which a chronic cough develops into a hypersensitivity syndrome [41].

In addition to motor effects, BTX also inhibits neurotransmitter release in sensory neurons, likely through the reduction in expression of neuropeptide transmitters, such as

SP and CGRP. TRPA1 and TRPV1 [42] are associated with CGRP-dependent pathways. Administration of BTX has been demonstrated to disrupt the transfer of TRP receptors to synaptic membranes [43,44]. Studies have previously demonstrated that BTX reduces pain and neurogenic inflammation caused by capsaicin, which is the antagonist of TRPV1 receptors [45]. As such, BTX sensory mechanism is at least partially via its effect on TRPV1 expression, with this modulation likely also interrupting the process of peripheral sensitization [46]. BTX is also thought to affect central sensitization; however, this remains controversial [46,47]. The interruption of these sensitivity pathways by peripheral administration of BTX is a potential way to modulate the symptoms experienced under the umbrella term laryngeal sensory dysfunction.

BTX was first used in the larynx by Blitzer in 1984 as a treatment for adductor spasmodic dysphonia [48] (a focal laryngeal dystonia). It has since become the gold standard for this condition. Injections are usually targeted to the involved intrinsic laryngeal adductor muscles to weaken them and prevent inappropriate contractions causing disruption of normal speech.

Several studies have reported the use of BTX targeted to the laryngeal adductor musculature for the treatment of chronic refractory cough [49–52]. Delivery of BTX into the supraglottic region is a more recent concept and was initially described by Young and Blitzer in 2007 as an adjunct treatment for patients with adductor spasmodic dysphonia who exhibited sphincteric closure of the supraglottic larynx during phonation [53]. In 2016, Simpson reported supraglottic BTX as an alternative primary treatment for adductor spasmodic dysphonia [54], showing improved voice outcomes with a favorable side effect profile compared with glottic BTX. To date, no study has examined the sensory effects of laryngeal BTX when delivered into the supraglottis rather than into the intrinsic laryngeal musculature.

1.6. Current Study Aims

The present study investigated a novel treatment of supraglottic BTX for LSD. The aims of the study were to: (1) describe the clinical characteristics of LSD in a cohort of patients referred for CRC and abnormal throat sensation (ATS); (2) describe a new treatment of supraglottic laryngeal botulinum toxin in the symptomatic management of laryngeal sensory dysfunction; (3) evaluate the efficacy of using botulinum toxin A in treatment of a pilot group of patients presenting with different phenotypes associated with laryngeal sensory dysfunction including CRC and ATS. We hypothesized that CRC and ATS can be manifestations of LSD and that treatment aimed at LSD would have therapeutic effects quantifiable using patient reported outcome measures of cough and throat sensation.

2. Materials and Methods

2.1. Study Design

This was a retrospective data review of an existing private specialized laryngology clinic database. The study was approved by the Human Research Ethics Committee of The University of Sydney (protocol number 2021/025).

2.2. Participants

A database search was implemented to identify all patients who underwent supraglottic BTX injections as part of treatment for clinical presentations associated with LSD.

Inclusion criteria were: (1) a history of sensory laryngeal symptoms (manifesting as CRC or ATS) for greater than 12 consecutive weeks despite assessment and treatment of potential/coexisting lower respiratory, sinonasal and laryngopharyngeal reflux pathology; (2) a Newcastle Laryngeal Hypersensitivity Questionnaire (LHQ) score of 17.1 or below [55].

Most patients had previously been offered neuromodulator medication and had either ceased this treatment due to poor response or negative side effects or remained on neuromodulators with partial symptom control whilst undergoing a trial of salvage laryngeal botulinum toxin treatment. All patients had been referred to a speech pathologist for behavioral treatment of their symptoms. Thirteen of the fourteen had seen a speech pathologist prior to BTX treatment. Speech pathology data was unavailable for one patient.

Fourteen patients were identified during the study period who underwent supraglottic BTX treatment for LSD, including six females and eight males. Mean age of patients was 54.9 years (standard deviation, SD = 12.5, range = 32–76).

Figure 1 shows diagram of study protocols. Table 2 presents information regarding demographics, onset, respiratory pathology, and neural modulator treatment for all patients.

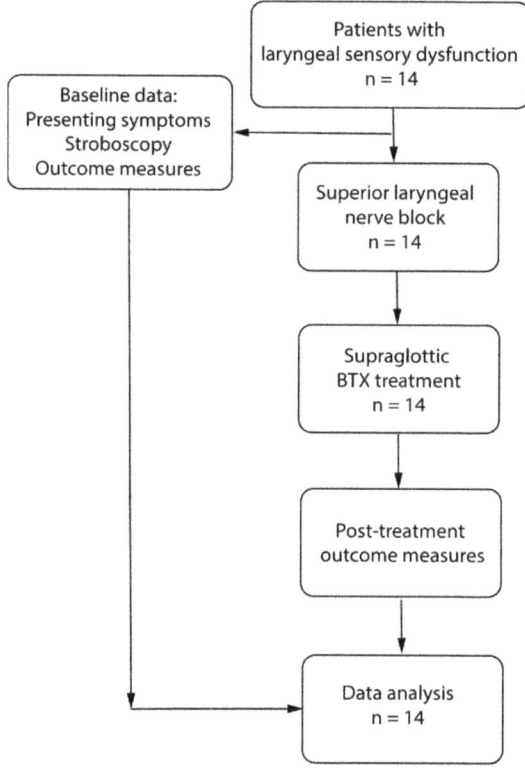

Figure 1. Flowchart of study protocols.

Table 2. Characteristics of the treatment cohort. NM, neuromodulator; SLN, superior laryngeal nerve; Gaba, gabapentin; PR, partial response; Ami, amitriptyline; NR, no response; URTI, upper respiratory tract infection; NS, nonsmoker, FS, former smoker.

Patient ID	Potential Preceding Factors Reported	Duration of Symptoms at Presentation (months)	Age, Gender	Smoking	Resp. Disease	Neuromodulator Treatment History
1	URTI	12	44, F	FS	Nil	Past Gaba—PR Ami current—PR
2	Occupational inhalational exposure	1	42, F	FS	Nil	Past Gaba—PR

Table 2. Cont.

Patient ID	Potential Preceding Factors Reported	Duration of Symptoms at Presentation (months)	Age, Gender	Smoking	Resp. Disease	Neuromodulator Treatment History
3	Intubation for hernia surgery	24	58, F	FS	Asthma, OSAS	Past Gaba—side effects
4	nil	5	76, M	FS	Asthma	Nil
5	Occupational inhalational exposure	14	56, M	FS	Nil	Past Gaba—side effects
6	Laryngeal trauma involving superior laryngeal nerve	11	48, M	FS	Nil	Ami current—PR, Past Gaba—side effects
7	URTI	120	32, M	FS	Nil	Declined
8	URTI	120	68, M	FS	Nil	Past Gaba—NR Ami current—PR
9	Occupational inhalational exposure	15	55, M	NS	Nil	Past Ami—side effects, Gaba current—PR
10	Intubation for cosmetic surgery	180	75, F	NS	Nil	Ami current—PR
11	nil	36	56, M	NS	Nil	Ami—side effects Gaba current—PR
12	nil	360	60, M	NS	Asthma (mild, controlled)	Nil
13	nil	240	44, F	NS	Nil	Past Gaba—NR
14	Thyroid surgery with Vocal fold palsy	7	54, F	NS	Nil	Past Ami—Side effects & NR Past Gaba—side effects & PR

2.3. Intervention: Supraglottic BTX Injection

Patients presenting with LSD who had persistent symptoms despite medical and behavioral (speech pathology) management underwent trial superior laryngeal nerve (SLN) block in the clinic. Immediate response to SLN block was measured using a 10-point Likert scale questionnaire based upon the patient's specific presenting symptoms which was developed using the Newcastle Laryngeal Hypersensitivity Questionnaire (LHQ) [55]. Immediate response was measured 20 min after SLN block and an improvement of their primary symptom by three or more points compared with baseline was considered a positive response. In the case of no response at 20 min, contralateral SLN block was offered, and response was assessed after a further 20 min. Patients who had symptomatic but short-term (<2 weeks) improvement after SLN block were offered subsequent botulinum toxin Type A (Botox™, Allergan, Irvine, CA, USA). Some patients who did not respond to SLN block elected to undergo a trial of supraglottic BTX treatment as salvage therapy after failed medical management including a trial of neuromodulator therapy.

BTX was usually given in an office-based outpatient setting. (In one patient with extreme hypersensitivity to flexible laryngoscopy, the BTX injection was given trans-orally during microlaryngoscopy under general anesthetic). Patients were seated semi-reclined with the head extended. Decongestant with local anesthesia was administered topically to the nasal cavity (5% lidocaine + phenylephrine) prior to the procedure. Bilateral SLN blocks were performed using 2% lidocaine, 0.5 cc on each side for the purpose of anesthesia during the procedure. BTX injection was performed using a 1 cc syringe coupled to a 23 or 25 G needle which was introduced into the larynx via a trans thyro-hyoid approach with the needle directed inferiorly, posteriorly and slightly laterally toward the targeted supraglottic region of the false vocal fold and posterosuperior larynx—where sensory receptor density is thought to be highest [18]. Flexible transnasal videolaryngoscopy was used to help guide the injection into the desired region and confirm placement. The injectate was delivered whilst keeping the needle in a submucosal plane without breaching the laryngeal airway and correct placement was confirmed via the presence of a visible bleb at the injection site (Figure 2). The BTX concentration was kept constant at 2.5 U per 0.1 cc of injectate with dosage adjusted by varying volume of injectate.

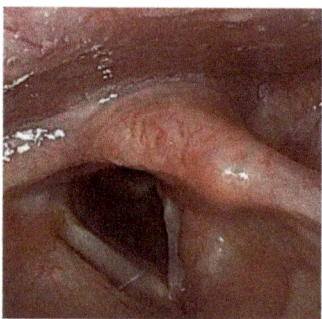 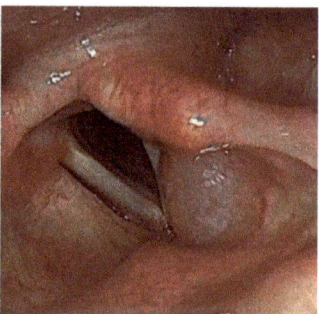

Figure 2. Endoscopic image of larynx before (**left**) and immediately after (**right**) supraglottic BTX injection showing visible submucosal bleb at injection site.

Nineteen treatments were given unilaterally and six bilaterally (2 synchronous, 4 staged). Mean dose for each supraglottic injection was 7.74 U (SD = 1.75 U). Mean time of post-treatment assessment was 7.1 weeks (SD = 3.2 weeks). The decision on which side to treat with BTX and whether to treat unilaterally or bilaterally was made based on a combination of the following factors: (i) the patient's self-perceived unilaterality of symptoms, (ii) laryngoscopic findings of motor asymmetry, particularly that of vertical height mismatch, with (iii) immediate response to SLN block on that side.

2.4. Data Extraction

One otolaryngologist and one registered nurse who were blind to the aims of the study performed data extraction from clinical records. The data described in the following subsection were collected during this review.

2.4.1. Demographic Characteristics and History

Demographic characteristics (age, gender). Smoking history. Symptom duration and potential preceding factors. Past investigation/treatment of significant co-morbidities including gastro-esophageal or laryngopharyngeal reflux, lower respiratory tract pathology, sinonasal conditions and obstructive sleep apnea. Current/past medications including ACE inhibitors and neuromodulators.

2.4.2. Videostrobolaryngoscopy Findings at Baseline

Videostrobolaryngoscopy is the gold standard clinical assessment for evaluating laryngeal structure and dynamic function [56]. All patients underwent neurolaryngological examination via trans nasal videostroboslaryngoscopy at baseline using a standardized clinical voice assessment protocol designed to identify potential features of laryngeal motor dysfunction [57]. Findings of vocal fold motion anomalies, glottic insufficiency and mucosal wave anomalies are the most reliable signs for the diagnosis of vocal fold paresis [56], a laryngeal motor impairment which may coexist with sensory dysfunction in some LSD patients where both efferent and afferent functions of the laryngeal nerve/s are affected.

All strobolaryngoscopy exams were extracted and blindly rated by two otolaryngologists using a tool developed in Bridge2practice, an online education and research platform developed for health and medical learning and practice of allied health professionals and students [58]. The following parameters were assessed: (1) vocal fold movement; (2) mucosal wave; (3) laryngeal muscle tension patterns.

Videos of eight strobolaryngoscopy exams were repeated, randomized and re-rated to evaluate intra-rater reliability. Ratings from the two blinded assessors were compared to calculate inter-rater reliability for stroboscopic parameters that are subject to low reliability of ratings such as vertical focal fold plane and phase symmetry [59]. Table 3 shows excellent intra-rater reliability and Table 4 shows good inter-rater reliability for key parameters.

Table 3. Intra-rater reliability (exact agreement in second rating/total repeated videos).

Parameters	Rater 1	Rater 2
Vocal fold movement	7/7	7/7
Abduction lag	7/7	6/7
Axis rotation on pitch glide	7/7	7/7
Phase symmetry	7/7	7/7
Amplitude	7/7	7/7

Table 4. Inter-rater reliability of strobolaryngoscopy ratings.

Parameters	Exact Agreement/Total Videos
Vocal fold movement	13/14
Abduction lag	8/14
Axis rotation on pitch glide	12/14
Vertical vocal fold mismatch	9/14
Phase symmetry	10/14

2.4.3. Outcome Measures

Several patient-reported outcome measures (PROMs) were used to evaluate laryngeal symptoms and were administered to all patients prior to BTX treatment and within 3 months of treatment. Where bilateral staged treatment was given, outcomes were measured after the second treatment.

(a) Newcastle Laryngeal Hypersensitivity Questionnaire (LHQ) [55].

The Newcastle Laryngeal Hypersensitivity Questionnaire (LHQ) scores 14 items across three specific domains: obstruction, pain/thermal and irritation, providing a robust measure of laryngeal sensory disturbance. This tool has proved useful in discriminating patients with laryngeal hypersensitivity from healthy people and in measuring changes in symptoms of laryngeal hypersensitivity following speech pathology treatment [55]. A normal score is considered to be 17.1 or above [55]. The clinically minimal important difference for this questionnaire is 1.7 [55].

(b) Cough Severity Index (CSI)

CRC is the context in which LSD has been most associated. The CSI [60] is a validated PROM commonly utilized in evaluating patients with CRC resulting from the upper airway and is proven to be sensitive in detecting treatment outcome [61,62]. A score of 3 or more is considered abnormal [60].

(c) Reflux Symptom Index (RSI)

The Reflux Symptom Index (RSI) is a validated PROM initially developed to measure symptom severity for laryngopharyngeal reflux (LPR) [63]. An RSI score >13 is considered abnormal [63]. Although not specific for LPR [64] it serves as a useful and commonly used marker of throat irritation with which it has been correlated [65] and a marker of symptomatic response to treatment [66].

(d) Voice Handicap Index 10 (VHI-10)

The Voice Handicap Index 10 is a validated PROM to assess patients' perception of their voice function [67]. This tool was used in the present study given that patients with LSD and CRC frequently present with voice problems, e.g., muscle tension dysphonia [3]. It also allowed assessment of the frequency and severity of potential voice change which is a recognized potential side effect of laryngeal BTX treatment [68]. A score of greater than 11 is considered abnormal [69] with 6 considered as the minimal important difference [70].

2.5. Statistical Analyses

Data were managed in Microsoft Excel 365 [71] and analyzed using IBM SPSS Statistics v.24.0 [72] and Prism v8.1.2 [73] for Windows. Descriptive statistics were used to describe the cohort's characteristics. Prior to analyses, normal distribution of the data was examined using Kolmogorov–Smirnov tests [74]. For continuous variables, mean, standard deviation (SD) and 95% confidence interval (normal distribution) or median and quartiles (non-normal distribution) were used. For categorical data, frequencies and percentages were used. Changes in outcome measures over the treatment period were analyzed using a linear mixed model with patients as random effects and time points (i.e., baseline and post-BTX injection) and gender as fixed effects. Interaction between 'time' (treatment) and the fixed factors was also calculated to determine the impact of included factors on treatment outcome. Association between categorical variables was examined using Chi-square test (χ^2). A significance level of two-tailed p of 0.05 was used. Where there were multiple calculations, Sidak-adjustment was applied to the p value. Effect sizes were calculated using Cohen's d (small = 0.2; medium = 0.5; large = 0.8) [75].

3. Results

3.1. Characteristics of LSD

Table 5 presents primary presenting symptoms and secondary symptoms for all included patients. Primary symptoms were abnormal throat sensation (ATS) (12/14), followed by chronic cough (12/14) with a mean (SD) duration of 81 (110) months (min = 1; max = 360). Other symptoms included dysphonia (5/14), choking sensation (5/14), laryngeal dyspnea (5/14) and dysphagia (2/14).

Table 5. Clinical characteristics. CC, chronic cough; ATS, abnormal throat sensation; LD, laryngeal dyspnea.

Patients	Primary Presenting Symptom/s	Secondary Symptoms
1	CC, ATS	Dysphonia, LD
2	Dysphonia, ATS	LD
3	LD, CC, ATS	Dysphagia
4	LD, choking	Dysphonia
5	ATS, dysphagia	CC, dysphonia
6	ATS, CC	Dysphonia, dysphagia, choking
7	ATS, CC	Choking
8	CC	Choking
9	CC, ATS, LD	Throat pain
10	CC, ATS	Dysphonia
11	CC, ATS	Choking
12	CC, ATS	
13	CC, ATS	
14	ATS, dysphonia	CC, choking

Table 6 lists the results of PROMs at baseline and normative cut-off values from the literature. This table showed that the score values for these scales were well within the pathological ranges.

Table 6. Descriptive statistics of patient reported outcome measures at baseline.

PROMs	Mean (SD)	95% CI	Abnormal Value
LHQ	12.81 (3.418)	11.16–14.45	<17.1 [55]
CSI	24.32 (8.870)	20.04–28.59	≥3 [60]
RSI	27.37 (6.946)	24.02–30.72	≥13 [63]
VHI 10	18.37 (10.308)	13.40–23.34	≥11 [69]

Table 7 shows findings for the relevant strobolaryngoscopy parameters. The predominant clinical feature on strobolaryngoscopy observed in 10/14 participants was vertical mismatch of the vocal folds, followed by some form of lateral or medial constriction of the supraglottic structures during phonation. Abduction lag and unilateral false vocal fold hyperfunction were observed in 6/14 participants and 5/14 participants were observed to have one vocal fold shorter than the other. Phase asymmetry and reduced mucosal wave amplitude were not features found in this population.

Table 7. Stroboscopy findings in LSD.

Parameters	Ratings	Number
Gross VF movement	Normal	11
	Decreased	2
	Absent	1
Abduction lag	Yes	6
	No	8
Axis Rotation on Pitch Glide	Yes	4
	None	10
VF length	Equal	9
	One VF shorter	5
Vertical Level on Phonation	On plane	4
	One VF lower	10
Phase symmetry	In phase	14
	Out of phase	0
Phase Closure	Normal	11
	Closed phase	3
Amplitude	Normal	14
	Abnormal	0
Periodicity	Regular	13
	Irregular	1
False Vocal Fold Hyperfunction	None	8
	Unilateral	6
Supraglottic lateral constriction	Severe	5
	Moderate	4
	Mild	5
Supraglottic AP constriction	Severe	1
	Moderate	2
	Mild	6
	None	5
Mucosal lesions	Yes	1
	No	13

3.2. Effects of Botox Injection on Outcome Measures

3.2.1. LHQ Score

Figure 3 shows LHQ score of all patients at baseline and post-BTX treatment. The majority of patients showed an improvement in LHQ following BTX treatment. Linear mixed model analysis was calculated with treatment ("time") and gender being the fixed factors and patients as random factors. There was a significant effect of the treatment on LHQ outcome ($F(1, 25) = 12.335$, $p = 0.002$). There was no significant effect of gender ($p = 0.265$) and no significant interaction effect between 'time' and gender ($p = 0.078$), indicating treatment effects were independent of gender. Parameter estimate showed that regression coefficient (b) for LHQ scores was statistically significant (b = -2.633, $t(25.0) = -3.423$, $p = 0.002$). After BTX treatment, mean LHQ score increased by 2.6 (95% CI = 1.1–4.2, Sidak-adjusted $p = 0.002$).

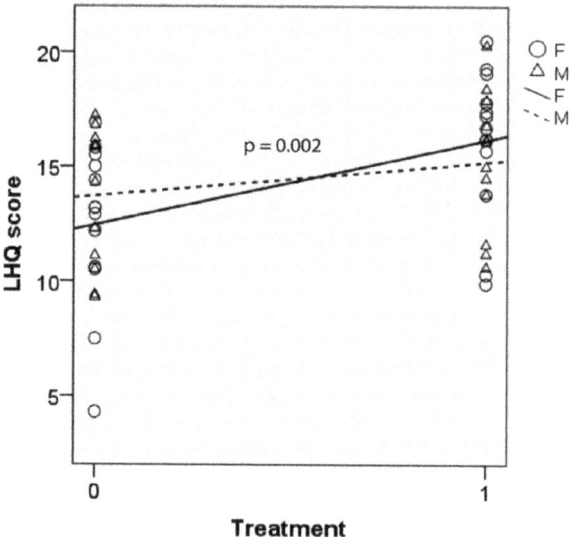

Figure 3. LHQ scores before and after BTX therapy with linear trend lines for male (M) and female (F). Higher score means better outcome. 0 = baseline; 1 = post-BTX treatment.

3.2.2. CSI

Figure 4 shows CSI scores for both genders at baseline and after BTX. There were significant fixed effects of treatment on CSI scores ($F(1, 18.998) = 15.068$, $p = 0.001$) and no significant interaction between treatment and gender ($p = 0.748$). Parameter estimate showed that CSI score decreased significantly after injection (b = 5.444, $t(18.998) = 2.900$, $p = 0.009$). Pairwise comparison showed that CSI score decreased by 5.0 after treatment (95% CI = 2.3–7.7, Sidak-adjusted $p = 0.001$).

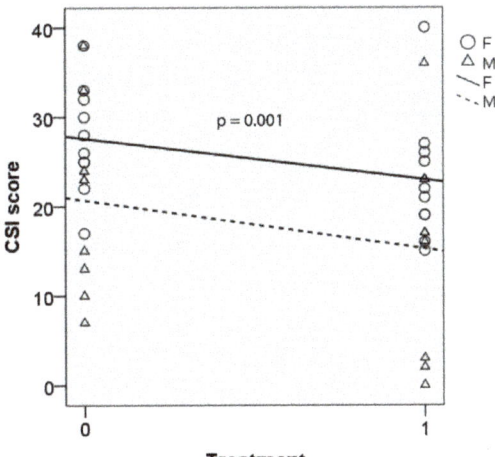

Figure 4. CSI scores before and after BTX therapy with linear trend lines for male (M) and female (F). Lower score indicates better outcome. 0 = baseline; 1 = post-BTX treatment.

3.2.3. RSI

Mixed model analysis was calculated for total RSI score which are shown for both males and females in Figure 5. There was significant fixed effect of treatment on total RSI score ($F(1, 25.001) = 19.766$, $p < 0.001$). There was no significant interaction between treatment and gender ($p = 0.219$). The decrease in RSI score after BTX injection was significant (b = 5.75, t (25.001) = 2.208, $p = 0.037$). Data from both genders showed that the mean RSI scores decreased by 8.0 after BTX injection (95% CI = 4.3–11.8, Sidak-adjusted $p < 0.001$).

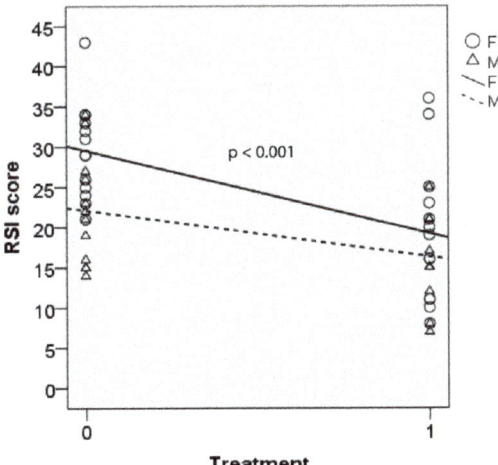

Figure 5. RSI scores before and after BTX therapy with linear trend lines for male (M) and female (F). Lower score indicates better outcome. 0 = baseline; 1 = post-BTX treatment.

Sub-score analysis of the RSI data was also performed using paired *t* test comparing scores of each of the RSI items between pre- and post-BTX. Results of comparisons are presented in Table 8, which showed significant differences with large effect sizes for sensory items related to cough and "breathing difficulties or choking episodes".

Table 8. Results of paired *t* test and effect size for RSI items (*n* = 25). All items were quoted verbatim from the original RSI scale by Belafsky et al. [63]. Cohen's d: small = 0.2; medium = 0.5; large = 0.8 [75]. MD, mean difference; (*), significant at *p* < 0.05.

RSI Items (from Reference [63])	MD	t	p	Cohen's D
"Hoarseness or a problem with your voice"	0.7	1.737	0.095	0.483
"Clearing your throat"	0.6	1.995	0.058	0.497
"Excess throat mucous or post-nasal drip"	0.6	2.777	0.010 *	0.388
"Difficulty swallowing food, liquids or pills"	1.0	3.062	0.005 *	0.560
"Coughing after you ate or after lying down"	0.8	3.199	0.004 *	0.942
"Breathing difficulties or choking episodes"	1.6	5.286	0.001 *	1.163
"Troublesome or annoying cough"	1.2	4.243	0.001 *	0.923
"Sensations of something sticking in your throat or a lump in your throat"	1.4	3.395	0.002 *	0.788
"Heartburn, chest pain, indigestion or stomach acid coming up"	0.2	0.451	0.656	0.093

3.2.4. VHI-10

There was no significant fixed effect of treatment on this outcome measure ($p = 0.734$) and there was also no significant interaction between treatment and gender ($p = 0.196$). Pairwise comparison showed that VHI-10 score dropped by 0.7 after BTX (95% CI = −3.6–5.1, Sidak-adjusted $p = 0.734$).

3.3. Effect Sizes of the Treatment

Table 9 shows mean differences, *p* value of the paired *t* test and Cohen's d for all outcome measures. This table shows that the treatment effect was large for the LHQ and RSI outcomes and medium for the CSI.

Table 9. Mean, mean difference, and effect sizes (Cohen's d: small = 0.2; medium = 0.5; large = 0.8). MID, minimal clinically important difference; (*), significant at *p* < 0.05.

Measures		Mean (SD)	N	Mean Difference	MID	p	d
LHQ	Pre	13.07 (3.288)	25	2.633	1.7	0.003 *	−0.800
	Post	15.70 (3.086)	25				
CSI	Pre	24.32 (8.870)	19	5.000	3 [60]	0.001 *	0.564
	Post	19.32 (10.193)	19				
RSI	Pre	25.96 (7.311)	25	8.120	4	0.001 *	1.111
	Post	17.84 (7.493)	25				
VHI-10	Pre	18.20 (9.916)	25	0.840	6	0.710	0.085
	Post	17.36 (8.850)	25				

3.4. Prediction of SLN Block Response on BTX Improvement

Short-term response to SLN block was evaluated using a 10-point Likert scale based upon the patient's specific presenting symptoms. Table 10 presents the number of patients who showed overall improvement after BTX injection versus those who responded to the SLN block. Responses to SLN block was significantly associated with improvement in LHQ scores ($\chi^2 (1) = 6.618$, $p = 0.01$).

Table 10. Overall BTX improvement versus outcome of SLN block.

		Overall BTX Improvement		Total	p
		No	Yes		
SLN block response	No	4 (16.0%)	1 (4.0%)	5 (20.0%)	
	Yes	4 (16.0%)	16 (64.0%)	20 (80.0%)	0.01
Total		8 (32.0%)	17 (68.0%)	25 (100%)	

3.5. Adverse Effects of BTX Treatment

Ten of the fourteen subjects experienced adverse effects of the BTX treatment. Dysphonia was the most common with weakness, breathiness or reduced volume and projection of the voice. These symptoms were mild and self-limiting, lasting for 2–3 weeks on average. There was no change in VHI-10 at reassessment. One person experienced mild dysphagia and a slower swallow mechanism which also resolved within three weeks.

3.6. Repeat Treatments

Six patients presented for repeat treatment. Two patients had a single repeat treatment at three months and five months respectively. One patient had a further two treatments at six and 9 months after the initial. One patient had a total of three treatments at approximately 3-month intervals. Two patients continue to present for repeat treatment with good effect at 3–6 monthly intervals.

4. Discussion

4.1. Clinical Presentation of Patients with LSD

Several disorders triggered by one or more sensory stimuli and manifested by hyperkinetic laryngeal dysfunction such as MTD, PVFM, globus and chronic cough have been grouped under "irritable larynx syndrome" [7]. However, the exact role of the dysfunctional sensory pathway in those conditions has not been confirmed by experimental evidence. Unlike motor function which can be examined using electromyography, there is currently no equivalent objective test for sensory function. This has made it challenging to define, explain and evaluate syndromes involving laryngeal hypersensitivity such as LSD. Explanations for these syndromes have been proposed using neuroplastic [7] or neuropathic models [4,76,77]. Examining sensory symptoms of patients with laryngeal sensitivity is therefore necessary to provide the main clinical clusters that may be useful for diagnosis and treatment follow-up.

Symptoms of LSD have been linked to several umbrella conditions in laryngeal hypersensitivity. Vertigan et al. [3] maintained that laryngeal hypersensitivity existed in the context of CRC, PVFM, MTD and globus. They found that laryngeal hypersensitivity was characterized by significantly higher symptom scores than controls in the breathing, cough, swallowing and phonation domains. They also found that within each clinical group of CRC, PVFM and MTD, the scores for the dominant domain were the highest, e.g., the CRC group had the highest cough score and PVFM had the highest breathing scores. Laryngeal paresthesia scores were significantly higher in these groups compared with controls and there were no significant differences in this score across the groups. Laryngeal sensory dysfunction was therefore investigated in the general pivotal syndromes related to phonation, cough, respiration and swallowing rather than in specific throat sensory profiles. However, they did not specifically describe sensory profiles in relevant PROM scales such as LHQ and RSI.

From case history data, the primary presenting symptoms in this cohort of patients were an abnormal throat sensation and CRC. Other symptoms observed with a lower frequency included choking sensation, voice problems, laryngeal dyspnea and problems with swallowing. PROM data were within the pathological ranges for LHQ, CSI, RSI and VHI-10 (Table 6). Videostrobolaryngoscopy was used to exclude other gross laryngeal pathology but was also useful in identifying signs of laryngeal motor impairment associated with sensory dysfunction in patients with vagal neuropathy [8]. Decreased gross vocal fold movement (3/14), abduction lag (6/14) and unequal vocal fold vertical height (10/14) were the main findings in these patients and gave some indication of laterality of peripheral neuropathy.

When examining potential preceding factors associated with onset, several patterns appear evident. Three of the fourteen people reported preceding URTI which has previously been suggested as a cause of vagal neuropathy [8,20]. Three of the fourteen reported preceding occupational inhalational exposure, a recognized trigger factor of irritable larynx syndrome [78]. Trauma to laryngeal nerves is another recognized cause of neuropathic symptoms [29] and was reported in 2/14 people (one iatrogenic during thyroid surgery and one due to external trauma), both of which exhibited motor signs of weakness on videostrobolaryngoscopy. Two of the fourteen reported preceding intubation, the relevance of this is unclear but local irritation of the larynx is one potential mechanism by which sensitization can take place. Four of the fourteen patients could not recall any preceding event.

Ten of the fourteen patients had a favorable response to a trial SLN block, supporting a diagnosis of sensory neuropathy. When considering a diagnosis of LSD, the majority of the following components should be present: ATS or CRC that has failed conventional medical/behavioral therapy; symptoms easily triggered by sensory stimuli; abnormal patient reported outcome measures of laryngeal sensory function (e.g., LHQ +/− RSI); signs of motor asymmetry on laryngeal stroboscopy; favorable response to a trial SLN block.

4.2. Treatment Effects of BTX on LSD

The present study is the first to describe the use and investigate the efficacy of supraglottic botulinum toxin type A injection for symptoms associated with Laryngeal Sensory Dysfunction. We postulated that BTX may affect the sensory afferent loop of the cough reflex via multiple mechanisms using a sensory neuropathic model [50,51]. The internal branch of the SLN is the primary laryngeal sensory afferent nerve contributing to a number of important reflexes including cough, swallow, respiration and laryngospasm [16]. It was thus hypothesized that targeting the peripheral sensory receptors in the distribution of this nerve would be a more effective and logical approach than targeting the intrinsic laryngeal musculature (previously described for the treatment of CRC [49–52]). Our hypothesis and treatment approach appears to be supported by the findings of this study.

There were statistically significant improvements in the primary patient reported outcome measures of LHQ (improving by 2.6 post-BTX) and CSI (improving by 5.0). The findings suggest a therapeutic effect of supraglottic BTX in the treatment of laryngeal sensory dysfunction. While not mechanistic proof, these findings are in support of the previously discussed peripheral and central sensitization model, and support the use of BTX in the treatment of neuropathic sensory dysfunction.

The findings relating to RSI score are noteworthy. Baseline RSI scores were within the abnormal range [63], despite ongoing medical and behavioral management of laryngopharyngeal reflux at the time of the BTX injection. Sub-item analysis (Table 8) showed significant improvement in the items relating to abnormal sensation; "excess throat mucous or post-nasal drip" and "sensation of something sticking in your throat or a lump in the throat" which are symptoms common to LSD. Improvement was also seen in the sub items relating to cough and breathing difficulties/choking episodes which are potential motor manifestations of laryngeal sensory dysfunction. These findings support the multi-faceted nature of LSD.

Despite RSI being developed as a tool for LPR symptoms [63], there is a lack of agreement between its score and laryngopharyngeal pH monitoring [79]. The findings of this study support the fact that symptoms reflected in the RSI are not always associated with LPR [80] and may be related to other etiologies including LSD. In light of this, the mechanism of action of BTX on ATS which resulted in improvement in RSI can be interpreted based upon findings from previous research on neuropathic pain involving peripheral nerve injury.

We found that CSI scores decreased significantly after supraglottic BTX injection, supporting its role as a potential treatment for CRC. The therapeutic effects of BTX on cough are thought to stem from its action upon the sensory pathways in modulating the cough and laryngeal adductor reflexes [50–52]. It is also possible that diffusion from the injection site into the intrinsic laryngeal adductor muscles may have occurred, producing the effects which have been reported and explained in some previous studies [50,51]; however, we would have expected an associated decrease in voice if this was the primary mechanism of action

In this study, VHI-10 scores did not change significantly despite the common reports of voice change after BTX treatment. This is in line with the mild and temporary nature of dysphonia after laryngeal BTX injections reported elsewhere in the literature [54,68].

4.3. The Role of SLN Nerve Block as Predictor of LSD, CRC and Efficacy of BTX

Recent work has explored SLN block as an office-based treatment for chronic refractory cough with a suspected neuropathic cause. In 2018, Simpson [62] reported improvement in cough severity index scores in a cohort of 23 patients where superior laryngeal nerve block was performed using local anesthesia with steroid. In total, 44% of patients had lasting improvement after one treatment but the mechanism of this extended effect remains unclear. Bupivicaine, considered to be the longest lasting local anesthetic, has an analgesic duration of action of only 4–8 h [81]. The addition of steroid to the local anesthetic could theoretically address any inflammation of the superior laryngeal nerve if it happens to be delivered to the site of the nerve inflammation. Twenty eight of the thirty patients treated by Dhillon reported at least a 50% reduction in symptoms along with significant improvement in CSI scores (the only outcome measure employed in this study) after a minimum of three injections [82,83]. Bradley et al. [84] described surgical section of the SLN as a viable option for treatment of selected patients with refractory neuropathic cough. They also however recognized dysphagia and aspiration as potential complications of this treatment.

In our practice we find SLN block a useful tool to assist with diagnosis of LSD and help guide treatment. Patients with laryngeal sensory symptoms persisting despite medical management of laryngeal irritants such as postnasal drip and laryngopharyngeal reflux are offered a trial unilateral SLN block based upon laterality of symptoms and any laryngeal stroboscopic findings that may suggest superior laryngeal nerve paresis. If there is no improvement in symptoms at 20 min compared with baseline, SLN block is offered on the contralateral side. Where symptom improvement is reported, this suggests that the anesthetized nerve or its peripheral receptors and nerve endings play a significant part in the patient's presentation, supporting a neuropathic diagnosis and offering a potential target for treatment. It is our experience that symptomatic improvement of LSD after SLN block is short term with most patients reporting a duration of effect in the order of hours rather than days before symptoms return.

In the present study, short term response to SLN block was a significant predictor of longer-term response to supraglottic botulinum toxin. Where laryngeal symptoms do not improve with SLN block, a diagnosis of sensory neuropathy is still possible but is likely to involve other sensory branches of the larynx such as the recurrent laryngeal nerve or may be referred from other sites of a neuropathic process in the vagal pathways.

4.4. Limitations of This Study

This was a retrospective study; however, we had a high level of data completeness with no patient loss to follow up. When performing supraglottic BTX treatment, it is our experience that the procedure is tolerated much better by the patient with the assistance of laryngeal anesthesia. We used SLN block at the time of BTX treatment for this purpose. Theoretically, some of the treatment effect may be related to the SLN block; however, all patients had reported only short-term response to prior SLN block performed as an independent procedure as part of workup for LSD and a much longer effect of treatment with concurrent BTX treatment. Finally, due to the retrospective nature of this study we were unable to include a separate control group. Future prospective studies investigating this novel treatment for LSD using a control treatment group (perhaps SLN block with BTX vs. SLN block alone) are indicated based on the promising results of the current study.

4.5. Recommendations for Assessment and Treatment of CRC

This study identified a sub-group of patients presenting with various symptoms within the LSD syndrome and provided preliminary data on the therapeutic effects of BTX administered into a novel supraglottic region of the larynx. This method of BTX administration can be safely performed as an office-based procedure that does not require complicated equipment and concurrent invasive procedures such as laryngeal electromyography. The recommended treatment planning for these patients can be summarized in a flowchart in Figure 6. Patients who present with LSD symptoms are offered superior laryngeal nerve block. If the symptoms improve, supraglottic BTX treatment is indicated. If LSD symptoms do not change after the block, patients will undergo alternative treatments such as medical treatment, neuromodulators, and speech pathology treatment. Those who do not respond to these alternative treatments can be indicated supraglottic BTX as a salvage treatment and they can revert to medical treatment and speech pathology treatment. It is important to mention that clinical trial designs are now required to validate the findings.

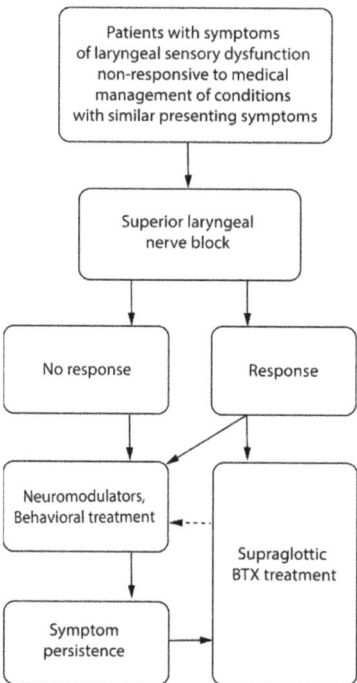

Figure 6. Recommendations of treatment plans for patients with LSD.

5. Conclusions

This study provided further evidence for defining, describing, and diagnosing a sub-group of patients presenting with various laryngeal symptoms related to altered laryngeal sensation. The major presenting symptoms for these patients were abnormal throat sensation and chronic cough. Diagnostic criteria for these patients should be based upon the onset and history of the sensory symptoms, resistance to medical and behavioral treatment, abnormal scores in PROMs evaluating abnormal laryngeal sensation including the LHQ and RSI, laryngeal videostroboscopy findings and responses to SLN block.

Symptomatic immediate response to SLN block supports the diagnosis of LSD affecting the supraglottic laryngeal afferent pathways. It was also a useful predictor of which patients were likely to respond to subsequent treatment with supraglottic BTX injection where the response to SLN block is short-lived.

Supraglottic BTX administration is a safe office-based procedure that effectively reduced sensory symptoms in a cohort of patients with various clinical presentations related to laryngeal sensory dysfunction. This treatment may be considered after the patient fails behavioral intervention and standard medical management for any related co-morbidities such as asthma, laryngopharyngeal reflux or sinonasal conditions including control of potential trigger factors. It can be used as an adjunct to neural modulators or as a standalone treatment to address neuropathic laryngeal symptoms related to LSD including reducing hypersensitivity of the laryngeal afferent pathways and protective reflexes manifesting as chronic refractory cough and throat clearing and reducing sensory symptoms of laryngeal paresthesia presenting as abnormal throat sensation.

Author Contributions: Conceptualization, D.N.; methodology, D.N., C.M. and D.D.N.; formal analysis, D.D.N.; investigation, D.N., M.S., T.S. and K.S.; data curation, T.S., A.C., K.S. and M.S.; writing—original draft preparation, D.N., D.D.N., A.C., M.S. and T.S.; writing—review and editing, D.N., D.D.N., C.M., A.C. and T.S.; project administration, D.N.; visualization, D.N.; funding acquisition, D.N. and C.M. All authors have read and agreed to the published version of the manuscript.

Funding: This research was funded by The Dr. Liang Voice Program at The University of Sydney.

Institutional Review Board Statement: This study was a retrospective cohort study conducted by medical record review of a private laryngology specialized clinic for the period from November 2019 to May 2021. The study was conducted according to the guidelines of the Declaration of Helsinki. The study was approved by the Human Research Ethics Committee of The University of Sydney (protocol number 2021/025).

Informed Consent Statement: Patient consent was waived due to it being impractical to seek consent for patients seen in the past and it was considered a threat to patient privacy to implement a process to locate and contact each individual participant to seek their consent. This waiver was approved by the Human Research Ethics Committee approval provided above.

Data Availability Statement: Data supporting reported results is retained by The University of Sydney in de-identified form and is confidential under the conditions of the Human Research Ethics Committee of The University of Sydney approval.

Acknowledgments: We acknowledge the clinicians referred to in the study and thank them for their rigorous data collection practices that supported this work.

Conflicts of Interest: First author D.N. is Director of Sydney Voice and Swallowing. C.M., D.D.N. and A.C. are employees of The University of Sydney and are partly or fully funded by the Dr. Liang Voice Program, a philanthropically funded program of research and post-graduate education in laryngology. The funders had no role in the design of the study; in the collection, analyses, or interpretation of data; in the writing of the manuscript, or in the decision to publish the results.

References

1. Sanders, I.; Mu, L. Anatomy of the human internal superior laryngeal nerve. *Anat. Rec.* **1998**, *252*, 646–656. [CrossRef]
2. Ludlow, C.L. Recent advances in laryngeal sensorimotor control for voice, speech and swallowing. *Curr. Opin. Otolaryngol. Head Neck Surg.* **2004**, *12*, 160–165. [CrossRef]
3. Vertigan, A.E.; Bone, S.L.; Gibson, P.G. Laryngeal sensory dysfunction in laryngeal hypersensitivity syndrome. *Respirology* **2013**, *18*, 948–956. [CrossRef]
4. Vertigan, A.E.; Gibson, P.G. Chronic refractory cough as a sensory neuropathy: Evidence from a reinterpretation of cough triggers. *J. Voice* **2011**, *25*, 596–601. [CrossRef]
5. Murry, T.; Branski, R.C.; Yu, K.; Cukier-Blaj, S.; Duflo, S.; Aviv, J.E. Laryngeal sensory deficits in patients with chronic cough and paradoxical vocal fold movement disorder. *Laryngoscope* **2010**, *120*, 1576–1581. [CrossRef]
6. Cukier-Blaj, S.; Bewley, A.; Aviv, J.E.; Murry, T. Paradoxical vocal fold motion: A sensory-motor laryngeal disorder. *Laryngoscope* **2008**, *118*, 367–370. [CrossRef]
7. Morrison, M.; Rammage, L.; Emami, A.J. The irritable larynx syndrome. *J. Voice* **1999**, *13*, 447–455. [CrossRef]

8. Amin, M.R.; Koufman, J.A. Vagal neuropathy after upper respiratory infection: A viral etiology? *Am. J. Otolaryngol.* **2001**, *22*, 251–256. [CrossRef] [PubMed]
9. Famokunwa, B.; Walsted, E.S.; Hull, J.H. Assessing laryngeal function and hypersensitivity. *Pulm. Pharmacol. Ther.* **2019**, *56*, 108–115. [CrossRef] [PubMed]
10. McGarvey, L.; Gibson, P.G. What Is Chronic Cough? Terminology. *J. Allergy Clin. Immunol. Pract.* **2019**, *7*, 1711–1714. [CrossRef] [PubMed]
11. Chung, K.F. Chronic 'cough hypersensitivity syndrome': A more precise label for chronic cough. *Pulm. Pharmacol. Ther.* **2011**, *24*, 267–271. [CrossRef]
12. O'Connell, F.; Thomas, V.E.; Pride, N.B.; Fuller, R.W. Capsaicin cough sensitivity decreases with successful treatment of chronic cough. *Am. J. Respir. Crit. Care Med.* **1994**, *150*, 374–380. [CrossRef] [PubMed]
13. Haque, R.A.; Usmani, O.S.; Barnes, P.J. Chronic idiopathic cough: A discrete clinical entity? *Chest* **2005**, *127*, 1710–1713. [CrossRef] [PubMed]
14. Mehdizadeh, O.B.; Dhar, S.I.; Evangelista, L.; Nativ-Zeltzer, N.; Bewley, A.F.; Belafsky, P.C. Prevalence of profound laryngeal sensory neuropathy in head and neck cancer survivors with feeding tube-dependent oropharyngeal dysphagia. *Head Neck* **2020**, *42*, 898–904. [CrossRef] [PubMed]
15. Jensen, T.S.; Finnerup, N.B. Allodynia and hyperalgesia in neuropathic pain: Clinical manifestations and mechanisms. *Lancet Neurol.* **2014**, *13*, 924–935. [CrossRef]
16. Ludlow, C.L. Laryngeal Reflexes: Physiology, Technique, and Clinical Use. *J. Clin. Neurophysiol.* **2015**, *32*, 284–293. [CrossRef]
17. Sinclair, C.F.; Téllez, M.J.; Tapia, O.R.; Ulkatan, S. Contralateral R1 and R2 components of the laryngeal adductor reflex in humans under general anesthesia. *Laryngoscope* **2017**, *127*, E443–E448. [CrossRef]
18. Sinclair, C.F.; Téllez, M.J.; Ulkatan, S. Human laryngeal sensory receptor mapping illuminates the mechanisms of laryngeal adductor reflex control. *Laryngoscope* **2018**, *128*, E365–E370. [CrossRef]
19. Gangadharan, V.; Kuner, R. Pain hypersensitivity mechanisms at a glance. *Dis. Model. Mech.* **2013**, *6*, 889–895. [CrossRef]
20. Rees, C.J.; Henderson, A.H.; Belafsky, P.C. Postviral vagal neuropathy. *Ann. Otol. Rhinol. Laryngol.* **2009**, *118*, 247–252. [CrossRef]
21. Avecillas-Chasin, J.; Kozoriz, M.G.; Shewchuk, J.R.; Heran, M.K.S.; Honey, C.R. Imaging and Surgical Findings in Patients with Hemi-Laryngopharyngeal Spasm and the Potential Role of MRI in the Diagnostic Work-Up. *AJNR Am. J. Neuroradiol.* **2018**, *39*, 2366–2370. [CrossRef] [PubMed]
22. Honey, C.R.; Kruger, M.T.; Morrison, M.D.; Dhaliwal, B.S.; Hu, A. Vagus Associated Neurogenic Cough Occurring Due to Unilateral Vascular Encroachment of Its Root: A Case Report and Proof of Concept of VANCOUVER Syndrome. *Ann. Otol. Rhinol. Laryngol.* **2020**, *129*, 523–527. [CrossRef] [PubMed]
23. Hu, A.; Morrison, M.; Honey, C.R. Hemi-laryngopharyngeal Spasm (HeLPS): Defining a New Clinical Entity. *Ann. Otol. Rhinol. Laryngol.* **2020**, *129*, 849–855. [CrossRef]
24. Altman, K.W.; Noordzij, J.P.; Rosen, C.A.; Cohen, S.; Sulica, L. Neurogenic cough. *Laryngoscope* **2015**, *125*, 1675–1681. [CrossRef] [PubMed]
25. Malek, N.; Pajak, A.; Kolosowska, N.; Kucharczyk, M.; Starowicz, K. The importance of TRPV1-sensitisation factors for the development of neuropathic pain. *Mol. Cell. Neurosci.* **2015**, *65*, 1–10. [CrossRef] [PubMed]
26. Mai, Y.; Fang, L.; Zhong, S.; de Silva, S.; Chen, R.; Lai, K. Methods for assessing cough sensitivity. *J. Thorac. Dis.* **2020**, *12*, 5224–5237. [CrossRef] [PubMed]
27. McCulloch, T.M.; Flint, P.W.; Richardson, M.A.; Bishop, M.J. Lidocaine effects on the laryngeal chemoreflex, mechanoreflex, and afferent electrical stimulation reflex. *Ann. Otol. Rhinol. Laryngol.* **1992**, *101*, 583–589. [CrossRef]
28. Shultz, E.H.; Chin, F.K.; Williams, J.D. Superior Laryngeal Nerve Block. *Radiology* **1970**, *97*, 94. [CrossRef]
29. Wani, M.K.; Woodson, G.E. Paroxysmal laryngospasm after laryngeal nerve injury. *Laryngoscope* **1999**, *109*, 694–697. [CrossRef]
30. Ryan, N.M.; Vertigan, A.E.; Birring, S.S. An update and systematic review on drug therapies for the treatment of refractory chronic cough. *Expert Opin. Pharmacother.* **2018**, *19*, 687–711. [CrossRef]
31. Ryan, N.M.; Birring, S.S.; Gibson, P.G. Gabapentin for refractory chronic cough: A randomised, double-blind, placebo-controlled trial. *Lancet* **2012**, *380*, 1583–1589. [CrossRef]
32. Wiffen, P.J.; Derry, S.; Bell, R.F.; Rice, A.S.; Tolle, T.R.; Phillips, T.; Moore, R.A. Gabapentin for chronic neuropathic pain in adults. *Cochrane Database Syst. Rev.* **2017**, *6*, CD007938. [CrossRef]
33. Lee, B.; Woo, P. Chronic cough as a sign of laryngeal sensory neuropathy: Diagnosis and treatment. *Ann. Otol. Rhinol. Laryngol.* **2005**, *114*, 253–257. [CrossRef]
34. Vertigan, A.E.; Theodoros, D.G.; Gibson, P.G.; Winkworth, A.L. Efficacy of speech pathology management for chronic cough: A randomised placebo controlled trial of treatment efficacy. *Thorax* **2006**, *61*, 1065–1069. [CrossRef] [PubMed]
35. Chamberlain, S.; Garrod, R.; Birring, S.S. Cough suppression therapy: Does it work? *Pulm. Pharmacol. Ther.* **2013**, *26*, 524–527. [CrossRef]
36. Vertigan, A.; Gibson, P.G. *Speech Pathology Management of Chronic Refractory Cough and Related Disorders*; Compton Publishing Ltd.: Oxford, UK, 2016.
37. Vertigan, A.E.; Haines, J.; Slovarp, L. An Update on Speech Pathology Management of Chronic Refractory Cough. *J. Allergy Clin. Immunol. Pract.* **2019**, *7*, 1756–1761. [CrossRef]
38. Wallace, H. Airway Pathogenesis Is Linked to TRP Channels. In *Neurobiology of Transient Receptor Potential Channels*; Rosenbaum Emir, T.L., Ed.; CRC Press: Boca Raton, FL, USA, 2017.
39. Groneberg, D.A.; Niimi, A.; Dinh, Q.T.; Cosio, B.; Hew, M.; Fischer, A.; Chung, K.F. Increased expression of transient receptor potential vanilloid-1 in airway nerves of chronic cough. *Am. J. Respir. Crit. Care Med.* **2004**, *170*, 1276–1280. [CrossRef] [PubMed]

40. Canning, B.J.; Chang, A.B.; Bolser, D.C.; Smith, J.A.; Mazzone, S.B.; McGarvey, L.; Panel, C.E.C. Anatomy and neurophysiology of cough: CHEST Guideline and Expert Panel report. *Chest* **2014**, *146*, 1633–1648. [CrossRef] [PubMed]
41. Chung, K.F. Advances in mechanisms and management of chronic cough: The Ninth London International Cough Symposium 2016. *Pulm. Pharmacol. Ther.* **2017**, *47*, 2–8. [CrossRef]
42. Fan, C.; Chu, X.; Wang, L.; Shi, H.; Li, T. Botulinum toxin type A reduces TRPV1 expression in the dorsal root ganglion in rats with adjuvant-arthritis pain. *Toxicon* **2017**, *133*, 116–122. [CrossRef]
43. Morenilla-Palao, C.; Planells-Cases, R.; Garcia-Sanz, N.; Ferrer-Montiel, A. Regulated exocytosis contributes to protein kinase C potentiation of vanilloid receptor activity. *J. Biol. Chem.* **2004**, *279*, 25665–25672. [CrossRef]
44. Shimizu, T.; Shibata, M.; Toriumi, H.; Iwashita, T.; Funakubo, M.; Sato, H.; Kuroi, T.; Ebine, T.; Koizumi, K.; Suzuki, N. Reduction of TRPV1 expression in the trigeminal system by botulinum neurotoxin type-A. *Neurobiol. Dis.* **2012**, *48*, 367–378. [CrossRef]
45. Xiao, L.; Cheng, J.; Zhuang, Y.; Qu, W.; Muir, J.; Liang, H.; Zhang, D. Botulinum toxin type A reduces hyperalgesia and TRPV1 expression in rats with neuropathic pain. *Pain Med.* **2013**, *14*, 276–286. [CrossRef]
46. Kumar, R. Therapeutic use of botulinum toxin in pain treatment. *Neuronal Signal.* **2018**, *2*, NS20180058. [CrossRef]
47. Park, J.; Park, H.J. Botulinum Toxin for the Treatment of Neuropathic Pain. *Toxins* **2017**, *9*, 260. [CrossRef] [PubMed]
48. Blitzer, A.; Brin, M.F.; Fahn, S.; Lange, D.; Lovelace, R.E. Botulinum toxin (BOTOX) for the treatment of "spastic dysphonia" as part of a trial of toxin injections for the treatment of other cranial dystonias. *Laryngoscope* **1986**, *96*, 1300–1301. [PubMed]
49. Sipp, J.A.; Haver, K.E.; Masek, B.J.; Hartnick, C.J. Botulinum toxin A: A novel adjunct treatment for debilitating habit cough in children. *Ear Nose Throat J.* **2007**, *86*, 570–572. [CrossRef] [PubMed]
50. Chu, M.W.; Lieser, J.D.; Sinacori, J.T. Use of botulinum toxin type A for chronic cough: A neuropathic model. *Arch. Otolaryngol. Head Neck Surg.* **2010**, *136*, 447–452. [CrossRef] [PubMed]
51. Sasieta, H.C.; Iyer, V.N.; Orbelo, D.M.; Patton, C.; Pittelko, R.; Keogh, K.; Lim, K.G.; Ekbom, D.C. Bilateral Thyroarytenoid Botulinum Toxin Type A Injection for the Treatment of Refractory Chronic Cough. *JAMA Otolaryngol. Head Neck Surg.* **2016**, *142*, 881–888. [CrossRef] [PubMed]
52. Cook, L.; Athanasiadis, T. Laryngeal Botox injection in recalcitrant cases of chronic cough. *Aust. J. Otolaryngol.* **2021**, *4*, 24. [CrossRef]
53. Young, N.; Blitzer, A. Management of supraglottic squeeze in adductor spasmodic dysphonia: A new technique. *Laryngoscope* **2007**, *117*, 2082–2084. [CrossRef]
54. Simpson, C.B.; Lee, C.T.; Hatcher, J.L.; Michalek, J. Botulinum toxin treatment of false vocal folds in adductor spasmodic dysphonia: Functional outcomes. *Laryngoscope* **2016**, *126*, 118–121. [CrossRef] [PubMed]
55. Vertigan, A.E.; Bone, S.L.; Gibson, P.G. Development and validation of the Newcastle laryngeal hypersensitivity questionnaire. *Cough* **2014**, *10*, 1. [CrossRef]
56. Estes, C.; Sadoughi, B.; Mauer, E.; Christos, P.; Sulica, L. Laryngoscopic and stroboscopic signs in the diagnosis of vocal fold paresis. *Laryngoscope* **2017**, *127*, 2100–2105. [CrossRef] [PubMed]
57. Nguyen, D.D.; Madill, C.; Chacon, A.; Novakovic, D. Laryngoscopy and stroboscopy. In *Manual of Clinical Phonetics*, 1st ed.; Ball, M.J., Ed.; Routledge: London, UK, 2021.
58. Madill, C.; So, T.; Corcoran, S. Bridge2practice: Translating Theory into Practice. Available online: https://bridge2practice.com/ (accessed on 7 March 2019).
59. Nawka, T.; Konerding, U. The interrater reliability of stroboscopy evaluations. *J. Voice* **2012**, *26*, 812.e1–812.e10. [CrossRef] [PubMed]
60. Shembel, A.C.; Rosen, C.A.; Zullo, T.G.; Gartner-Schmidt, J.L. Development and validation of the cough severity index: A severity index for chronic cough related to the upper airway. *Laryngoscope* **2013**, *123*, 1931–1936. [CrossRef] [PubMed]
61. Crawley, B.K.; Murry, T.; Sulica, L. Injection Augmentation for Chronic Cough. *J. Voice* **2015**, *29*, 763–767. [CrossRef]
62. Simpson, C.B.; Tibbetts, K.M.; Loochtan, M.J.; Dominguez, L.M. Treatment of chronic neurogenic cough with in-office superior laryngeal nerve block. *Laryngoscope* **2018**, *128*, 1898–1903. [CrossRef]
63. Belafsky, P.C.; Postma, G.N.; Koufman, J.A. Validity and reliability of the reflux symptom index (RSI). *J. Voice* **2002**, *16*, 274–277. [CrossRef]
64. Pontes, P.; Tiago, R. Diagnosis and management of laryngopharyngeal reflux disease. *Curr. Opin. Otolaryngol. Head Neck Surg.* **2006**, *14*, 138–142. [CrossRef]
65. Mozzanica, F.; Robotti, C.; Lechien, J.R.; Pizzorni, N.; Pirola, F.; Mengucci, A.; Dell'Era, A.; Ottaviani, F.; Schindler, A. Vocal Tract Discomfort and Dysphonia in Patients Undergoing Empiric Therapeutic Trial with Proton Pump Inhibitor for Suspected Laryngopharyngeal Reflux. *J. Voice* **2020**, *34*, 280–288. [CrossRef] [PubMed]
66. Francis, D.O.; Patel, D.A.; Sharda, R.; Hovis, K.; Sathe, N.; Penson, D.F.; Feurer, I.D.; McPheeters, M.L.; Vaezi, M.F. Patient-Reported Outcome Measures Related to Laryngopharyngeal Reflux: A Systematic Review of Instrument Development and Validation. *Otolaryngol. Head Neck Surg.* **2016**, *155*, 923–935. [CrossRef]
67. Rosen, C.A.; Lee, A.S.; Osborne, J.; Zullo, T.; Murry, T. Development and validation of the voice handicap index-10. *Laryngoscope* **2004**, *114*, 1549–1556. [CrossRef]
68. Novakovic, D.; Waters, H.H.; D'Elia, J.B.; Blitzer, A. Botulinum toxin treatment of adductor spasmodic dysphonia: Longitudinal functional outcomes. *Laryngoscope* **2011**, *121*, 606–612. [CrossRef] [PubMed]
69. Arffa, R.E.; Krishna, P.; Gartner-Schmidt, J.; Rosen, C.A. Normative values for the Voice Handicap Index-10. *J. Voice* **2012**, *26*, 462–465. [CrossRef]
70. Misono, S.; Yueh, B.; Stockness, A.N.; House, M.E.; Marmor, S. Minimal Important Difference in Voice Handicap Index-10. *JAMA Otolaryngol. Head Neck Surg.* **2017**, *143*, 1098–1103. [CrossRef] [PubMed]

71. Microsoft. Microsoft Excel. Available online: https://www.microsoft.com/en-us/microsoft-365/excel (accessed on 2 June 2021).
72. IBM Corp. IBM SPSS Software. Available online: https://www.ibm.com/analytics/data-science/predictive-analytics/spss-statistical-software (accessed on 1 February 2018).
73. GraphPad Software. Prism 8. Available online: https://www.graphpad.com/scientific-software/prism/ (accessed on 20 April 2018).
74. Massey, F.J. The Kolmogorov-Smirnov Test for Goodness of Fit. *J. Am. Stat. Assoc.* **1951**, *46*, 68–78. [CrossRef]
75. Cohen, J. A power primer. *Psychol. Bull.* **1992**, *112*, 155–159. [CrossRef]
76. Chung, K.F.; McGarvey, L.; Mazzone, S.B. Chronic cough as a neuropathic disorder. *Lancet Respir. Med.* **2013**, *1*, 414–422. [CrossRef]
77. Niimi, A.; Chung, K.F. Evidence for neuropathic processes in chronic cough. *Pulm. Pharmacol. Ther.* **2015**, *35*, 100–104. [CrossRef]
78. Denton, E.; Hoy, R. Occupational aspects of irritable larynx syndrome. *Curr. Opin. Allergy Clin. Immunol.* **2020**, *20*, 90–95. [CrossRef]
79. Wang, J.Y.; Peng, T.; Zhao, L.L.; Feng, G.J.; Liu, Y.L. Poor consistency between reflux symptom index and laryngopharyngeal pH monitoring in laryngopharyngeal reflux diagnosis in Chinese population. *Ann. Transl. Med.* **2021**, *9*, 25. [CrossRef] [PubMed]
80. Nacci, A.; Bastiani, L.; Barillari, M.R.; Lechien, J.R.; Martinelli, M.; Bortoli, N.; Berrettini, S.; Fattori, B. Assessment and Diagnostic Accuracy Evaluation of the Reflux Symptom Index (RSI) Scale: Psychometric Properties using Optimal Scaling Techniques. *Ann. Otol. Rhinol. Laryngol.* **2020**, *129*, 1020–1029. [CrossRef] [PubMed]
81. Swerdlow, M.; Jones, R. The duration of action of bupivacaine, prilocaine and lignocaine. *Br. J. Anaesth.* **1970**, *42*, 335–339. [CrossRef] [PubMed]
82. Dhillon, V.K. Superior laryngeal nerve block for neurogenic cough: A case series. *Laryngoscope Investig. Otolaryngol.* **2019**, *4*, 410–413. [CrossRef]
83. Dhillon, V.K. Longitudinal Follow-up of Superior Laryngeal Nerve Block for Chronic Neurogenic Cough. *OTO Open* **2021**, *5*, 2473974X21994468. [CrossRef] [PubMed]
84. Bradley, J.P.; Gross, J.; Paniello, R.C. Superior laryngeal nerve transection for neuropathic cough: A pilot study. *Auris Nasus Larynx* **2020**, *47*, 837–841. [CrossRef]

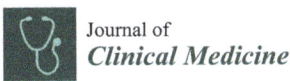

Article

Active Ingredients of Voice Therapy for Muscle Tension Voice Disorders: A Retrospective Data Audit

Catherine Madill [1,*], Antonia Chacon [1], Evan Kirby [1], Daniel Novakovic [1,2] and Duy Duong Nguyen [1]

1. Voice Research Laboratory, Discipline of Speech Pathology, Faculty of Medicine and Health, The University of Sydney, Sydney, NSW 2006, Australia; antonia.chacon@sydney.edu.au (A.C.); evan.kirby@sydney.edu.au (E.K.); daniel.novakovic@sydney.edu.au (D.N.); duong.nguyen@sydney.edu.au (D.D.N.)
2. Faculty of Medicine and Health, Central Clinical School, The University of Sydney, Sydney, NSW 2006, Australia
* Correspondence: cate.madill@sydney.edu.au

Abstract: Background: Although voice therapy is the first line treatment for muscle-tension voice disorders (MTVD), no clinical research has investigated the role of specific active ingredients. This study aimed to evaluate the efficacy of active ingredients in the treatment of MTVD. A retrospective review of a clinical voice database was conducted on 68 MTVD patients who were treated using the optimal phonation task (OPT) and sob voice quality (SVQ), as well as two different processes: task variation and negative practice (NP). Mixed-model analysis was performed on auditory–perceptual and acoustic data from voice recordings at baseline and after each technique. Active ingredients were evaluated using effect sizes. Significant overall treatment effects were observed for the treatment program. Effect sizes ranged from 0.34 (post-NP) to 0.387 (post-SVQ) for overall severity ratings. Effect sizes ranged from 0.237 (post-SVQ) to 0.445 (post-NP) for a smoothed cepstral peak prominence measure. The treatment effects did not depend upon the MTVD type (primary or secondary), treating clinicians, nor the number of sessions and days between sessions. Implementation of individual techniques that promote improved voice quality and processes that support learning resulted in improved habitual voice quality. Both voice techniques and processes can be considered as active ingredients in voice therapy.

Keywords: Sob Voice Therapy; Optimal Phonation Task; Negative Practice; auditory-perceptual analysis; acoustic voice analysis

1. Introduction

A muscle-tension voice disorder (MTVD) is a commonly occurring dysphonia that results from disorganisation or dysfunction of the laryngeal musculature [1]. It can occur as a primary condition without organic changes to the vocal folds or as a secondary, compensatory condition to underlying organic or neurological laryngeal pathology. The aetiology of MTVD can be multifactorial and includes phonotrauma, excessive vocal load, glottic incompetence (vocal fold paresis and atrophy), psychological stress, and co-occurring medical conditions such as upper respiratory tract infection, laryngopharyngeal reflux, and sinusitis with post-nasal drip [2,3]. Within the voice-disordered population, functional dysphonia has documented prevalence rates of between 20.5 to 41%, while the prevalence of phonotraumatic lesions (e.g., vocal nodules and polyps) is 12–15% [4,5]. The majority of MTVDs are preventable [2] and early intervention is recommended to mitigate the negative impact of the disorder [6].

1.1. Behavioural Voice Therapy Is the First-Line Treatment for MTVD

Treatment of MTVD requires voice therapy as the first line of treatment [7], alongside the medical management of co-existing or contributing medical conditions. Both indirect and direct voice therapies are utilised in the treatment of MTVD in adults and children [8–10]. Indirect voice therapy, also termed vocal hygiene, aims to facilitate an individual's vocal rehabilitation by identifying and eliminating poor vocal behaviours or other constraints to good vocal health, while promoting vocal health. Direct voice therapy describes a large range of individual vocal techniques and structured programs designed to change the habitual movement of the vocal system during phonation [8] such that the vocal needs of the individual are met without deterioration in the sound or sensation of phonation. Numerous systematic reviews and an increasing body of evidence have demonstrated that voice therapy is effective for the majority of patients with MTVD [11]; however, there is insufficient evidence to determine if one treatment is more effective than another. While some research has demonstrated that speech and language pathologists (SLPs) use a common approach to therapy [12], it is also well documented that SLPs use more than one MTVD therapy technique at a time [9,10]. This prevents clear identification of the therapeutic effect of each component of the treatment regime prescribed by the clinician. Therapies for MTVD are also very heterogenous and target different aspects of voice production. In addition, different therapies employ different conceptual approaches and there is a paucity of outcome data on the individual treatment components thought to modify voice production towards more optimal function.

There is a pressing need to ensure that the most cost-effective treatments are used, that is, treatments that provide evidence-based treatment effects with the maximum therapeutic effect in the minimum amount of time. Average treatment times for dysphonia across 140 research publications were documented as approximately consisting of 11 sessions of mostly 30 or 60-min durations, with average clinician-to-client face-to-face time estimated at 8.17 h [13]. The authors acknowledge that this was a conservative analysis, with many studies using fixed-treatment designs and others documenting clinical outcomes in North America, in which health insurance rules may influence intervention length and cost. If treatment efficacy can be improved, time and health-care costs may be reduced without compromising treatment outcomes, nor patient-centred care [14].

1.2. What Is an Active Ingredient in Voice Therapy?

The definition of an active ingredient has been recently considered in allied health and speech language pathology (SLP), specifically in [15–17]. Nevertheless, behaviours that generate a therapeutic effect can be difficult to identify in behavioural therapies due to a number of challenges. These include the lack of clarity surrounding rehabilitation ingredients, the fact that rehabilitation treatments often attempt to change multiple interacting patient functions, and a lack of standard nomenclature and definitions for specific treatment ingredients [18]. The treatment of voice disorders is one area in which significant efforts are being made to identify active ingredients in detail.

Quantifiable ingredients such as dosage, frequency, and intensity were initially proposed as active ingredients in SLP [16]. In recent times, a more expansive consideration of those components of a therapy that may have a therapeutic effect has been modelled in the Taxonomy of Voice Therapy [19]. This model proposes that treatment components may be classified into direct interventions (subdivided into auditory, somatosensory, musculoskeletal, respiratory, and vocal function), intervention delivery models (extrinsic and intrinsic), and indirect interventions (pedagogy and counselling) with more specific interventions listed under each sub-category [14]. The Rehabilitation Specification System (RTSS) [18] describes a simpler theoretical framework and proposed methodology by which treatments can be described according to a singular treatment target (the patient function that is to be changed by the ingredient(s)); one or more ingredients (what the clinician does to modify the target); and the mechanism(s) of action of the treatment [16]. Both the Taxonomy of Voice Therapy and the broader RTSS provide complex and detailed theoretical models that can inform our understanding; however, these models defining active ingredients are yet to be tested in clinic-based research.

Verdolini provides a simpler conceptualisation of the mechanisms of action as being divisible by the 'what' (the vocal technique) and the 'how' (the modality by which the change of function is learned) [20]. Across different voice therapies, the 'what' can vary from a single technique, such as Conversation Training Therapy (CTT) (use a clear voice) and Resonant Voice Therapy (RVT) (feel the buzz and notice the ease of phonation), to multiple technique therapies, such as Vocal Function Exercises (VFE) [21] (four distinct exercises targeting the whole vocal system), stretch and flow therapy [22], and the Accent Method [23,24]. The 'how' of learning to habituate the new vocal technique is remarkably homogenous across voice therapies [25] and involves processes originally described in motor learning research, such as task variation (hierarchical or end goal target) and negative practice.

There is little existing research on voice-disordered populations investigating the effectiveness of specific techniques and/or processes, as most research designs have evaluated the impact of the whole therapy rather than its component parts or stages. Most voice therapy programs that aim to provide a standardised series of voice exercises have been evaluated in controlled clinical trials [21–24,26,27]. All of these programs consist of multiple exercises that may be hierarchical in nature (e.g., Lessac Madsen Resonant Voice Therapy and RVT) or address different aspects of vocal function (e.g., VFE and the Accent Method). All have demonstrated efficacy with a range of effect sizes demonstrated across a variety of voice outcome measures; however, none have systematically evaluated the effect of each component or 'ingredient' in the treatment provided. Preliminary research investigating individual effects of components of VFE has isolated the therapeutic effects of practise dosage and the use of a semi-occluded vocal tract (nasal sound) [28,29]; however, this research was conducted in controlled experimental conditions with non-voice-disordered volunteers.

1.3. VoiceCraft® Sob Voice Therapy

VoiceCraft® Sob Voice Therapy (SVT) [30] is a direct voice therapy program whereby discrete individual techniques and processes are introduced at specific times and thus provides an opportunity to isolate possible effects of individual ingredients. Voicecraft® is an SLP-directed voice therapy treatment model developed in the 1980s based on the work of numerous voice-science researchers and clinicians [31]. Described as a differentiated vocal tract model of vocal training that aims to develop the control of specific muscular movements in the larynx [32], it consists of a range of treatment programs for different patient populations (e.g., Yell Well for children with vocal nodules) that can be adjusted to the individual presentation of the patient depending on the type of voice condition, their individual muscular function in the larynx, and/or awareness of perceptual outcomes of phonation. This approach to the remediation of functional voice disorders has not been documented previously. Voicecraft training has proven to be effective in improving voice quality in healthy subjects [33] and to 'fatigue proof' the voice under conditions of sleep deprivation [33]. Despite being used across Australasia, Singapore, Europe, and the UK to treat voice and resonance disorders in adults and children, efficacy of Voicecraft® programs, such as Sob Voice Therapy, has not been reported in voice-disordered populations.

Sob Voice Therapy is used to treat adolescent and adult patients with MTVD with or without organic change. The program consists of up to four techniques (as required) and utilises two common learning processes to support the generalisation and maintenance of the new voice techniques, namely task variation and negative practice (Table 1). It follows a hierarchical progression from an initial exercise utilising the most common features of voice therapy exercises, namely the optimal phonation task (OPT), followed by the introduction of sob voice quality (SVQ), the so-called heartbroken voice quality, and then habitual speech quality. Twang voice quality can be taught to assist in the production of loud voicing without effort, should the patient require this skill to meet their vocal needs. Task variance and negative practice are used in between the introduction of each technique. The difference between each technique can be physiologically and perceptually described according to the targeted activation of muscle groups that result in measurable movement outcomes. For example, the difference between OPT and SVQ involves targeting a lower larynx potion and some degree of laryngeal tilt in SVQ compared to OPT.

Table 1. Name and brief description of each of the first four Sob Voice Therapy components.

Component	Description
Optimal phonation task (OPT)	The patient is instructed to breathe in and out, then produce a clear, effortless, and quiet /m/ using the sound we make when we mean 'yes'. Instructions are given to prime the vocal system for low effort and low impact phonation including a gradual start (simultaneous onset). Focus is on ensuring the sound has communicative intent and is not produced as in singing. The patient is cued to notice how the sound feels and sounds. Explicit instruction is provided if whole-task modelling and imitation is insufficient for the patient to acquire the task. Home practise is recommended, ten repetitions/hour for 10 h during the day.
Sob voice quality (SVQ)	The patient is instructed to produce a clear, quiet, and effortless /ŋ/ using a gradual start to the sound and a sad, mournful expression (similar to a puppy whimper). Explicit instruction is provided to cue increased accessory muscle activation if whole-task modelling and imitation is insufficient for the patient to acquire the task. The patient is cued to notice how their voice feels and sounds. Home practise is recommended from six to eight repetitions/hour for 10 h during the day.
SVQ task variation (SVQ variants)	The patient is instructed to produce all voice carrier phrases beginning with a momentary /ŋ/ using SVQ. Phrases begin with all voiced sounds and then phrases with voiceless sounds are introduced. The patient is taught to produce a siren using a clear, quiet, and effortless /ŋ/ using SVQ, slowly, smoothly, evenly, and effortlessly sliding the pitch up and down in the middle of their comfortable vocal range. Siren extensions that gradually increase and decrease pitch in the siren are also introduced. The patient is cued to notice how their voice feels and sounds. Home practise is recommended with six phrases/hour and two to three sirens/hour for 10 h during the day.
Negative practice (NP)	The patient is instructed to imitate the voice quality they presented with at assessment by listening to their initial voice recording. They are instructed to use this 'old voice' quality in carrier phrases used in SVQ task variation and then compare this with SVQ carrier phrases (still initiated with a momentary /ŋ/), which is the 'new voice'. They are then asked to describe the differences between the two voice qualities with a focus on the sound and feeling of the voice. Home practise is recommended using three to four negative practice pairs (old way/new way) of SVQ phrases/hour for 10 h during the day.

NB: Practise recommendations are cumulative over the four components. Patients are instructed to randomise practise tasks in hourly practise sessions as different tasks are introduced.

VoiceCraft® and SVT describe voice therapy techniques that are based on a dynamical systems approach which acknowledges that the vocal system, like other complex movement systems, is self-organising [34]. Identifying the component of vocal function that is the most disorganised is the focus of the treatment and in the case of MTVD, it relates to some aspect of laryngeal function; for example, differentiated control of the adduction of the true vocal folds and retraction of the false vocal folds, and/or lowering of the larynx. Specifically, primary movements are targeted as these are implicated across a number of presenting symptoms (e.g., supraglottic constriction is associated with degraded voice quality and increased vocal effort). In this way, targeting a single movement, such as the widening of the supraglottic area via the release of laryngeal constriction manoeuvres, that then may address multiple aims, presents an efficient process of treatment, as multiple symptoms are addressed in one movement adjustment. Other aspects of the phonatory system such as breathing and resonance are de-emphasized unless they are the primary source of dysfunction, as it is presumed the neural system will automatically reorganise these functions around the biomechanical movement that is reorganised/optimised. For example, breathing is assumed to be mediated by communicative intent [35,36]. Different learning processes may have greater effect in the learning of the new, more optimal movement.

1.4. Retrospective Cohort Analysis vs. Randomised Control Trial

Given the value of voice therapy programs as the first line of treatment for commonly occurring MTVDs, understanding which treatment programs are effective and estimating their potential 'active ingredients' is essential. Despite being considered the highest level of evidence, the use of randomized controlled trials (RCTs) in investigating the treatment efficacy of voice therapies on voice disorders presents certain difficulties. Firstly, it is ethically challenging to allocate patients into different study arms given the need to recover the voice of professional voice users. Secondly, cost-effectiveness is a barrier to both clinicians and their patients, as most voice therapy programs require a course of weeks to months to complete. Lastly, patient compliance and the impact of various co-factors and comorbidities/medical conditions are amongst the burdens that can interfere with the intervention outcomes and how these are interpreted. A retrospective review of existing clinical databases had advantages of bringing evidence from 'real-world' scenarios to help clinicians and researchers determine (1) whether a particular therapy program is effective and, in standardised treatment programs, (2) to compare different therapy components with respect to their treatment efficacy.

The aims of the present study were to:

(1) evaluate the overall treatment effects of the Sob Voice Therapy program on MTVD with and without mucosal lesions of the vocal folds;
(2) investigate the effects of ingredients within the Sob Voice Therapy program on treatment outcomes for patients with MTVD; and
(3) identify any diagnostic or service delivery factors that influence the efficacy of a specific technique or process.

It was hypothesized that: (1) Sob Voice Therapy, which includes two vocal techniques (OPT and SVQ) and two training processes (SVQ variant and NP), would be effective in the treatment of MTVD; (2) processes (task variation and negative practice) rather than techniques (OPT and SVQ) would demonstrate statistically significant treatment effects; and (3) session number, treatment duration, and diagnostic and service delivery factors would have significant effects on treatment outcomes.

2. Materials and Methods

2.1. Study Design

This was a retrospective file audit of an existing private practice speech pathology clinical database. This study was approved by the Human Research Ethics Committee of the University of Sydney (protocol number: 2019/529).

2.2. Participants

2.2.1. Selection Criteria

Participants were included if they had received a diagnosis of primary or secondary MTVD from an Ear, Nose and Throat specialist (ENT). 'Primary' referred to MTVD without visible vocal fold mucosal lesions and 'secondary' referred to MTVD with slight associated mucosal changes related to vocal trauma, such as pre-nodular and swelling lesions.

Inclusion criteria included: (1) over 18 years of age; (2) diagnosis of MTVD by an ENT report based on laryngoscopy; (3) had attended at least one voice assessment and one voice therapy session, enabling pre and post-acoustic data baseline recordings prior to and following both the teaching and practise of the OPT; (4) received only Sob Voice Therapy components as described above; and (5) reported to have done some practise of the therapy component (technique or process) as recommended by the clinician.

Exclusion criteria included: (1) under 18 years of age; (2) missing an ENT laryngoscopy report/diagnosis; (3) had undergone surgery of the larynx or surrounding structures (e.g., thyroid surgery) throughout their voice intervention period; (4) neurological voice and speech problems (e.g., dysarthria) or predominant mucosal lesions (e.g., cysts, polyps, and neoplasms); (5) types of functional dysphonia not related to vocal trauma, e.g., puberphonia, presbyphonia, and transgender voice; (6) missing voice recordings for more than one data point other than the initial and final session; (7) voice recordings with severely aperiodic signals (type 3 and type 4 signals) [37], precluding fundamental frequency-based measures; (8) received instruction in another voice therapy technique or process not described in Sob Voice Therapy; and (9) patients who could not detect any change in the sound or sensation of their voice production regardless of their success in achieving voice change during the OPT trial therapy task in the initial assessment, as this would suggest a possible undiagnosed neurosensory or cognitive impairment.

2.2.2. Sample Size Calculation

The required number of patients for the retrospective review was estimated using an online sample calculation tool called GLIMMPSE [38], as this has been recommended for calculating samples for repeated-measures study designs [39]. Parameters used included: power = 90%; Geisser-greenhouse corrected test; Type I error rate $\alpha = 0.05$; outcome measures = harmonics-to-noise ratio (HNR); number of measurements = 3 (baseline and two post-therapy assessments); predictor variables = type of muscle-tension voice disorders (primary and secondary); treatment effects = [MTD type x harmonics-to-noise ratio interaction]; mean scale factor = 2; and variability scale factor = 1. Regarding the mean values to put into the formula, we used baseline HNR values taken from baseline data in a randomized control clinical trial by Nguyen and Kenny [21], in which HNR pre-treatment of primary MTD was 18.6 decibels (dB). Considering there has been no similar study design in the literature, we assumed the first treatment and second treatment resulted in a 3.8 dB improvement in HNR for the primary MTD group as observed in the Nguyen and Kenny study [21]. Mean baseline HNR for secondary MTD was taken from Wenke et al. [40] in which baseline HNR was 16.6 dB as their study used participants with both primary MTD and MTD with lesions such as vocal nodules. We assumed the first and second treatments resulted in a 2.9 dB improvement in HNR for the secondary MTD group as observed in their standard treatment protocols [40]. Standard deviation (SD) of HNR for the formula was set at 4.5 dB according to the study of Wenke et al. [40]. The calculation resulted in a sample size of 74 (patients).

2.3. Voice Therapy Programs under Review: Sob Voice Therapy

Sob Voice Therapy was delivered to the patients by six different SLPs who had completed a 4-day workshop in VoiceCraft® and SVT [30]. All were certified practicing speech pathologists with experience in treating patients with MTVD ranging from 1 to 15 years. Therapy was delivered in a face-to-face, one-on-one service delivery model across six different sites in an office setting. Patients were charged a fee for service in all cases. Eighteen out of sixty-eight participants were treated by more than one clinicians. Patients were taught the specific technique or process and required to perform the technique or task to 80% accuracy as judged by the clinician before moving onto the next phase. All sessions were documented as being 60 min long (according to the clinical hour of 50 min face-to-face time and 10 min of note taking/administration). Patients were recommended to undertake a specific amount of daily practise in each technique and/or process. Recommendations were based on motor learning principles of high frequency, distributed variable, and randomised and context-variable practise [41]. Typically, patients were recommended to practise once an hour for between 1 and 3 min, aiming for 10 practise sessions/day. As the therapy is based on hierarchical additive fractionation, patients were required to add practise in a new technique or process to that of their previous practise, which also allowed for task variation and randomisation. Individual specific practise data was not collected routinely from patients; however, all patients reported some level of practise. The number of sessions required to meet 80% correctness in the technique/process ranged from 1.3 to 2.4, with the number of days between each technique/process ranging from 27.8–37.5.

Extracted data was collected at five time points: (1) at the initial session (baseline) after which the OPT was taught in the same session; (2) at the subsequent session in which it was judged by the clinician whether the OPT had been acquired and the next technique

(SVQ) was taught (OPT-SVQ); (3) at the subsequent session in which the clinician judged that SVQ had been acquired and sob variants were taught (SVQ-SVQ variants); (4) at the subsequent session in which the clinic judges whether the SVQ variants had been acquired and NP was taught (SVQ variants-NP); and (5) at the beginning of the session following the introduction of the NP process (NP post-NP). The number of sessions and days between each of the time points varied due to variation in clinic attendance and time taken to acquire each technique/process. The modal number of sessions between each technique/process was 1 and modal number of days was 14 (Table 2).

Table 2. Number of sessions and days between each technique and process of the Sob Voice Therapy. Abbreviations: SD, standard deviation, and CI, confidence interval.

	OPT-SVQ $n = 64$		SVQ-SVQ Variants $n = 43$		SVQ Variant-NP $n = 33$		NP Post-NP $n = 24$		Total OPT Post-NP	
	Sessions	Days	Sessions	Days	Sessions	Days	Sessions	Days	Sessions	Days
Mean (SD)	1.3 (0.6)	28.5 (27.6)	1.5 (0.9)	38.3 (48.2)	2.5 (2.3)	37.3 (27.0)	1.2 (0.5)	24.0 (17.0)	4.0 (3.0)	83.1 (59.2)
95% CI	1.2–1.5	21.5–35.5	1.2–1.8	24.0–52.6	1.6–3.3	27.0–47.6	1.0–1.4	16.7–31.4	3.2–4.8	68.1–98.1
Min–max	1.0–4.0	4.0–173.0	1.0–5.0	6.0–248.0	1.0–11.0	7.0–105.0	1.0–3.0	7.0–84.0	1.0–15.0	7.0–283.0
Median	1.0	21.0	1.0	23.5	2.0	26.0	1.0	23.0	3.0	72.5

2.4. Data Extraction

2.4.1. Demographic Characteristics

During the initial voice assessment, a thorough case history interview was conducted. This supplemented the referral and case history information collected by a comprehensive case history questionnaire [42] and the patient reported outcomes (PROMS) data collected prior to the assessment session including both the Voice Handicap Index-10 (VHI-10) [43] and Reflux Symptom Index (RSI) [44] as a standard (data not reported here). Data about age, gender, occupation, MTVD type (primary and secondary), vocal load, lifestyle, and history of comorbidities were extracted.

2.4.2. Extraction of Voice Recordings

Patient data was extracted and de-identified by authors AC and EK to ensure the first author was blinded to the identification of patient data to remove any risk of bias. All patients included in this review had high-quality audio recordings of a comprehensive voice assessment undertaken at baseline including the reading of the Rainbow Passage [45], the Consensus Auditory Perceptual Evaluation–Voice (CAPE-V) phrases [46], and the prolonged vowel (/a/). All voice signals were captured using an AKG C520 cardioid ear-mounted microphone [47] placed at a constant distance of 6 cm, 45° off the mouth axis, and were analogue-to-digital converted using a professional external sound card (Roland Quadcapture [48]) at 44.1 kHz and 16-bit resolution. The signals were processed and saved to a laptop computer using the Audacity sound editing software [49] in *.wav format. Calibration of the sound level in the voice signals was not undertaken. In subsequent treatment sessions, audio recordings were made at the beginning of each session of the Rainbow Passage, CAPE-V phrases, and prolonged vowel/a/for a minimum of 3 s.

2.5. Auditory–Perceptual Outcome Measures

This retrospective review used four auditory–perceptual parameters for outcome measures, including overall severity of dysphonia, roughness, breathiness, and strain. These outcome measures were evaluated using auditory–perceptual analysis, which is considered the gold standard for clinical voice assessment [50].

2.5.1. Listeners

Two certified practicing SLPs (2 and 3.5 years of experience in clinical voice assessment, respectively) and one ENT surgeon (19 years of experience in voice assessment) participated in the perceptual analyses. The raters reported normal hearing and vision at the time of the study.

2.5.2. Stimuli

Voice samples were edited to include the middle three seconds of the second attempt of the sustained /a/ vowel production, the third CAPE-V phrase (CAPEV3), and the Rainbow Passage ('When the sunlight . . . . . . at the end of the rainbow'). These tasks were combined into a single file in Audacity. To avoid variabilities related to unequal sound pressure levels/hearing levels of the samples, all stimuli were normalized for loudness using the command 'Loudness Normalization' in the program to ensure that the perceived loudness of stimuli was 23 loudness units full-scale (LUFS). The intensity level of stimuli ranged from 70 to 72 dB as measured in Praat [51] using default intensity settings. Stimuli from 35 patients were randomly repeated for testing intra-rater reliability. In total, 285 samples were used.

2.5.3. Procedure

Raters judged the level of the four voice dimensions, including overall severity, roughness, breathiness, and strain, using a 100-point visual analogue scale (VAS) based on the items described in the CAPE-V protocol [46] and embedded in an online auditory–perceptual rating tool called Bridge2practice, which is an education and research platform developed for audio–perceptual learning and practise of speech pathology students [52]. Judgments were made by moving a slider between 1 and 100, representing the minimum and maximum level of the quality being rated, respectively. Listeners were required to listen to the voice tasks as many times as they wished using a headphone and to make a judgment by changing the position of the slider on the VAS line mentioned above. All voice tasks were randomized. Responses were registered in the rating platform and exported to an Excel spreadsheet. The CAPE-V rating includes other perceptual rating features such as pitch, volume, and resonance, as well as additional features such as fry and diplophonia; however, features were not rated in this dataset.

2.5.4. Reliability of Auditory–Perceptual Analyses

Reliability was assessed using SPSS 24.0 [53]. Intraclass correlation coefficients (ICC) [54] were used to determine the level of agreement between the first and second (repeated) ratings (intra-rater reliability) and across listeners (inter-rater reliability). ICC was calculated using a two-way mixed model, consistency type, and single measure analysis [ICC (3,1)]. To assess the level of correlation, ICC < 0.5 indicates poor correlation, 0.5–0.75 indicates moderate correlation, 0.75–0.9 indicates good correlation, and >0.9 indicates excellent correlation [55]. Table 3 shows good to excellent intra-rater reliability for most of the rated voice dimensions. Table 4 shows moderate to good inter-rater reliability for all rated voice dimensions.

Table 3. Intra-rater reliability of the perceptual analysis ($p < 0.001$ for all measures).

Rater	Types of Measures	ICC			
		Severity	Roughness	Breathiness	Strain
Rater 1	Single measures	0.854	0.869	0.738	0.862
	Average measures	0.921	0.930	0.849	0.926
Rater 2	Single measures	0.977	0.889	0.948	0.896
	Average measures	0.988	0.941	0.974	0.945
Rater 3	Single measures	0.822	0.812	0.810	0.829
	Average measures	0.903	0.896	0.895	0.906

Table 4. Inter-rater reliability of the perceptual analysis.

Voice Measure	ICC Measures	ICC	95% CI	p
Overall severity	Single measures	0.703	0.547–0.824	0.000
	Average measures	0.876	0.783–0.933	0.000
Roughness	Single measures	0.696	0.537–0.819	0.000
	Average measures	0.873	0.777–0.932	0.000
Breathiness	Single measures	0.659	0.490–0.795	0.000
	Average measures	0.853	0.743–0.921	0.000
Strain	Single measures	0.691	0.531–0.816	0.000
	Average measures	0.870	0.772–0.930	0.000

2.6. Acoustic Outcome Measures

Voice samples were edited in Audacity to extract the middle three seconds (s) of the sustained /a/ vowels, CAPEV3, and the second and third sentences of the Rainbow Passage (RP23). RP23 is a standard task in the analysis of dysphonia in speech and voice (ADSV) [56], which was used for the acoustic analysis in the present study. The use of RP23 would allow for cepstral measures to be comparable with the previous studies that used this task [57]. The quality of audio recordings for all samples was checked using the signal-to-noise ratio (SNR) using a Praat script called 'Speech-to-noise ratio/voice-to-noise ratio v.01.01' [58]. Only samples with a SNR $\geq$ 30 dB were used for the acoustic analyses [59].

2.6.1. Harmonics-to-Noise Ratio (HNR)

HNR quantifies the level of noise in the voice signals and intensifies it in pathological voices [60]. It has been found that HNR is correlated with the perceptual assessment of hoarseness [60] and vocal clarity [61]. HNR has been an important and commonly used outcome measure of voice treatment [62,63]. Praat 6.1.40 [51] was used to measure HNR from the middle 3-s segments from three trials of vowel samples and the averaged result (in dB) was used for the statistical analysis.

2.6.2. Fundamental Frequency (F0)

F0 remains one of the most important frequency-based measures that has been extensively used to reflect voice changes associated with different laryngeal configurations, e.g., vocal fold dimension [64] and vocal fold stiffness [65]. F0 was measured in Praat from CAPEV3 and the full Rainbow Passage. The standard deviation of F0 (F0SD), which represent vocal stability [66], was measured from the sustained vowel /a/. All voice data with severely aperiodic signals (signal types 3 and 4) [37] were excluded from the F0 and HNR measurements. F0 settings in Praat are presented in Appendix A.1.

2.6.3. Cepstral Peak Prominence: Non-Smoothed (CPP) and Smoothed (CPPS)

A voice cepstrum is measured using a Fourier transform of the logarithm power spectrum [67]. A cepstral peak is identified within the dominant 'rahmonic' corresponding to the fundamental period from which the cepstral peak prominence (CPP) is calculated as the amplitude between the peak and the regression line directly below it [68]. A signal with a highly periodic waveform and a clear harmonic structure would have a higher cepstral peak than aperiodic signals [68]. CPP has been shown to have stronger weighted correlations with overall voice quality than any other acoustic measure [69]. It has also been considered a significant predictor of dysphonic severity [70].

The acoustic analysis program ADSV [56] was used to measure cepstral peak prominence (CPP) in dB for the vowel, CAPEV3, and RP23 vocal tasks. CPP settings in ADSV are presented in Appendix A.2. CPPS was measured in Praat using recommended settings [71,72], which are shown in Appendix A.3. Smoothing before calculating the cepstral peak can improve the accuracy of estimation [73]. In Praat, the smoothing of the cepstral measurement followed the procedures by Hillenbrand and Houde [73] using 20-ms (10-frame) time-smoothing windows and 1-ms (10-bin) quefrency smoothing [51]. The first step involves averaging cepstral values over time, while the second step involves cepstra being averaged across the quefrency [51]. Both CPP and CPPS were used to allow the data to be comparable to the other studies that used either of these measures. We also expected that CPPS was more sensitive than CPP in detecting treatment outcome due to its smoothing algorithm.

2.6.4. Cepstral/Spectral Index of Dysphonia

The Cepstral/Spectral Index of Dysphonia (CSID) reflects overall voice quality [57,74] and has been shown to have high sensitivity and specificity [57] in discriminating pathological aspects from normal voice quality [75]. CSID data were obtained automatically in ADSV for the vowel and CAPEV3 task, and were manually calculated for RP23 samples based on CPP, low/high spectral ratio (LH), and low/high spectral ratio standard deviation (SDLH) values measured in ADSV using the following formula [57]:

$$\text{CSID of Rainbow Passage} = 154.59 - 10.39 \times \text{CPP} - 1.08 \times \text{LH} - 3.71 \times \text{SDLH}$$

2.6.5. Vocal Intensity

Vocal intensity was measured in Praat from the /a/ vowel, CAPEV3, and the whole Rainbow Passage. It was used to validate the cepstral measures as previous research has found CPP measures to be affected by vocal intensity: CPP would increase when vocal intensity was elevated [76].

2.6.6. Reliability Analysis of Acoustic Measurements

Baseline acoustic data for 30 patients were reanalysed for two acoustic measures that involved the manual selection of the analysis samples (HNR of the vowel and F0 of CAPEV3). Results from the two analyses were compared using ICC statistics. The results showed that, for HNR, ICC values were 1 for both single measures and average measures ($p < 0.001$). For F0 of CAPEV3, ICC = 0.999 for single measures ($p < 0.001$) and ICC = 1 for average measures ($p < 0.001$). These results demonstrated excellent inter-rater reliability of the acoustic analysis. CPP, CPPS, and CSID measures were analysed using the entire edited vocal samples, which involved no manual selection of the waveform. Therefore, reliability analyses were deemed not necessary for those measures.

2.7. Statistical Analyses

Data were managed in Microsoft Excel [77] and analysed using IBM SPSS Statistics v.24.0 [53]. Descriptive statistics were used to describe cohort characteristics. Prior to the analyses, normal distribution of the data was examined using Kolmogorov–Smirnov tests [78]. For continuous variables, mean, standard deviation (SD), range, median, and the interquartile range were used. For categorical data, frequencies and percentages were used. Changes in outcome measures over the treatment period were analysed using a linear mixed model with patients representing random effects and time point (baseline and the four treatment technique points) representing fixed effects. Gender, diagnosis (MTVD primary vs. secondary), and treating clinicians also represented fixed effects. Interaction between time and the fixed factors was calculated to determine the impact of the factors on the treatment outcome. Significant fixed effects of time were further tested using pairwise comparison with the Sidak adjustment for p values. One-way repeated-measures analysis of variance (ANOVA) was used to examine the effects of each individual treatment ingredient on auditory–perceptual and acoustic outcome measures by comparing data between baseline and after each treatment. Effect size was calculated using partial Eta squared (η^2) with the values of 0.01, 0.1, and 0.25 indicating small, medium, and large effects, respectively [79].

Pearson's correlation coefficient (r) was used to calculate the correlation between the number of therapy sessions and treatment duration, as well as the treatment outcome in which r = 0.1, 0.3, and 0.5 indicated small, medium, and large effects, respectively [80]. Where there were multiple calculations, the Bonferroni adjustment was applied to the p value. In all statistical analyses, a significance of $p < 0.05$ was used.

3. Results

3.1. Characteristics of the Study Population

In total, 68 participants were included in this study. Of these, there were 60 females (88.7%) with a mean age of 34.5 years (SD = 13.0, range = 20–84). There were eight males (11.3%) with mean age of 43.6 years (SD = 16.3, range = 25–70). In brief, 11 were vocal performers (16.2%), 49 were professional voice users (72.1%), and 8 belonged to other occupations (11.8%). Twenty-six had a history of vocal training (38.2%), 36 had not had voice training before (52.9%), and 6 did not provide information about voice training history (8.8%). Laryngeal assessment via ENT was reported to have been conducted on all 68 patients, which showed that 34 had primary MTD and 34 had MTD with mucosal lesions. The mean duration of voice problems was 19.2 months (SD = 26.5; 95% CI for mean = 12.5–25.9; minimum = 1.0; maximum = 132.0; median = 12.0; interquartile range = 18.0). The mean VHI-10 score was 17.8 (SD = 9.4; 95% CI = 15.5–20.1; minimum = 1; maximum = 38; median = 18.0; and interquartile range = 14.0). The study cohort was therefore considered typical of previously documented treatment-seeking populations with voice disorders reported in other studies [81,82]. Data on vocal load, history of comorbidities, and lifestyle are presented in Tables A1–A3 in Appendix B.

Figure 1 shows the number of patients who underwent all four components of Sob Voice Therapy. For all participants (*n* = 68), the OPT was taught as the initial therapy exercise/laryngeal posture. Sixty-four participants (94.1%) went on to be taught SVQ as their second voice therapy exercise. Three (4.7%) were taught SVQ in addition to a SVQ variant (i.e., sob phrases or sob sirens) simultaneously in their second appointment. Of the 61 patients who were taught the OPT followed by SVQ, 43 (70.5%) were then taught SVQ variants, with most of these participants (*n* = 33) first being taught SVQ phrases. Fourteen out of sixty-one (22.9%) did not attend any further sessions following the successive teaching of the OPT and SVQ. Following teaching of the OPT, SVQ, and SVQ variants, 55.8% (*n* = 24/43) of participants were then taught the generalisation technique of negative practice, with the remaining 19 participants being lost to follow up or having incomplete data sets.

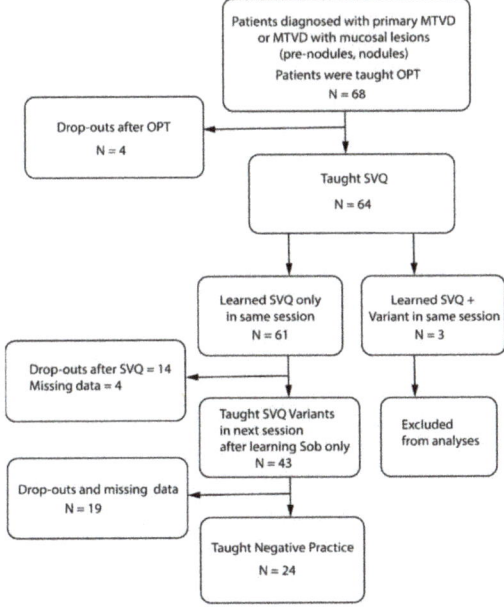

Figure 1. Flowchart of the treatment techniques.

3.2. Treatment Effects of Sob Voice Therapy on MTVD

3.2.1. Auditory-Perceptual Outcomes

The changes in perceptual outcome measures over time were calculated using a linear mixed model. Patients were treated as random effects and treatment (i.e., baseline and the four technique points) as fixed effects. Diagnosis (primary MTD and secondary MTD) was also a fixed factor to examine the interaction with treatment. The estimate of the fixed effects was based on the regression coefficient (b) for each effect associated with its 95% CI and the p value. Changes of the outcome measures over time were evaluated using multiple pairwise testing in which the Sidak adjustment for p values was applied.

- Overall severity ratings

Figure 2 shows rating scores of the overall severity of dysphonia for all time points. The overall progression, as indicated by the trend line, was that the rating scores were lower towards the final technique point (NP) for both diagnostic groups. There were significant fixed effects of treatment [$F(4, 170.706) = 12.142, p < 0.001$]. There was no significant effect of diagnosis ($p = 0.125$) and no significant interaction between treatment and diagnosis ($p = 0.431$). Parameter estimates showed a significant decrease in the overall severity ratings at the final technique point (NP) compared to baseline (b = 5.603, t = 3.047, $p = 0.003$). Compared with baseline, the mean (95% CI, Sidak-adjusted p) of the overall severity rating score decreased by 3.2 (0.4–5.9, $p = 0.013$), 6.9 (3.7–10.2, $p < 0.001$), 5.4 (1.7–9.0, $p < 0.001$), and 7.2 (3.0–11.4, $p < 0.001$) after treatments with OPT, SVQ, the SVQ variants, and NP, respectively.

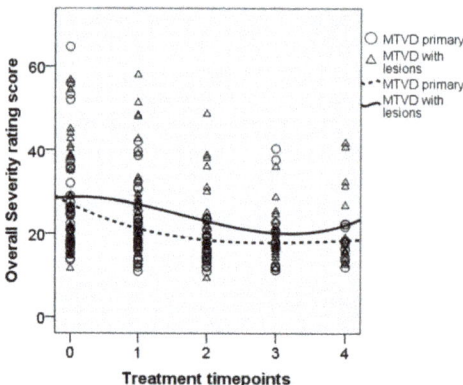

Figure 2. Longitudinal plot of data for the overall severity ratings. Trend line is shown for each subgroup. 0 = baseline, 1 = OPT, 2 = SVQ, 3 = SVQ variant, and 4 = NP.

- Roughness ratings

Figure 3 shows the changes of roughness rating scores over time with a steady decrease towards the end of the treatment program. The effects of the fixed factor 'treatment' on this outcome measure were significant [$F(4, 171.467) = 10.082, p < 0.001$]. The effect of diagnosis ($p = 0.090$) and interaction effects between treatment and diagnosis ($p = 0.231$) were not significant. Parameter estimates showed a significant decrease in the rating score of roughness after NP as compared to baseline (b = 4.842, t = 2.493, $p = 0.014$). The mean (95% CI, Sidak-adjusted p) of the roughness rating scores decreased by 3.5 (0.6–6.4, $p = 0.007$), 5.7 (2.3–9.2, $p < 0.001$), 6.4 (2.5–10.2, $p < 0.001$), and 7.3 (2.9–11.7, $p < 0.001$) after OPT, SVQ, the SVQ variants, and NP, respectively.

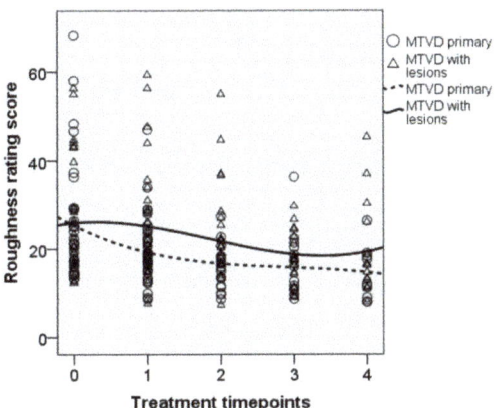

Figure 3. Longitudinal plot of data for the roughness ratings. Trend line is shown for each subgroup. 0 = baseline, 1 = OPT, 2 = SVQ, 3 = SVQ variant, and 4 = NP.

- Breathiness ratings

Changes in the breathiness rating scores over the treatment period are presented in Figure 4, which shows a similar trend of decrease across the treatment techniques. There were significant effects of treatment [$F(4, 170.294) = 5.482$, $p < 0.001$], no significant effect of diagnosis ($p = 0.102$), and no significant interaction between treatment and diagnosis ($p = 0.715$). The decrease in breathiness rating scores after NP was significant as compared with baseline ($b = 4.27$, $t = 2.13$, $p = 0.035$). The mean (95% CI, Sidak-adjust p) ratings of breathiness decreased by 2.1 (-0.9–5.1, $p = 0.367$), 4.7 (1.2–8.2, $p = 0.002$), 4.1 (0.1–8.0, $p = 0.040$), and 5.8 (1.3–10.3, $p = 0.004$) after OPT, SVQ, the SVQ variants, and NP, respectively.

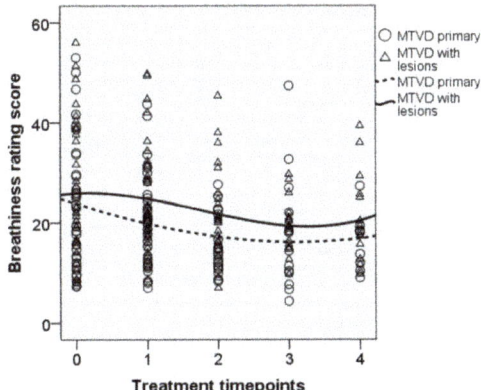

Figure 4. Longitudinal plot of data for the breathiness ratings. Trend line is shown for each subgroup. 0 = baseline, 1 = OPT, 2 = SVQ, 3 = SVQ variant, and 4 = NP.

- Strain ratings

Figure 5 shows the changes in the rating scores for strain quality after each technique. Overall, rating scores of this voice dimension decreased over the technique points. The trajectory of the trend lines shows that the rating scores for primary MTD decreased immediately at OPT while the decrease was not so obvious for MTD with lesions. There were significant effects of the fixed factors 'treatment' [$F(4, 171.739) = 9.743$, $p < 0.001$]

and 'diagnosis' [F(1, 73.367) = 5.033, p = 0.028], and marginally significant interaction between treatment and diagnosis [F(4, 171.739) = 2.422, p = 0.05]. There was a significant improvement in this voice quality after the last time point (NP) as compared to baseline (b = 5.01, t = 2.643, p = 0.009). There were decreases in the mean (95% CI, Sidak-adjusted p) of 3.8 (0.9–6.6, p = 0.002), 3.7 (0.3–7.0, p = 0.021), 6.6 (2.9–10.4 p < 0.001), and 7.4 (3.1–11.7, p < 0.001) after OPT, SVQ, the SVQ variants, and NP, respectively.

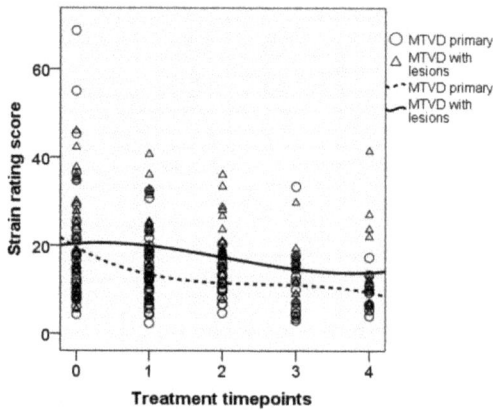

Figure 5. Longitudinal plot of data for the strain ratings. Trend line is shown for each subgroup. 0 = baseline, 1 = OPT, 2 = SVQ, 3 = SVQ variant, and 4 = NP.

3.2.2. Acoustic Outcomes

- Harmonics-to-noise Ratio

Figure 6 shows the mean HNR (dB) at baseline and at all the treatment time points. Significant effects of the treatment were found [F(4, 168.921) = 3.672, p = 0.007], while no significant interaction between treatment and diagnosis was present (p = 0.327), meaning that the effects of the treatment did not depend upon MTD type (primary or with mucosal lesions). The improvement in HNR between baseline and NP was significant (b = −2.82, t = −2.470, p = 0.014). The mean (95% CI, Sidak-adjusted p) of HNR (dB) increased by 1.6 (−0.2–3.3, p = 0.099), 1.7 (−0.3–3.7, p = 0.141), 2.5 (0.2–4.8, p = 0.022), and 2.4 (−0.3–5.2, p = 0.11) after OPT, SVQ, the SVQ variants, and NP, respectively.

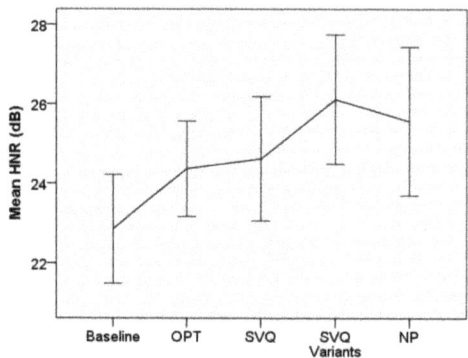

Figure 6. Mean harmonics-to-noise ratio. Error bars indicate 95% CI for the mean.

- Fundamental frequency

Table 5 presents F0 data at baseline for all three vocal tasks. For F0 of CAPEV3, there were no significant fixed effects of treatment ($p = 0.585$) and no significant interaction between treatment and diagnosis ($p = 0.358$). There were also no significant effects of treatment ($p = 0.276$) and no significant interaction between treatment and diagnosis ($p = 0.523$) for the F0 of the Rainbow Passage.

Table 5. Fundamental frequency data (Hz) of the cohort at baseline ($n = 68$).

		Norms	Mean (SD)	95% CI	Min–Max
F0 of CAPEV3	Male	108.94 [83]	137.5 (31.2)	111.5–163.6	107.3–199.7
	Female	235.07 [83]	189.2 (17.7)	184.5–193.8	148.1–232.9
F0 of RP	Male	84–178 [40]	140.6 (43.3)	104.4–176.7	97.6–236.9
	Female	127–275 [40]	185.8 (14.7)	181.9–189.7	148.9–219.6
F0SD	Male	3.3 [84]	1.8 (1.0)	1.0–2.6	0.8–4.0
	Female	20–29y: 3.8 [85] 30–40y: 2.5 [86] 40–50y: 2.8 [86] 60–69y: 4.3 [85]	2.3 (1.4)	2.0–2.7	0.7–8.2

F0SD (vowel) also showed significant effects of treatment ($p = 0.716$) and no significant interaction between treatment and diagnosis ($p = 0.111$).

- CPP

Figure 7 shows CPP data for all three vocal tasks. A significant effect of treatment was found for the CPP of CAPEV3 [$F(4, 168.369) = 4.721$, $p = 0.001$] but there was no interaction between treatment and diagnosis ($p = 0.737$). The improvement of CPP at NP as compared to baseline was significant (b = -0.915, t = -2.726, $p = 0.007$). Compared to baseline, the CPP of CAPEV3 only improved by 0.5dB after OPT (95% CI = -0.04–0.96, $p = 0.088$). After SVQ, the SVQ variants, and NP, the mean (95% CI, Sidak-adjusted p) of this measure (in dB) increased by 0.62 (0.04–1.21, $p = 0.03$), 0.8 (0.2–1.5, $p = 0.006$), and 0.8 (0.05–1.5, $p = 0.03$), respectively.

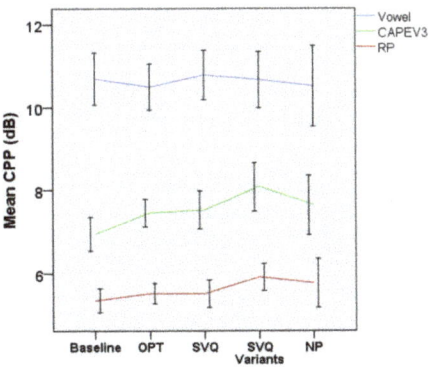

Figure 7. Cepstral peak prominence (CPP) of all vocal tasks. Error bars indicate 95% CI for the mean. Abbreviations: CAPEV3, third CAPEV phrase and RP, Rainbow Passage.

There was marginal fixed effect of treatment on the CPP of the Rainbow Passage [$F(4, 171.130) = 2.312$, $p = 0.06$]. Significant improvement in this measure was found after NP as compared to baseline (b = -0.442, t = -2.137, $p = 0.034$). Pairwise comparisons with baseline showed that the mean (95% CI, Sidak-adjusted p) of the CPP (dB) of the Rainbow Passage increased by 0.14 (-0.17–0.45, $p = 0.912$), 0.17 (-0.2–0.54, $p = 0.879$), 0.31

(−0.1–0.72, $p = 0.284$), and 0.45 (−0.02–0.92, $p = 0.069$) after OPT, SVQ, the SVQ variants, and NP, respectively.

There was no significant fixed effect of treatment ($p = 0.849$) and no significant interaction between treatment and diagnosis ($p = 0.227$) on the CPP of the vowel.

- CPPS

Figure 8 shows CPPS data for all treatment time points. The CPPS of CAPEV3 demonstrated a steady increase from OPT towards the final technique (NP). There was a significant effect of treatment on this measure [$F(4, 171.649) = 14.921$, $p < 0.001$] but there was no significant interaction between treatment and diagnosis ($p = 0.673$), i.e., the changes in this measures over time were similar between primary MTD and MTD with lesions. The increase in the CPPS of CAPEV3 at NP as compared to baseline was significant (b = −1.985, t = −4.286, $p < 0.001$). The mean (95% CI, Sidak-adjusted p) of this measure (in dB) increased by 1.02 (0.33–1.7, $p < 0.001$), 1.43 (0.63–2.23, $p < 0.001$), 2.06 (1.17–2.95, $p < 0.001$), and 1.91 (0.88–2.94, $p < 0.001$) after OPT, SVQ, the SVQ variants, and NP, respectively.

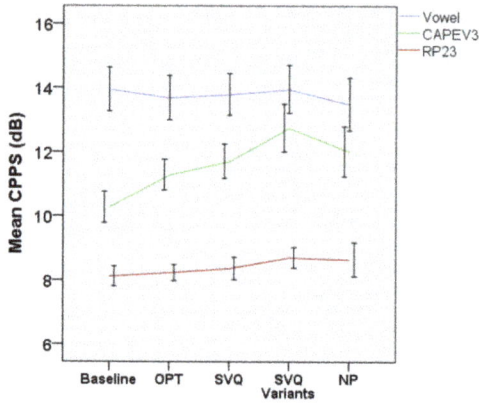

Figure 8. Smoothed cepstral peak prominence of all vocal tasks. Error bars indicate 95% CI for the mean. Abbreviations: CAPEV3, third CAPEV phrase and RP, Rainbow Passage.

The CPPS of vowels and RP23 are also shown in Figure 8. No significant effects of treatment were found for the CPPS of the vowel ($p = 0.819$) and RP23 ($p = 0.156$).

- CSID

Figure 9 shows the CSID of all tasks. There was a significant effect of treatment on the CSID of the Rainbow Passage [$F(4, 170.887) = 2.859$, $p = 0.025$]. No significant interaction effect between treatment and diagnosis was found ($p = 0.161$). The model showed a significant decrease in CSID after NP as compared with baseline (b = 6.04, t = 2.327, $p = 0.021$). Pairwise comparisons across time points showed that the mean (95% CI, Sidak-adjusted p) of CSID decreased by 2.82 (−1.07–6.7, $p = 0.344$), 2.51 (−2.11–7.13, $p = 0.736$), 4.33 (−0.8–9.47, $p = 0.164$), and 6.03 (0.16–11.89, $p = 0.04$) after OPT, SVQ, the SVQ variants, and NP, respectively.

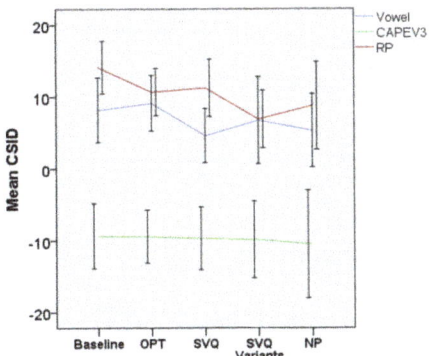

Figure 9. Mean CSID of all vocal tasks. Error bars indicate 95% CI for the mean. Abbreviations: CAPEV3, third CAPEV phrase and RP, Rainbow Passage.

The effects of the treatment for the CSID of the vowel ($p = 0.683$) and CAPEV3 ($p = 0.935$) were not statistically significant ($p > 0.05$).

- Vocal intensity

There were no significant fixed effects of treatment on the intensity of the vowel ($p = 0.557$), CAPEV3 ($p = 0.357$), and Rainbow Passage ($p = 0.777$).

3.3. Estimates of Active Ingredients within the Sob Voice Therapy Program

Apart from evaluating the treatment outcome of the whole Sob Voice Therapy program, we were also interested in estimating the effects of each of the individual therapy components (OPT, SVQ, the SVQ variants, and NP). This was evaluated via effect sizes, which were calculated as the Eta squared (η^2) using one-way repeated-measures ANOVA for the differences in the outcome measures between baseline and after each technique point. This calculation was performed for auditory–perceptual and acoustic measures with statistically significant fixed effects of treatment. The data set for this calculation was $n = 24$ patients who had completed voice recordings at all mentioned time points. Patients with any missing data points were excluded from this analysis.

3.3.1. Effect Size for Auditory–Perceptual Outcomes

Table 6 shows the mean (SD) and mean differences between baseline and each of the voice therapy techniques for all auditory–perceptual parameters. This table also presents the effect sizes corresponding to the results for the repeated-measures ANOVA. Overall, findings for auditory–perceptual ratings of overall severity, roughness, and breathiness showed that SVQ, the SVQ variants, and NP were active ingredients with large effect sizes. OPT did not demonstrate therapeutic effects. For strain ratings, only the SVQ variants and NP were the active ingredients.

Table 6. Auditory–perceptual outcomes after four stages of Sob Voice Therapy. Partial $\eta^2 = 0.01, 0.1$, and 0.25 indicate small, medium, and large effects, respectively. Abbreviation: MD, mean difference; (*), significance at $p < 0.05$.

Measures	Time Point	Mean (SD)	95% CI for Mean	MD	F	p	Partial η^2
	Baseline	26.8 (13.7)	20.2–33.4				
	OPT	25.8 (11.3)	20.4–31.3	1.0	0.376	0.546	0.018
Overall severity	SVQ	20.0 (7.9)	16.2–23.8	6.8	12.001	0.003 *	0.387
	SVQ variant	20.9 (7.2)	17.4–24.4	5.9	12.381	0.002 *	0.360
	NP	21.6 (8.9)	17.3–25.9	5.2	11.312	0.003 *	0.340

Table 6. Cont.

Measures	Time Point	Mean (SD)	95% CI for Mean	MD	F	p	Partial η²
Roughness	Baseline	24.1 (12.8)	17.9–30.3				
	OPT	22.8 (12.4)	16.8–28.8	1.3	0.865	0.363	0.041
	SVQ	19.5 (9.2)	15.1–23.9	4.6	7.069	0.016 *	0.271
	SVQ variant	18.8 (8.8)	14.5–23.0	5.3	12.289	0.002 *	0.358
	NP	19.4 (9.7)	14.7–24.1	4.7	10.471	0.004 *	0.322
Breathiness	Baseline	23.4 (13.8)	16.8–30.1				
	OPT	23.6 (11.1)	18.5–28.6	0.2	0.007	0.936	0.001
	SVQ	18.6 (8.2)	14.6–22.5	4.9	6.859	0.017 *	0.265
	SVQ variant	18.9 (5.9)	16.0–21.7	4.6	6.375	0.019 *	0.225
	NP	19.8 (8.1)	15.9–23.7	3.6	5.444	0.029 *	0.198
Strain	Baseline	18.4 (11.6)	12.8–23.9				
	OPT	16.8 (9.5)	12.2–21.3	1.6	1.526	0.231	0.071
	SVQ	17.0 (6.6)	13.8–20.2	1.3	1.085	0.311	0.054
	SVQ variant	12.3 (7.0)	8.9–15.7	6.1	17.713	0.001 *	0.446
	NP	13.6 (9.2)	9.2–18.0	4.8	9.409	0.006 *	0.300

3.3.2. Effect Size for Acoustic Outcomes

Table 7 shows effect sizes associated with the outputs of the repeated-measures ANOVA for the changes in acoustic measures after each voice therapy ingredient as compared with baseline. Findings on the CPPS of CAPEV3 showed that SVQ, the SVQ variants, and NP were the active ingredients, and the last two ingredients (SVQ variant and NP) were associated with large effect sizes. Data of the CPP of CAPEV3 and CSID of the Rainbow Passage suggested that NP was an active ingredient.

Table 7. Acoustic outcomes after four stages of Sob Voice Therapy. Partial η² = 0.01, 0.1, and 0.25 indicate small, medium, and large effects, respectively. Abbreviations: MD, mean difference and NA, not available; (*), significance at $p < 0.05$.

Measure	Normative Cut-Off	Time Point	Mean (SD)	95% CI	MD	F	p	Partial η²
HNR	20 dB [51]	Baseline	23.6 (5.4)	21.1–26.1				
		OPT	23.5 (6.1)	20.7–26.4	0.1	0.001	0.976	0.000
		SVQ	24.7 (4.9)	22.4–270.0	1.1	1.203	0.286	0.060
		SVQ variant	25.3 (4.7)	23.1–27.5	1.7	2.153	0.157	0.093
		NP	25.6 (4.2)	23.6–27.6	20.0	2.574	0.124	0.114
CPP of CAPEV3	>7.8 dB [87]	Baseline	7.1 (1.3)	6.5–7.7				
		OPT	7.2 (1.5)	6.5–80.0	0.2	1.147	0.296	0.052
		SVQ	7.4 (1.7)	6.6–8.1	0.3	0.995	0.331	0.050
		SVQ variant	7.4 (1.8)	6.6–8.3	0.4	1.563	0.224	0.064
		NP	7.7 (1.7)	6.9–8.5	0.6	50.098	0.034 *	0.188
CPPS of CAPEV3	NA	Baseline	10.6 (1.6)	9.9–11.4				
		OPT	11.2 (2.4)	10.2–12.3	0.6	1.752	0.200	0.077
		SVQ	11.6 (2.1)	10.6–12.6	10.0	6.208	0.022 *	0.237
		SVQ variant	120.0 (20.0)	11.1–12.9	1.4	10.587	0.003 *	0.315
		NP	12.1 (1.8)	11.3–12.9	1.5	17.629	0.001 *	0.445

Table 7. Cont.

Measure	Normative Cut-Off	Time Point	Mean (SD)	95% CI	MD	F	p	Partial η²
CPP RP23	6.6 dB [87]	Baseline	5.6 (0.9)	5.1–60.0				
		OPT	5.5 (0.8)	5.1–5.9	0.1	1.126	0.292	0.017
		SVQ	5.8 (1.1)	5.3–6.4	0.2	0.806	0.375	0.019
		SVQ variant	5.9 (10.0)	5.3–6.4	0.3	50.009	0.032 *	0.135
		NP	60.0 (10.0)	5.5–6.5	0.4	3.577	0.071	0.135
CSID of CAPEV3	NA	Baseline	−130.0 (15.5)	(−20.2)–(−5.7)				
		OPT	−7.3 (17.3)	−15.4–0.9	5.7	50.096	0.035 *	0.195
		SVQ	−9.1 (14.6)	(−15.9)–(−2.2)	3.9	1.490	0.237	0.073
		SVQ variant	−8.7 (16.2)	(−16.2)–(−1.1)	4.3	2.416	0.134	0.095
		NP	−11.5 (16.4)	(−19.2)–(−3.8)	1.5	1.157	0.294	0.050
CSID of RP23	<24.27 [57]	Baseline	12.5 (12.3)	6.9–18.1				
		OPT	15.3 (13.9)	90.0–21.7	2.8	1.339	0.260	0.057
		SVQ	11.2 (14.7)	4.6–17.9	1.3	0.247	0.624	0.012
		SVQ variant	9.8 (14.4)	3.3–16.4	2.7	1.382	0.252	0.057
		NP	8.9 (13.5)	2.7–150.0	3.7	4.396	0.047 *	0.160

Other acoustic measures did not show significant changes after the treatment techniques as compared with baseline. The effect sizes for acoustic measures with non-significant fixed effects of treatment are shown in Table A4 in Appendix C.

3.4. Impact of Service Delivery Factors on the Treatment Outcome

3.4.1. Number of Sessions and Duration of Sob Voice Therapy

Bivariate correlation coefficients were calculated to examine the relationship between the treatment dose and the differences in the outcome measure values for each technique. For example, for OPT, the differences between baseline and post-OPT data were calculated, which were then used to calculate the correlation with the number of sessions and treatment duration. For OPT, there was no significant correlation between the number of therapy sessions, duration of voice therapy (weeks), and any of the pre/post differences in the auditory–perceptual and acoustic measures ($p > 0.05$). For SVQ and SVQ variants, there was no significant correlation between the number of sessions, duration of voice therapy, and the pre/post differences in the auditory–perceptual and acoustic outcome measures ($p > 0.05$). For NP, there were correlations between the number of sessions and the pre/post differences in both the roughness ratings ($r = -0.49$, $p = 0.024$) and strain ratings ($r = -0.49$, $p = 0.024$). After Bonferroni's adjustment for multiple correlation calculations, a significant p value would be 0.0035. Therefore, these were deemed not statistically significant.

3.4.2. Clinician Effects

Due to the involvement of six SLPs in the treatment process across patients, the effects of the treating clinicians were examined using a factorial two-way ANOVA test [clinician × treatment] with repeated measures on 'treatment' (baseline, OPT, SVQ, SVQ variants, and NP). Main effects were calculated for the 'clinician × treatment' interaction. The results showed that there were no significant interaction effects between clinicians and the treatment for all perceptual and acoustic variables ($p > 0.05$). This suggested that all clinicians contributed the same amount of variance in the treatment outcome over time.

3.5. Drop-Out Rate

Ten out of 68 (14.7%) did not attend further therapy following their second appointment. Twelve participants (17.6%) did not attend further sessions after their third appointment. Eleven participants (16.2%) did not return to therapy following their fourth session.

4. Discussion

Voice therapy is a major therapeutic intervention that can be delivered as a stand-alone treatment or in combination with medical and/or surgical treatment. Early and effective voice therapy outcomes can prevent more complicated pathologies within the larynx that require costly treatment regimes. The purpose of this study was to retrospectively review clinical data from an SLP voice database to investigate the clinical outcomes of four components of a standardised voice therapy program (Sob Voice Therapy) and to provide preliminary data on the effects of its 'active ingredients'. Statistical analyses involved the use of a linear mixed model, which allowed for the robust estimation of the treatment effects, given that patients were treated as random effects [88]. Patient factors such as history of comorbidities, voice use, and previous training were therefore considered random and were not specifically analysed. Treatment outcomes were evaluated using CAPE-V auditory–perceptual analysis, which is the "gold standard" of voice evaluation, and acoustic analysis including spectral-based measures (CPP/CPPS and CSID), which is an objective, non-invasive, and reliable evaluation with great sensitivity and specificity to voice changes [57,69,89]. These were believed to accurately reflect the treatment effects of the Sob Voice Therapy. Treatment sessions and timeframes were comparable to averages reported in the literature [13].

4.1. Treatment Effects of Sob Voice Therapy on Patients with MTVD

The first aim in the present study was to evaluate the treatment effects of SVT on MTVD. The study population consisted of typical treatment-seeking patients with primary MTVD (without obvious vocal fold mucosal lesions) or secondary MTVD (with mild mucosal changes deemed related to vocal hyperfunction, such as pre-nodules swellings and mucosal thickening) as these are the most common voice disorder types, representing approximately 40% of the case load in voice clinics [90]. The findings showed significant treatment effects in all auditory–perceptual measures for the whole treatment when compared to pre-treatment levels. There was a significant positive effect of SVT as measured by the decreased auditory–perceptual ratings of overall severity, roughness, breathiness, and strain between baseline and NP. Significant effects of treatment were also observed for acoustic measures such as HNR (vowel), CPP (CAPEV3 and Rainbow Passage), CPPS (CAPEV3), and CSID (Rainbow Passage). Notably, the HNR (vowel) value post-treatment is likely to have been judged perceptually clear compared to being not clear prior to treatment, based on [61]. However, no significant changes were found for F0, F0SD, and intensity ($p > 0.05$). These suggested that this voice therapy program was more effective in improving voice quality than in modifying pitch and loudness. The non-significant effects on F0SD also stemmed from the findings that the values of this measure were within normal ranges for both genders (Table 5).

For both auditory–perceptual and acoustic measures, the treatment effects did not depend upon the MTVD type, whether being primary or secondary. The significant effects of diagnosis observed for the auditory–perceptual ratings of breathiness and strain accurately reflected the MTVD type, with primary MTVD showing lower rating scores than secondary MTVD. This is expected with persistent associated laryngeal pathology that may affect voice quality.

Baseline values across outcome measures were indicative of predominantly mild MTVD in the cohort. For example, the mean auditory–perceptual rating score ranged from 18.7 for strain to 26.8 for overall severity (Table 6). Mean acoustic measure values were only marginally below cut-off values for voice disorder for CPP, while CSID values at baseline were within normative ranges (Table 7). The effects of the SVT on patients with more severe MTVD and on patients with predominantly mucosal lesions remain unclear and would need future studies to investigate if the same therapy components are 'active ingredients' in this cohort; signal typing as an outcome measure would be recommended in that case. Home practise dosage and frequency data was not collected, which precluded the analysis of home practise as an active ingredient. This study also lacked long-term follow-up, which impacts on the inference of the maintenance/sustainability of the outcome for this voice disorder. This study did not directly measure specific muscle-tension parameters or provide patient-reported outcome measures as outcome data, and not all participants were diagnosed by examination using videostrobolaryngoscopy. Prospective designs would address these issues.

4.2. Active Ingredients of the Sob Voice Therapy Program

Each technique within the SVT has a specific role. In OPT and SVQ, patients practised different techniques that targeted at a clear and effortless voice. In the SVQ variants and NP, patients practise specific exercises for generalising a clear and effortless voice to connected speech with intonation variation. We hypothesised that treatment effects in habitual voice quality would be observed after the SVQ variants and NP were introduced, that is, after the patient had practised exercises designed to facilitate generalisation of improved vocal function to habitual, connected speech contexts. The findings revealed that the SVQ, SVQ variants, and NP were the most active ingredients with small to medium effect sizes across the auditory–perceptual and acoustic measures of voice quality.

4.2.1. Effects of OPT

As hypothesized, the findings showed that OPT was not a statistically significantly active ingredient to change voice quality in the habitual phonation of the cohort, despite resulting in improved voice outcome measures after this component was introduced. Auditory–perceptual outcome measures (Table 6) and acoustic measures, except the CSID of CAPEV3 (Table 7), demonstrated that the effects of OPT were not significant. The data on OPT may be explained by a range of factors. Firstly, the task is taught at the end of the initial assessment session with the purpose of raising perceptual awareness to the auditory–perceptual and kinaesthetic features of the voice, as well as providing cues to prime improved laryngeal function. The sound produced, however, is brief (less than 2 s as modelled) and may not be sufficient for the generalisation of improved vocal function in habitual connected speech. As it is described, it is the 'sound we make when we say yes', ergo, it is cueing a habitual phonatory task, while cueing only subtle muscular or physiological improvements in phonation. The use of features that prime improved vocal function, including a semi-occluded vocal tract [29], voice onset at resting expiratory level [91], and cueing for a clear and effortless voice [19], may not be sufficient in this technique as gross changes in voice quality and increased activation of muscles not usually activated in habitual phonation (e.g., low larynx and cricothyroid activation) are not cued. These features are, however, repeated in SVQ in which increased muscle activation and re-posturing of the larynx is also cued.

The finding of improved voice quality measures after OPT (/m/) and SVQ (/ŋ/) were taught and practised as single sounds was unexpected, as these tasks are individual sounds designed to assist the patient to re-posture the larynx for more optimal phonation, which is acquired (or re-acquired) as a new voice motor skill. They were not trained in connected speech and were not habitual speech task targets, and as such were not expected to generalise to habitual speaking after having just acquired the task (and met the target in a single sound). Consideration of these two techniques as active ingredients is therefore warranted. It is important to note that the effect size was calculated with $n = 24$, a rather small sample size. Significant findings in the CSID of the CAPEV3 phrase may be due to the increased sensitivity of CSID as a measure of voice quality. Therefore, the findings on OPT need further investigation in future studies.

4.2.2. Effects of SVQ

The significant effect of SVQ (as measured in auditory-perceptual ratings and the CPPS of CAPEV3) on the habitual speaking voice of patients after practising the SVQ in isolation was not predicted, given that the task itself was to acquire (not immediately generalise) the desired laryngeal adjustments of the technique and practise in preparation for the next exercise, which was task variation using SVQ. The improved voice quality in habitual speech was observed after the practising of an isolated sound suggests that the postural adjustments cued by the SVQ are possibly primary muscular movements of optimal phonation that could be considered active ingredients in themselves. Alternatively, the likely increased activation of both muscular and neural systems may also be implicated.

SVQ requires the production of a clear, quiet, and effortless 'ng' sound, descending as if imitating a puppy whimper, to refine control of the optimal posture for phonation [30]. First described as 'light' registration by Vennard [92] and defined as "Falsetto break, expressive of grief" (p. 251) and "whine: Prolonged nasal or twangy sound, usually light in production, on descending portamento, expressing pain or disappointment" (p. 251), SVQ has subsequently been investigated as a voice quality mode named 'cry', compared to three other voice quality modes (speech, twang, and opera) [93]. Biomechanical and postural features observed in cry include low larynx position, increased space between the hyoid and thyroid, pharyngeal/supraglottic widening, increased aryepiglottic space, elongation of vocal folds, arytenoids not being tightly adducted, gentle and brief vocal fold closure, and possible increased activity of the cricothyroid and posterior crico-arytenoid [93]. Nearly all of these muscular parameters have been implicated in MTVD, including a raised larynx position, narrow supraglottic region, hyperadduction of the true vocal folds [94], and decreased hyoid/thyroid 'visor' [95].

This physiological description of SVQ suggests that all three biomechanical dimensions of the larynx are manipulated concurrently (medio-laterally, anterio-posteriorly, and inferior-superior) to correct the common biomechanical features of MTVD, with the added element of possibly activating the secondary neurological vocal pathway responsible for emotional vocalisation, as described by Simonyan [96]. Auditory–perceptual and kinaesthetic training is provided and encouraged in practice to link perception and production links in the vocal system [97,98]. More efficient learning and re-organisation of motor movements has been demonstrated in other domains to require maximal tolerable task complexity [99,100] and ability to recognise the target so that an internal reference of correctness is established for effective practice [41]. SVQ is a complex muscular task, the sound of which does not resemble habitual phonation (often a criticism of patients) but is perceptually recognizable and distinct from habitual phonation. This may promote increased recognition of the target (clear and effortless voicing) more readily than voicing in habitual conversation speech, in which the suboptimal phonation automatically occurs, assisting in generalisation.

4.2.3. Effects of SVQ Task Variation

Task variation of carrier phrases and sirening in SVQ was used in this treatment to generalise the features of clear voice quality and the perceptions of effortless phonation to contexts other than /ŋ/. Results confirmed, as hypothesised, that task variation was effective in improving habitual voice quality across auditory–perceptual and acoustic analysis outcome measures. This was hypothesised based on a large body of previous research in voice therapy and motor learning, as task variation is considered essential in the learning, generalisation, and maintenance of all motor skills [101,102], despite the use of SVQ in the task. Task variation using connected speech tasks such as phrases and conversational speech is common across voice therapy approaches [25]. The explicit vocal target, use of connected speech contexts with a communicative intent, and practise regimes of SVQ are similar to other voice therapies, e.g., CTT (clear speech), but the physiological mechanism by which it is achieved is extremely different. This suggests that the mechanism of action [18] as a concept could be expanded to include the physiological description of movement as well as the acquisition and learning processes.

4.2.4. Effects of Negative Practice

The NP component of SVT was highly effective across outcome measures based on results from both the mixed model and the ANOVA analysis of effect size. This was observed in auditory–perceptual outcomes in patients with primary and secondary MTVD, and across the whole cohort in acoustic measures. Negative practice (also called old way/new way) is thought to be a form of proactive interference that promotes forgetting of the old movement [103] and is commonly used in SLP and voice therapy [25,104,105]. The plateau in outcome from SVQ variants and NP may be explained by the function of NP to maintain the improvements resulting from SVQ variants, which may have resulted in a reduction in performance in the short term in some cases. As NP reintroduces the 'old' pre-treatment movement pattern, it is also possible that the performance parameters of the 'new way' are temporarily shifted until a clear differentiation between the generalised motor program for the two voice modes are well established. It is therefore conceivable that one session of NP with subsequent practise may have temporarily destabilised consistent access to the improved technique, resulting in temporary reduction in voice quality. As NP is designed to assist with generalisation and maintenance of a newly acquired skill and to extinguish access to the old suboptimal movement, an improvement in voice quality may not occur but rather a stabilisation of improvement may be more likely, as was observed in this study. Analysis of subsequent sessions is required to evaluate if habitual voice quality returned to post-SVQ levels and was retained in the long term.

4.3. Effect of Diagnosis and Service Delivery

Diagnosis of primary or secondary MTVD had a significant effect on auditory–perceptual voice ratings of strain only and was consistent over the four stages of the treatment. The clinical population in this study was typical of other MTVD cohorts reported in the literature, with retention rates also similar to other studies in which therapy was provided at no charge. There is significant evidence across RCTs and clinical studies that the retention of clients in voice therapy is generally poor [106]. Although the consequence of this is undocumented, high attrition runs the risk of ineffective treatment outcomes if the session dosage for the therapeutic effect is insufficient. In this study, positive therapeutic effects were observed across multiple voice outcomes within one to two sessions of 60-min durations with minimum durations of 1–2 weeks. If positive effects can be measured and demonstrated to patients within these short time frames, it is hoped that this would reduce attrition and increase compliance with further therapy recommendations.

Researchers have speculated that clinicians can have a therapeutic effect independent of the treatment type [107]. This is the first study to evaluate whether therapy delivered by multiple clinicians has a significant effect on voice outcomes. In this study, neither clinician, length of time, nor number of sessions had a significant effect on efficacy. This suggests that the active ingredients and overall efficacy of SVT are independent of the clinician, number of sessions, and length of treatment.

4.4. Comparison with Other Voice Therapy Outcomes Research

Comparison of effects found in this study with other treatments for patients with MTVD are difficult to make given the large range of outcome measures and different statistical analyses used across studies [11]. Numerous RCTs and prospective studies report a reduction in auditory–perceptual rating scores and improved acoustic analysis measures of voice quality including HNR, CPP, and CSID. Two retrospective cohort studies were found investigating the efficacy of VFE on patients with age-related dysphonia [108,109], only one of which documented the therapeutic outcome on voice quality auditory–perceptual and acoustic measures [109]. Small to medium effect sizes using Hedge's 'h' were reported across a number of prospective and retrospective studies for improvements in voice quality outcome measures (shimmer and jitter only) after therapy, utilising VFE in patients with voice disorders [110]. Only one voice therapy treatment study reported using a mixed-model statistical analysis to measure voice outcomes across multiple time points in a prospective study of CTT with patients with mild MTVD who were stimulable for CTT [106]. This study reported significant effects of 4 weekly sessions, conducted no more than 10 days apart, using CTT. Five outcome measures were comparable with our study, including auditory–perceptual ratings using the CAPE-V, mean F0, CPP and CSID of a prolonged vowel, and CSID on the third CAPE-V phrase (amongst other outcome measures). Increases in mean F0 and reductions in CAPE-V ratings of the six CAPE-V phrases were reported. Effect sizes for significant effects were not reported, however. Baseline measures of the cohort in the CTT study were similar for mean F0 and the CPP vowel; however the CSID of the vowel and the third CAPE-V phrase were lower in our study. Significant improvements in habitual phonation as measured by acoustic voice analyses (CPP and CSID) were measured during and 1 week after the CTT therapy, but was not retained at 3 months. While the average number of sessions, average time between sessions, and practise recommendations were similar between the two studies, the retrospective nature of our study and the use of multiple clinicians meant that there was less control of the treatment variables, as it occurs in real-life clinical contexts.

We used both CPP (measured from ADSV) and CPPS (measured from Praat) to ensure that researchers can compare their data with the present study depending upon which software is available to them. Although ADSV is a commercial specialized software for clinical application, it is not accessible/available to many users, especially the non-clinicians, while Praat is a freeware. The discrepancy between the CPP and CPPS results for the CAPEV3 task (Table 7) probably resulted from the slight differences in the algorithms between these two programs rather than from the effects of the data distribution. CPPS showed more significant effects of treatment as the smoothing is believed to improve the cepstral estimation accuracy [73]; therefore, it would be more likely to detect finer changes in the voices given the mild dysphonic severity of the study cohort.

5. Conclusions

SVT was effective in reducing the signs and symptoms of mild MTVD in a typical treatment-seeking cohort, as measured by auditory–perceptual and acoustic voice outcomes. Three out of four individual components of the therapy program demonstrated statistically significant positive therapeutic effects, independent of the session number, duration of therapy, and clinician. This provides preliminary evidence that the SVQ technique and both the SVQ task variation and NP can be considered as active ingredients in the treatment of patients with MTVD.

Author Contributions: Conceptualisation, C.M.; methodology, C.M. and D.D.N.; formal analysis, D.D.N.; investigation, C.M.; data curation, A.C. and E.K.; writing—original draft preparation, C.M. and D.D.N.; writing—review and editing, C.M., D.D.N., A.C., E.K. and D.N.; project administration, C.M.; visualisation, D.N.; funding acquisition, C.M. and D.N. All authors have read and agreed to the published version of the manuscript.

Funding: This research was funded by the Dr. Liang Voice Program at the University of Sydney.

Institutional Review Board Statement: The study was conducted according to the guidelines of the Declaration of Helsinki and was approved by the Human Research Ethics Committee of the University of Sydney, protocol number: 2019/529.

Informed Consent Statement: Patient consent was waived due to it being impractical to seek consent for patients seen in the past and it was considered a threat to patient privacy to implement a process to locate and contact each individual participant to seek their consent. This waiver was approved by the Human Research Ethics Committee and the approval is provided above.

Data Availability Statement: Data supporting the reported results are retained by the University of Sydney in a deidentified form and is confidential under the conditions of the Human Research Ethics Committee of the University of Sydney approval.

Conflicts of Interest: The first author, C.M., is the director and sole shareholder of Voicecraft International Pty Ltd., the legal entity retaining ownership of the intellectual property of Voicecraft®. C.M., D.D.N., D.N., A.C. and E.K. are employees of the University of Sydney and are partly or fully funded by the Dr. Liang Voice Program, a philanthropically funded program of research and post-graduate education in laryngology. The funders had no role in the design of the study; in the collection, analyses, or interpretation of data; in the writing of the manuscript, or in the decision to publish the results.

Abbreviations

MD, mean difference; CAPEV3, the third CAPEV phrase; RP, Rainbow Passage; RP23, second and third sentences of the Rainbow Passage; CPP, cepstral peak prominence; CPPS, cepstral peak prominence smoothed; and CSID, Cepstral/Spectral Index of Dysphonia.

Appendix A. Settings for Acoustic Measurements

Appendix A.1. Settings for the Fundamental Frequency Measurement in Praat

F0 range = 75–500 Hz, cross-correlation method, maximum number of candidates = 15, silence threshold = 0.03, voicing threshold = 0.45, octave cost = 0.01, octave-jump cost = 0.35, and voice/unvoiced cost = 0.14. The check box of "very accurate" was checked.

Appendix A.2. Settings for the CPP Measurement in the Analysis of Dysphonia in Speech and Voice (ADSV)

Resampling rate = 25 kHz, spectral window size (pts) = 1024, maximum frequency for regression line calculation = 10,000, frame overlap = 75%, cepstral time-averaging (frames) = 7, CPP threshold (dB) = 0, and cepstral peak extraction range minimum–maximum = 60–300 Hz. Low/high spectral ratio cut-off = 4000 Hz.

Appendix A.3. Settings for the CPPS Measurement in Praat

Pitch floor (Hz) = 60, time steps (s) = 0.002, maximum frequency (Hz) = 5000, pre-emphasis from (Hz) = 50, time-averaging window (s) = 0.01, quefrency-averaging window (s) = 0.001, peak search pitch range (Hz) = 60–330, tolerance (0–1) = 0.05, interpolation = parabolic, subtract tilt before smoothing = no, tilt line quefrency range (s) = 0.001–0.0 (=end), line type = straight, and fit method = robust.

Appendix B

Table A1. Vocal load (missing data: $n = 6$).

Vocal Load	Frequency	Percent
Below 2 h	4	6.5
2–4 h	9	14.5
4–6 h	16	25.8
Above 6 h	33	53.2
Total	62	100.0

Table A2. History of voice-related comorbidities.

Comorbidities		Frequency	Percent
Reflux	No	37	54.4
	Yes	31	45.6
Sinusitis	No	52	76.5
	Yes	16	23.5
Asthma	No	57	83.8
	Yes	11	16.2
Cough	No	33	48.5
	Yes	35	51.5
Stress (missing data $n = 4$)	No	22	34.4
	Yes	42	65.6

Table A3. Lifestyle information.

Factors		Frequency	Percent
Caffein (missing data $n = 2$)	No	7	10.6
	Yes	59	89.4
Alcohol (missing data $n = 1$)	No	14	20.9
	Yes	53	79.1
Smoking (missing data $n = 1$)	No	65	97.0
	Yes	2	3.0

Appendix C

Table A4. Changes in the acoustic outcomes before and after the four stages of Sob Voice Therapy. Partial $\eta^2 = 0.01, 0.1,$ and 0.25 indicate small, medium, and large effects, respectively.

Measure	Normative Cut-Off	Time Point	Mean (SD)	95% CI	MD	F	p	Partial η^2
CPP vowel	11.74 dB [87]	Baseline	11.4 (2.6)	10.0–12.7				
		OPT	9.7 (2.6)	8.4–11.1	1.7	0.722	0.399	0.011
		SVQ	10.3 (2.3)	9.0–11.5	1.1	0.096	0.759	0.002
		SVQ variant	10.4 (2.1)	9.2–11.4	1.0	0.514	0.479	0.017
		Post NP	10.9 (2.1)	9.7–12.0	0.5	0.599	0.448	0.029
CPPS vowel	14.45 dB [111]	Baseline	14.5 (3.2)	12.8–16.1				
		OPT	13.3 (3.9)	11.4–15.3	1.2	0.658	0.420	0.010
		SVQ	13.4 (2.6)	12.1–14.7	1.1	1.215	0.277	0.029
		SVQ variant	13.6 (1.8)	12.6–14.5	0.9	0.197	0.661	0.007
		NP	13.7 (1.8)	12.8–14.6	0.8	1.054	0.317	0.050
CPPS RP23	9.33 dB [111]	Baseline	8.4 (1.0)	7.9–8.9				
		OPT	8.4 (1.0)	8.0–8.9	0.0	0.497	0.483	0.007
		SVQ	8.7 (1.3)	8.1–9.3	0.3	0.647	0.426	0.015
		SVQ variant	8.6 (1.1)	7.7–8.8	0.2	2.622	0.115	0.076
		NP	8.8 (1.2)	8.2–9.4	0.4	3.108	0.091	0.119
CSID vowel	NA	Baseline	3.8 (16.6)	−5.1–12.6				
		OPT	12.7 (17.3)	3.5–22.0	8.9	0.287	0.594	0.004
		SVQ	6.1 (11.5)	0.0–12.2	2.3	0.094	0.760	0.002
		SVQ variant	6.2 (12.8)	−0.6–13.0	2.4	0.935	0.341	0.030
		NP	3.4 (11.1)	−2.6–9.3	0.4	0.001	0.973	0.000

Table A4. *Cont.*

Measure	Normative Cut-Off	Time Point	Mean (SD)	95% CI	MD	F	p	Partial η²
Intensity vowel	73.42 dB [76]	Baseline	57.0 (7.0)	53.4–60.6				
		OPT	56.4 (7.5)	52.6–60.3	0.6	1.147	0.288	0.018
		SVQ	57.9 (6.4)	54.6–61.2	0.9	0.253	0.618	0.006
		SVQ variant	58.0 (6.4)	54.7–61.3	1.0	0.118	0.734	0.004
		NP	56.8 (6.9)	53.3–60.4	0.2	0.055	0.817	0.003
Intensity CAPEV3	NA	Baseline	56.6 (5.3)	53.9–59.2				
		OPT	57.0 (6.8)	53.6–60.4	0.4	0.474	0.494	0.007
		SVQ	56.8 (6.0)	53.8–59.8	0.2	0.837	0.366	0.020
		SVQ variant	56.8 (5.6)	54.1–59.6	0.2	0.034	0.854	0.001
		NP	54.9 (6.3)	51.8–58.0	1.7	1.155	0.294	0.050
Intensity of RP	68.37 dB [112]	Baseline	47.9 (6.7)	44.7–51.1				
		OPT	49.3 (6.0)	46.4–52.2	1.4	0.369	0.545	0.006
		SVQ	49.5 (5.4)	46.9–52.1	1.6	0.035	0.852	0.001
		SVQ variant	49.0 (6.5)	45.9–52.1	1.1	0.036	0.851	0.001
		NP	47.8 (7.8)	44.0–51.6	0.1	0.006	0.938	0.000

References

1. Baker, J.; Ben-Tovim, D.I.; Butcher, A.; Esterman, A.; McLaughlin, K. Development of a modified diagnostic classification system for voice disorders with inter-rater reliability study. *Logop. Phoniatr. Vocol.* **2007**, *32*, 99–112. [CrossRef]
2. Oates, J.; Winkworth, A. Current knowledge, controversies and future directions in hyperfunctional voice disorders. *Int. J. Speech-Lang. Pathol.* **2008**, *10*, 267–277. [CrossRef]
3. Dabirmoghaddam, P.; Rahmaty, B.; Erfanian, R.; Taherkhani, S.; Msc, S.H.; Satariyan, A. Voice Component Relationships with High Reflux Symptom Index Scores in Muscle Tension Dysphonia. *Laryngoscope* **2021**, *131*. [CrossRef]
4. Martins, R.H.G.; Amaral, H.A.D.; Tavares, E.L.M.; Martins, M.G.; Gonçalves, T.M.; Dias, N.H. Voice Disorders: Etiology and Diagnosis. *J. Voice* **2016**, *30*, 761.e1–761.e9. [CrossRef] [PubMed]
5. Van Houtte, E.; Van Lierde, K.; Claeys, S. Pathophysiology and Treatment of Muscle Tension Dysphonia: A Review of the Current Knowledge. *J. Voice* **2011**, *25*, 202–207. [CrossRef]
6. Nanjundeswaran, C.; Li-Jessen, N.; Chan, K.M.; Wong, K.S.R.; Yiu, E.M.-L.; Verdolini-Abbott, K. Preliminary Data on Prevention and Treatment of Voice Problems in Student Teachers. *J. Voice* **2012**, *26*, 816.e1–816.e12. [CrossRef] [PubMed]
7. Mathieson, L. *The Voice and Its Disorders*, 6th ed.; Whurr Publishers: London, UK, 2001.
8. Carding, P. *Evaluating Voice Therapy. Measuring the Effectiveness of Treatment*; Whurr Publishers: London, UK, 2000.
9. Chan, A.K.; McCabe, P.; Madill, C. The implementation of evidence-based practice in the management of adults with functional voice disorders: A national survey of speech-language pathologists. *Int. J. Speech-Lang. Pathol.* **2013**, *15*, 334–344. [CrossRef]
10. Signorelli, M.E.; Madill, C.; McCabe, P. The management of vocal fold nodules in children: A national survey of speech-language pathologists. *Int. J. Speech-Lang. Pathol.* **2011**, *13*, 227–238. [CrossRef]
11. Eastwood, C.; Madill, C.; Mccabe, P. The behavioural treatment of muscle tension voice disorders: A systematic review. *Int. J. Speech-Lang. Pathol.* **2015**, *17*, 287–303. [CrossRef]
12. Gartner-Schmidt, J.L.; Roth, D.F.; Zullo, T.G.; Rosen, C.A. Quantifying Component Parts of Indirect and Direct Voice Therapy Related to Different Voice Disorders. *J. Voice* **2013**, *27*, 210–216. [CrossRef] [PubMed]
13. De Bodt, M.; Patteeuw, T.; Versele, A. Temporal Variables in Voice Therapy. *J. Voice* **2015**, *29*, 611–617. [CrossRef] [PubMed]
14. Zanca, J.M.; Turkstra, L.S.; Chen, C.; Packel, A.; Ferraro, M.; Hart, T.; Van Stan, J.H.; Whyte, J.; Dijkers, M.P. Advancing Rehabilitation Practice Through Improved Specification of Interventions. *Arch. Phys. Med. Rehabil.* **2019**, *100*, 164–171. [CrossRef] [PubMed]
15. Roy, N. Optimal dose–response relationships in voice therapy. *Int. J. Speech-Lang. Pathol.* **2012**, *14*, 419–423. [CrossRef]
16. Baker, E. Optimal intervention intensity in speech-language pathology: Discoveries, challenges, and unchartered territories. *Int. J. Speech-Lang. Pathol.* **2012**, *14*, 478–485. [CrossRef] [PubMed]
17. Turkstra, L.S.; Norman, R.; Whyte, J.; Dijkers, M.P.; Hart, T. Knowing What We're Doing: Why Specification of Treatment Methods Is Critical for Evidence-Based Practice in Speech-Language Pathology. *Am. J. Speech-Lang. Pathol.* **2016**, *25*, 164–171. [CrossRef]
18. Van Stan, J.H.; Whyte, J.; Duffy, J.R.; Barkmeier-Kraemer, J.M.; Doyle, P.B.; Gherson, S.; Kelchner, L.; Muise, J.; Petty, B.; Roy, N.; et al. Rehabilitation Treatment Specification System: Methodology to Identify and Describe Unique Targets and Ingredients. *Arch. Phys. Med. Rehabil.* **2021**, *102*, 521–531. [CrossRef]
19. Van Stan, J.H.; Roy, N.; Awan, S.; Stemple, J.; Hillman, R.E. A taxonomy of voice therapy. *Am. J. Speech-Lang. Pathol.* **2015**, *24*, 101–125. [CrossRef]
20. Verdolini-Abbott, K. *Lessac-Madsen Resonant Voice Therapy Clinician Manual*; Plural Publishing: San Diego, CA, USA, 2008.

21. Nguyen, D.D.; Kenny, D.T. Randomized controlled trial of vocal function exercises on muscle tension dysphonia in Vietnamese female teachers. *J. Otolaryngol. Head Neck Surg.* **2009**, *38*, 261–278. [PubMed]
22. Stone, R.E.; Casteel, R.I. Restoration of voice in nonorganically based dysphonia. In *Phonatory Voice Disorders in Children*; Filter, M., Ed.; Charles C Thomas: Springfield, IL, USA, 1982.
23. Bassiouny, S. Efficacy of the accent method of voice therapy. *Folia Phoniatr. Logop.* **1998**, *50*, 146–164. [CrossRef] [PubMed]
24. Fex, B.; Fex, S.; Shiromoto, O.; Hirano, M. Acoustic analysis of functional dysphonia: Before and after voice therapy (accent method). *J. Voice* **1994**, *8*, 163–167. [CrossRef]
25. Iwarsson, J. Facilitating behavioral learning and habit change in voice therapy—Theoretic premises and practical strategies. *Logop. Phoniatr. Vocol.* **2015**, *40*, 179–186. [CrossRef]
26. S.L. Hunter Speechworks. Resonant Voice Therapy. 2008. Available online: https://www.slhunterspeechworks.com/Therapy-Services/Voice-Therapy/Resonant-Voice-Therapy (accessed on 12 August 2021).
27. Watts, C.R.; Diviney, S.S.; Hamilton, A.; Toles, L.; Childs, L.; Mau, T. The Effect of Stretch-and-Flow Voice Therapy on Measures of Vocal Function and Handicap. *J. Voice* **2015**, *29*, 191–199. [CrossRef]
28. Bane, M.; Angadi, V.; Dressler, E.; Andreatta, R.; Stemple, J. Vocal function exercises for normal voice: The effects of varying dosage. *Int. J. Speech-Lang. Pathol.* **2019**, *21*, 37–45. [CrossRef]
29. Bane, M.; Brown, M.; Angadi, V.; Croake, D.J.; Andreatta, R.D.; Stemple, J.C. Vocal function exercises for normal voice: With and without semi-occlusion. *Int. J. Speech-Lang. Pathol.* **2019**, *21*, 175–181. [CrossRef] [PubMed]
30. Madill, C.; Bagnall, A.D.; Beatty, J. *Voicecraft Essentials Workshop Manual*; Voicecraft International: Adelaide, SA, Australia, 2015.
31. Bagnall, A.D. *Voicecraft Workshop Manual*; Voicecraft International: Adelaide, SA, Australia, 1997.
32. Madill, C.; Sheard, C.; Heard, R. Differentiated Vocal Tract Control and the Reliability of Interpretations of Nasendoscopic Assessment. *J. Voice* **2010**, *24*, 337–345. [CrossRef] [PubMed]
33. Bagnall, A.D.; McCulloch, K. The Impact of Specific Exertion on the Efficiency and Ease of the Voice: A Pilot Study. *J. Voice* **2005**, *19*, 384–390. [CrossRef] [PubMed]
34. Kelso, J.A.S.; Schöner, G. Self-organization of coordinative movement patterns. *Hum. Mov. Sci.* **1988**, *7*, 27–46. [CrossRef]
35. Winkworth, A.L.; Davis, P.J.; Adams, R.D.; Ellis, E. Breathing Patterns During Spontaneous Speech. *J. Speech Lang. Hear. Res.* **1995**, *38*, 124–144. [CrossRef]
36. Winkworth, A.L.; Davis, P.J.; Ellis, E.; Adams, R.D. Variability and Consistency in Speech Breathing During Reading. *J. Speech Lang. Hear. Res.* **1994**, *37*, 535–556. [CrossRef]
37. Sprecher, A.; Olszewski, A.; Jiang, J.J.; Zhang, Y. Updating signal typing in voice: Addition of type 4 signals. *J. Acoust. Soc. Am.* **2010**, *127*, 3710–3716. [CrossRef]
38. GLIMMPSE. General Linear Mixed Model Power and Sample Size. Available online: https://glimmpse.samplesizeshop.org/ (accessed on 2 January 2021).
39. Guo, Y.; Logan, H.L.; Glueck, D.H.; Muller, K.E. Selecting a sample size for studies with repeated measures. *BMC Med. Res. Methodol.* **2013**, *13*, 493–498. [CrossRef]
40. Wenke, R.; Coman, L.; Walton, C.; Madill, C.; Theodoros, D.; Bishop, C.; Stabler, P.; Lawrie, M.; O'Neill, J.; Gray, H.; et al. Effectiveness of Intensive Voice Therapy Versus Weekly Therapy for Muscle Tension Dysphonia: A Noninferiority Randomised Controlled Trial with Nested Focus Group. *J. Voice* **2021**. [CrossRef] [PubMed]
41. Maas, E.; Robin, D.A.; Hula, S.N.A.; Freedman, S.E.; Wulf, G.; Ballard, K.; Schmidt, R.A. Principles of Motor Learning in Treatment of Motor Speech Disorders. *Am. J. Speech-Lang. Pathol.* **2008**, *17*, 277–298. [CrossRef]
42. Sataloff, R.T. *Professional Voice: The Science and Art of Clinical Care*; Plural Publishing: San Diego, CA, USA, 2017.
43. Rosen, C.A.; Lee, A.S.; Osborne, J.; Zullo, T.; Murry, T. Development and Validation of the Voice Handicap Index-10. *Laryngoscope* **2004**, *114*, 1549–1556. [CrossRef]
44. Belafsky, P.C.; Postma, G.N.; Koufman, J.A. Validity and Reliability of the Reflux Symptom Index (RSI). *J. Voice* **2002**, *16*, 274–277. [CrossRef]
45. Fairbanks, G. *Voice and Articulation Drillbook*, 2nd ed.; Harper & Row: New York, NY, USA, 1960.
46. Kempster, G.B.; Gerratt, B.R.; Verdolini-Abbott, K.; Barkmeier-Kraemer, J.; Hillman, R.E. Consensus Auditory-Perceptual Evaluation of Voice: Development of a Standardized Clinical Protocol. *Am. J. Speech-Lang. Pathol.* **2009**, *18*, 124–132. [CrossRef]
47. AKG Acoustics. C520. Available online: https://www.akg.com/Microphones/Headset%20Microphones/C520.html (accessed on 1 June 2018).
48. Roland Corp. Quad-Capture—USB 2.0. Audio Interface. Available online: https://www.roland.com/au/products/quad-capture/ (accessed on 7 March 2019).
49. Audacity Team. Audacity(R): Free Audio Editor and Recorder [Computer Application]. Available online: https://www.audacityteam.org/ (accessed on 16 March 2021).
50. Kreiman, J.; Gerratt, B.R.; Kempster, G.B.; Erman, A.; Berke, G.S. Perceptual Evaluation of Voice Quality. *J. Speech Lang. Hear. Res.* **1993**, *36*, 21–40. [CrossRef]
51. Boersma, P.; Weenink, D. Praat: Doing Phonetics by Computer. Available online: http://www.fon.hum.uva.nl/praat/ (accessed on 1 January 2018).
52. Madill, C.; So, T.; Corcoran, S. Bridge2practice: Translating Theory into Practice. Available online: https://bridge2practice.com/ (accessed on 7 March 2019).

53. IBM Corp. IBM SPSS Software. Available online: https://www.ibm.com/analytics/data-science/predictive-analytics/spss-statistical-software (accessed on 1 February 2018).
54. Shrout, P.E.; Fleiss, J.L. Intraclass correlations: Uses in assessing rater reliability. *Psychol. Bull.* **1979**, *86*, 420–428. [CrossRef] [PubMed]
55. Koo, T.K.; Li, M.Y. A Guideline of Selecting and Reporting Intraclass Correlation Coefficients for Reliability Research. *J. Chiropr. Med.* **2016**, *15*, 155–163. [CrossRef] [PubMed]
56. Pentax Medical. Analysis of Dysphonia in Speech and Voice—ADSV [Computer Application]. Available online: https://www.pentaxmedical.com/pentax/en/99/1/Analysis-of-Dysphonia-in-Speech-and-Voice-ADSV (accessed on 1 March 2018).
57. Awan, S.N.; Roy, N.; Zhang, D.; Cohen, S. Validation of the Cepstral Spectral Index of Dysphonia (CSID) as a Screening Tool for Voice Disorders: Development of Clinical Cutoff Scores. *J. Voice* **2016**, *30*, 130–144. [CrossRef]
58. Maryn, Y. Recording Quality: Speech-To-Noise Ratio and Voice-To-Noise Ratio. Available online: https://www.phonanium.com/product/recording-quality/ (accessed on 24 November 2020).
59. Deliyski, D.D.; Shaw, H.S.; Evans, M.K. Adverse Effects of Environmental Noise on Acoustic Voice Quality Measurements. *J. Voice* **2005**, *19*, 15–28. [CrossRef] [PubMed]
60. Yumoto, E.; Gould, W.J.; Baer, T. Harmonics-to-noise ratio as an index of the degree of hoarseness. *J. Acoust. Soc. Am.* **1982**, *71*, 1544–1550. [CrossRef]
61. Warhurst, S.; Madill, C.; McCabe, P.; Heard, R.; Yiu, E. The Vocal Clarity of Female Speech-Language Pathology Students: An Exploratory Study. *J. Voice* **2012**, *26*, 63–68. [CrossRef]
62. Desuter, G.; Dedry, M.; Schaar, B.; Van Lith-Bijl, J.; Van Benthem, P.P.; Sjögren, E.V. Voice outcome indicators for unilateral vocal fold paralysis surgery: A review of the literature. *Eur. Arch. Oto-Rhino-Laryngol.* **2018**, *275*, 459–468. [CrossRef] [PubMed]
63. Hassan, M.M.; Yumoto, E.; Kumai, Y.; Sanuki, T.; Kodama, N. Vocal outcome after arytenoid adduction and ansa cervicalis transfer. *Arch. Otolaryngol. Head Neck Surg.* **2012**, *138*, 60–65. [CrossRef]
64. Hollien, H. Vocal Fold Dynamics for Frequency Change. *J. Voice* **2014**, *28*, 395–405. [CrossRef]
65. McKenna, V.S.; Murray, E.S.H.; Lien, Y.-A.S.; Stepp, C.E. The Relationship Between Relative Fundamental Frequency and a Kinematic Estimate of Laryngeal Stiffness in Healthy Adults. *J. Speech Lang. Hear. Res.* **2016**, *59*, 1283–1294. [CrossRef] [PubMed]
66. Linville, S.E. Intraspeaker variability in fundamental frequency stability: An age-related phenomenon? *J. Acoust. Soc. Am.* **1988**, *83*, 741–745. [CrossRef] [PubMed]
67. Noll, A.M. Cepstrum pitch determination. *J. Acoust. Soc. Am.* **1967**, *41*, 293–309. [CrossRef]
68. Hillenbrand, J.; Cleveland, R.A.; Erickson, R.L. Acoustic Correlates of Breathy Vocal Quality. *J. Speech Lang. Hear. Res.* **1994**, *37*, 769–778. [CrossRef]
69. Maryn, Y.; Roy, N.; Bodt, M.; Cauwenberge, P.; Corthals, P. Acoustic measurement of overall voice quality: A meta-analysis. *J. Acoust. Soc. Am.* **2009**, *126*, 2619–2634. [CrossRef] [PubMed]
70. Awan, S.N.; Roy, N. Toward the development of an objective index of dysphonia severity: A four factor acoustic model. *Clin. Linguist. Phon.* **2006**, *20*, 35–49. [CrossRef] [PubMed]
71. Watts, C.R.; Awan, S.N.; Maryn, Y. A Comparison of Cepstral Peak Prominence Measures from Two Acoustic Analysis Programs. *J. Voice* **2017**, *31*, 387.e1–387.e10. [CrossRef]
72. Phadke, K.V.; Laukkanen, A.-M.; Ilomäki, I.; Kankare, E.; Geneid, A.; Švec, J.G. Cepstral and Perceptual Investigations in Female Teachers with Functionally Healthy Voice. *J. Voice* **2018**, *34*, 485.e33–485.e43. [CrossRef]
73. Hillenbrand, J.M.; Houde, R.A. Acoustic Correlates of Breathy Vocal Quality: Dysphonic Voices and Continuous Speech. *J. Speech Lang. Hear. Res.* **1996**, *39*, 311–321. [CrossRef]
74. Awan, S.N.; Roy, N.; Jette, M.E.; Meltzner, G.S.; Hillman, R.E. Quantifying dysphonia severity using a spectral/cepstral-based acoustic index: Comparisons with auditory-perceptual judgements from the CAPE-V. *Clin. Linguist. Phon.* **2010**, *24*, 742–758. [CrossRef] [PubMed]
75. Watts, C.R.; Awan, S.N. Use of Spectral/Cepstral Analyses for Differentiating Normal from Hypofunctional Voices in Sustained Vowel and Continuous Speech Contexts. *J. Speech Lang. Hear. Res.* **2011**, *54*, 1525–1537. [CrossRef]
76. Awan, S.N.; Giovinco, A.; Owens, J. Effects of Vocal Intensity and Vowel Type on Cepstral Analysis of Voice. *J. Voice* **2012**, *26*, 670.e15–670.e20. [CrossRef] [PubMed]
77. Microsoft. Microsoft Excel. Available online: https://www.microsoft.com/en-us/microsoft-365/excel (accessed on 2 June 2021).
78. Massey, F.J. The Kolmogorov-Smirnov Test for Goodness of Fit. *J. Am. Stat. Assoc.* **1951**, *46*, 68–78. [CrossRef]
79. Murphy, K.R. *Statistical Power Analysis: A Simple and General Model. for Traditional and Modern Hypothesis Tests*, 4th ed.; Routledge: New York, NY, USA, 2014.
80. Cohen, J. A power primer. *Psychol. Bull.* **1992**, *112*, 155–159. [CrossRef]
81. Roy, N.; Merrill, R.M.; Gray, S.D.; Smith, E.M. Voice Disorders in the General Population: Prevalence, Risk Factors, and Occupational Impact. *Laryngoscope* **2005**, *115*, 1988–1995. [CrossRef]
82. Roy, N.; Merrill, R.M.; Thibeault, S.; Parsa, R.A.; Gray, S.D.; Smith, E.M. Prevalence of Voice Disorders in Teachers and the General Population. *J. Speech Lang. Hear. Res.* **2004**, *47*, 281–293. [CrossRef]
83. Procter, T.; Joshi, A. Cultural Competency in Voice Evaluation: Considerations of Normative Standards for Sociolinguistically Diverse Voices. *J. Voice* **2020**. [CrossRef] [PubMed]

84. Snidecor, J.C. A comparative study of the pitch and duration characteristics of impromptu speaking and oral reading. *Speech Monogr.* **1943**, *10*, 50–56. [CrossRef]
85. Stoicheff, M.L. Speaking Fundamental Frequency Characteristics of Nonsmoking Female Adults. *J. Speech Lang. Hear. Res.* **1981**, *24*, 437–441. [CrossRef]
86. Saxman, J.H.; Burk, K.W. Speaking Fundamental Frequency Characteristics of Middle-Aged Females. *Folia Phoniatr. Logop.* **1967**, *19*, 167–172. [CrossRef]
87. Garrett, R. Cepstral- and Spectral-Based Acoustic Measures of Normal Voices. Ph.D. Thesis, University of Wisconsin-Milwaukee, Milwaukee, WI, USA, 2013.
88. Diaz, F.J. Measuring the individual benefit of a medical or behavioral treatment using generalized linear mixed-effects models. *Stat. Med.* **2016**, *35*, 4077–4092. [CrossRef]
89. Maryn, Y.; Weenink, D. Objective Dysphonia Measures in the Program Praat: Smoothed Cepstral Peak Prominence and Acoustic Voice Quality Index. *J. Voice* **2015**, *29*, 35–43. [CrossRef] [PubMed]
90. Koufman, J.A.; Isaacson, G. The Spectrum of Vocal Dysfunction. *Otolaryngol. Clin. N. Am.* **1991**, *24*, 985–988. [CrossRef]
91. Madill, C.; Lee, R.; Heard, R.; Roarke, R.; McCabe, T. Impact of breathing instructions on voice onset time. In Proceedings of the Voice Foundation 45th Annual Symposium, Philadelphia, PA, USA, 1–5 June 2016.
92. Vennard, W. *Singing: The Mechanism and the Technic*, 5th ed.; Fischer: New York, NY, USA, 1968.
93. Colton, R.H.; Estill, J. Elements of Voice Quality: Perceptual, Acoustic, and Physiologic Aspects. In *Speech and Language: Advances in Basic Research and Practice*; Lass, N.J., Ed.; Academic Press: Cambridge, MA, USA, 1981; Volume 5, pp. 311–401.
94. Roy, N.; Whitchurch, M.; Merrill, R.M.; Houtz, D.; Smith, M.E. Differential Diagnosis of Adductor Spasmodic Dysphonia and Muscle Tension Dysphonia Using Phonatory Break Analysis. *Laryngoscope* **2008**, *118*, 2245–2253. [CrossRef]
95. Harris, T.; Harris, S.; Rubin, J.S.; Howard, D.M. *The Voice Clinic Handbook*; Wiley: Chichester, UK, 1997.
96. Simonyan, K.; Ackermann, H.; Chang, E.F.; Greenlee, J.D. New Developments in Understanding the Complexity of Human Speech Production. *J. Neurosci.* **2016**, *36*, 11440–11448. [CrossRef]
97. Nikjeh, D.A.; Lister, J.J.; Frisch, S.A. The relationship between pitch discrimination and vocal production: Comparison of vocal and instrumental musicians. *J. Acoust. Soc. Am.* **2009**, *125*, 328–338. [CrossRef] [PubMed]
98. Estis, J.M.; Dean-Claytor, A.; Moore, R.E.; Rowell, T.L. Pitch-Matching Accuracy in Trained Singers and Untrained Individuals: The Impact of Musical Interference and Noise. *J. Voice* **2011**, *25*, 173–180. [CrossRef]
99. Carey, J.R.; Bhatt, E.; Nagpal, A. Neuroplasticity promoted by task complexity. *Exerc. Sport Sci. Rev.* **2005**, *33*, 24–31. [PubMed]
100. Kantak, S.S.; Zahedi, N.; McGrath, R. Complex Skill Training Transfers to Improved Performance and Control of Simpler Tasks After Stroke. *Phys. Ther.* **2017**, *97*, 718–728. [CrossRef] [PubMed]
101. Braun, D.A.; Aertsen, A.; Wolpert, D.M.; Mehring, C. Motor Task Variation Induces Structural Learning. *Curr. Biol.* **2009**, *19*, 352–357. [CrossRef] [PubMed]
102. Dhawale, A.K.; Smith, M.A.; Ölveczky, B.P. The Role of Variability in Motor Learning. *Annu. Rev. Neurosci.* **2017**, *40*, 479–498. [CrossRef]
103. Vecchione, J.; Madill, C.; Hodges, N. Modifying Technique in Self-Paced Motor Tasks. In *Psychology of Closed Self-Paced Motor Tasks*; Ziv, G.L.R., Ed.; Routledge: Philadelphia, PA, USA, 2021.
104. Rutherford, B.R. The Use of Negative Practice in Speech Therapy with Children Handicapped by Cerebral Palsy, Athetoid Type. *J. Speech Disord.* **1940**, *5*, 259–264. [CrossRef]
105. Lyndon, E.H.; Malcolm, B. The effects of proactive and retroactive inhibition: The Old Way/New Way methodology and its application to speech pathology. In *Proceedings of the Annual Conference of the Australian Association of Speech and Hearing: Beyond 1984*; University of Adelaide: Adelaide, SA, Australia, 1984.
106. Gillespie, A.I.; Yabes, J.; Rosen, C.A.; Gartner-Schmidt, J.L. Efficacy of Conversation Training Therapy for Patients with Benign Vocal Fold Lesions and Muscle Tension Dysphonia Compared to Historical Matched Control Patients. *J. Speech Lang. Hear. Res.* **2019**, *62*, 4062–4079. [CrossRef] [PubMed]
107. Colloca, L. How do placebo effects and patient-clinician relationships influence behaviors and clinical outcomes? *PAIN Rep.* **2019**, *4*, e758. [CrossRef]
108. Berg, E.E.; Hapner, E.; Klein, A.; Johns, M.M., 3rd. Voice Therapy Improves Quality of Life in Age-Related Dysphonia: A Case-Control Study. *J. Voice* **2008**, *22*, 70–74. [CrossRef] [PubMed]
109. Kaneko, M.; Hirano, S.; Tateya, I.; Kishimoto, Y.; Hiwatashi, N.; Fujiu-Kurachi, M.; Ito, J. Multidimensional Analysis on the Effect of Vocal Function Exercises on Aged Vocal Fold Atrophy. *J. Voice* **2015**, *29*, 638–644. [CrossRef]
110. Angadi, V.; Croake, D.; Stemple, J. Effects of Vocal Function Exercises: A Systematic Review. *J. Voice* **2019**, *33*, 124.e13–124.e34. [CrossRef]
111. Murton, O.; Hillman, R.; Mehta, D. Cepstral Peak Prominence Values for Clinical Voice Evaluation. *Am. J. Speech-Lang. Pathol.* **2020**, *29*, 1596–1607. [CrossRef] [PubMed]
112. Belsky, M.A.; Rothenberger, S.D.; Gillespie, A.I.; Gartner-Schmidt, J.L. Do Phonatory Aerodynamic and Acoustic Measures in Connected Speech Differ Between Vocally Healthy Adults and Patients Diagnosed with Muscle Tension Dysphonia? *J. Voice* **2020**, *35*, 663.e1–663.e7. [CrossRef] [PubMed]

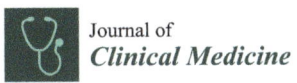 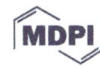

Article

Effect of Progressive Head Extension Swallowing Exercise on Lingual Strength in the Elderly: A Randomized Controlled Trial

Jin-Woo Park *, Chi-Hoon Oh, Bo-Un Choi, Ho-Jin Hong, Joong-Hee Park, Tae-Yeon Kim and Yong-Jin Cho

Department of Physical Medicine and Rehabilitation, Dongguk University Ilsan Hospital, Goyang-si 10326, Gyeonggi-do, Korea; chejuoh@hanmail.net (C.-H.O.); moongirl33@naver.com (B.-U.C.); frischen@naver.com (H.-J.H.); s65271@hanmail.net (J.-H.P.); tinaccjj@naver.com (T.-Y.K.); pigboom@hanmail.net (Y.-J.C.)
* Correspondence: jinwoo.park.md@gmail.com; Tel.: +82-31-961-7484

Citation: Park, J.-W.; Oh, C.-H.; Choi, B.-U.; Hong, H.-J.; Park, J.-H.; Kim, T.-Y.; Cho, Y.-J. Effect of Progressive Head Extension Swallowing Exercise on Lingual Strength in the Elderly: A Randomized Controlled Trial. *J. Clin. Med.* **2021**, *10*, 3419. https://doi.org/10.3390/jcm10153419

Academic Editor: Renee Speyer

Received: 13 July 2021
Accepted: 29 July 2021
Published: 31 July 2021

Publisher's Note: MDPI stays neutral with regard to jurisdictional claims in published maps and institutional affiliations.

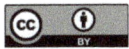

Copyright: © 2021 by the authors. Licensee MDPI, Basel, Switzerland. This article is an open access article distributed under the terms and conditions of the Creative Commons Attribution (CC BY) license (https://creativecommons.org/licenses/by/4.0/).

Abstract: Lingual strengthening training can improve the swallowing function in older adults, but the optimal method is unclear. We investigated the effects of a new progressive resistance exercise in the elderly by comparing with a conventional isometric tongue strengthening exercise. Twenty-nine participants were divided into two groups randomly. One group performed forceful swallow of 2 mL of water every 10 s for 20 min, and a total of 120 swallowing tasks per session at 80% angle of maximum head extension. The other group performed five repetitions in 24 sets with a 30 s rest, and the target level was settled at 80% of one repetition maximum using the Iowa Oral Performance Instrument (IOPI). A total of 12 sessions were carried out by both groups over a 4-week period. Blinded measurements (for maximum lingual isometric pressure and peak pressure during swallowing) were obtained using IOPI before exercise and at four weeks in both groups. After four weeks, both groups showed a significant improvement in lingual strength involving both isometric and swallowing tasks. However, there was no significant difference between the groups in strength increase involving both tasks. Regardless of the manner, tongue-strengthening exercises substantially improved lingual pressure in the elderly with equal effect.

Keywords: deglutition disorders; tongue; exercise; deglutition; ageing

1. Introduction

Presbyphagia means characteristic alteration in the deglutition mechanism of healthy older adults [1]. Aging worsens motor swallowing mechanism, which, in turn, leads to weakness in tongue muscle [2]. It is significant that the tongue is the main source of propelling oropharyngeal swallowing [3], and abnormal tongue strength and coordination can decrease the safety and efficiency of swallowing [4,5].

Fortunately, tongue exercises can increase tongue strength and improve swallowing ability in older people. In this way, exercise using an air bulb or pushing against hard palate as a resistive isometric exercise can improve tongue strength and swallowing function [6,7]. Real swallowing exercise can also improve tongue strength in the elderly [8]. However, the method that is the best for increasing tongue strength is currently unclear.

We know that the training method based on the basic principle of exercise is the best [9]. Training specificity means that improvement in performance is most dramatic when movements closely coincide with the exercise. When applied to the tongue, the tongue strength is improved during swallowing. According to the overload principle, exercise resistance should be gradually increased as the individual capabilities improve throughout the training. Exercises using an air bulb or tongue depressor [6,10,11] are resistive isometric exercises and appropriate for the overload principle but are not based on training specificity. Actual swallowing exercises such as effortful swallow [12] are based on training specificity, but they do not adhere to the overload principle because the exercise intensity cannot be adjusted.

However, head extension swallowing exercises can increase lingual swallowing pressure and endurance in an older adult population [13]. Even though this exercise is based on the work of a single research group involving a limited number of people which has yet to be replicated elsewhere, it can be easily performed anytime and anywhere without the need for additional equipment, especially given the benefits of resistance exercise. We thought that it might conform to training specificity and overload principle, and effectively improve tongue strength. We modified this exercise by adjusting the angle of head extension in order to control and increase the intensity of the exercise (progressive resistance exercise). We hypothesized that this new exercise is effective in increasing tongue strength in older adults, and that the exercise is superior to the lingual elevation exercise. Therefore, in this study, we analyzed the effects of a new progressive resistance exercise for performance by older adults, and we compared the results with conventional isometric tongue-strengthening exercises.

2. Materials and Methods

2.1. Participants

Thirty-five healthy older volunteers were eligible for this study, which was conducted from August 2019 to February 2020. The inclusion criteria were: (1) healthy older people aged above 65 years without dysphagia, and (2) sufficient cognitive function to perform tongue-strengthening exercises (mini-mental status exam ≥ 26). Thus, the exclusion criteria were: (1) history of odynophagia or dysphagia, (2) drugs that influence swallowing, and (3) history of cervical spine disease that prohibits head extension. Before attending this study, all of the participants were examined by a doctor. This study adheres to CONSORT guidelines, and the Institutional Review Board approved this study. Informed consent was obtained from each subject. Twenty-nine volunteers participated in this study, and 26 of the 29 participants who completed the 12 sessions of the exercise were included in this analysis (Figure 1). Three of the 29 participants dropped out after performing the exercise 2 to 3 times because they either had no time to visit the hospital or their place of residence was located too far from the hospital. The mean age of the study group was 72.9 ± 6.4 years, and the study included 5 males and 21 females. The general characteristics of these volunteers are shown in Table 1.

Table 1. General characteristics of participants in this study.

	Tongue Progressive Resistance Exercise; G1 ($n = 13$)	Tongue Isometric Exercise; G2 ($n = 13$)	p-Value
Age (years)	72.7 ± 7.3 (65–87)	73.2 ± 5.7 (65–82)	0.835
Sex			0.135
Male	4	1	
Female	9	12	
Mini-mental status exam	28.6 ± 1.3 (26–30)	28.2 ± 1.3 (26–30)	0.387
Baseline maximum head extension angle (degrees)	39.6 ± 9.9 (25–55)		
4th week maximum head extension angle (degrees)	57.7 ± 7.8 (40–70)		
Baseline maximum isometric pressure (kPa)	40.5 ± 9.2 (22–56)	43.5 ± 10.4 (29–62)	0.455
Baseline peak pressure during swallowing (kPa)	26.1 ± 12.4 (10–54)	31.3 ± 12.6 (17–59)	0.297

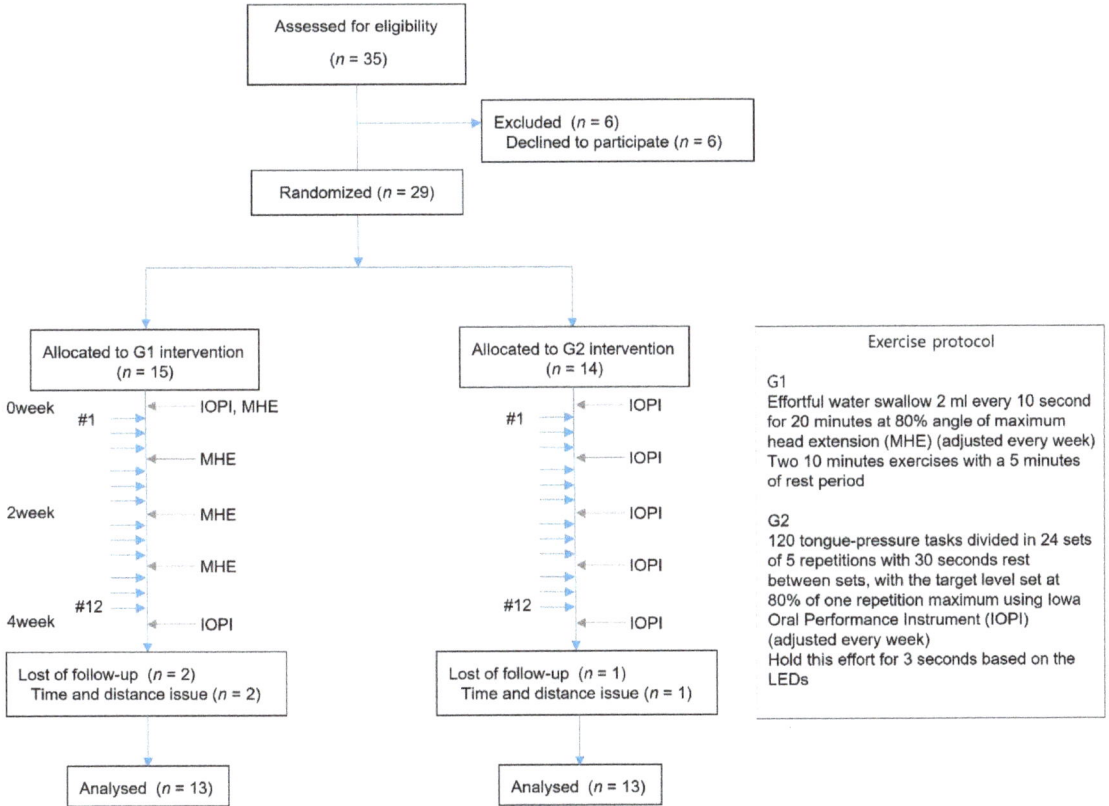

Figure 1. Flow diagram and exercise protocol.

2.2. Experimental Protocol

This study was designed as a randomized, controlled study and was scheduled for a total of 4 weeks. The study participants were randomly allocated to two groups with a 1:1 ratio: tongue progressive resistance exercise group (G1) or tongue isometric exercise group (G2) using a randomization computer program. The assessor and statistical analyst were unaware of the group assignment. Before strengthening training, we measured the baseline data including maximum lingual isometric pressure and peak pressure during swallowing using Iowa Oral Performance Instrument (IOPI) (model 2.1; IOPI Medical LLC, Carnation, WA, USA), which is a handheld tool for measuring the pressure on a small air-filled bulb [14]. Each strengthening program was then administered to the participants over a course of 4 weeks, followed by reassessment of strength to evaluate the training effects of the tongue-strengthening exercise.

2.3. Tongue Strengthening Training

The G1 group performed an effortful swallow of 2 mL of water every 10 s for 20 min with a total of 120 swallowing tasks per session at 80% angle of maximum head extension (MHE). One session consisted of two 10 min period exercises with a 5 min period rest between exercises to avoid muscle fatigue. All participants received instruction to maintain the same posture by staring at one point during the swallowing attempts. The point was determined to ensure that the participants looked comfortable by staring at the grid on the wall 1 m away while maintaining the determined head extension angle. Next, the G2 group did an exercise, which consisted of five repetitions, 24 sets, 30 s rest between sets and a total of 120 lingual pressing tasks per session, with the target level set at 80% of one repetition maximum (RM) using an IOPI. Participants hold the bulb for 3 s based on the light-emitting diode (LED). MHE and one RM were repeatedly measured every week and the exercise levels were readjusted. Three sessions were performed by both groups each week over a 4-week duration (total 12 sessions). All exercises were carried out in the University Hospital under supervision.

2.4. Head Extension Measurements

Each participant in the G1 group sat on a chair ensuring that the thoracic vertebrae were in constant contact with the back of the chair, and the lumbar vertebrae filled the gap between the seat and the back. The participant's feet were placed flat on the floor and arms were placed freely at their sides. Next, the inclinometer (Baseline® Bubble Inclinometer, FEI, White Plains, NY, USA) was mounted over the participant's vertex of the head. Next, the tester instructed each participant to extend his or her head until they could not swallow volitionally, and then measured the MHE angle using the inclinometer (Figure 2).

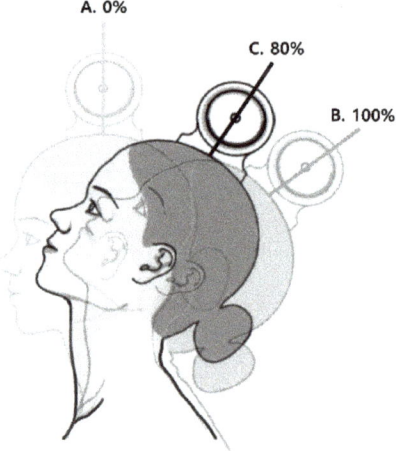

Figure 2. Head extension angle. A. neutral position B. maximal head extension (MHE) C. 80% of MHE.

2.5. Tongue Strength Measurements

In the study, the blinded lingual pressures were measured using IOPI with participants seated comfortably in an upright position during two different tasks: (1) maximum isometric pressure and (2) peak pressure during saliva swallowing [15]. The bulb was positioned at 10 mm anterior to the most posterior circumvallate and pressures (expressed in kPa) were displayed on a liquid crystal display (LCD) panel on the device. For the isometric task, volunteers received instruction to press the bulb against the "roof of the mouth" with the tongue as "hard as possible." For the swallowing task, the participants were instructed to swallow saliva as they would normally with the bulb in place. Three trials to generate maximal pressures were attempted and the highest pressure was used to measure the tongue strength.

2.6. Statistical Analysis

The statistical analysis was carried out using SPSS version 12.0 (SPSS, Inc., Chicago, IL, USA). For determining the sample size, the predicted difference (d) of IOPI was set to 5 and the standard deviation S was set to 5. An alpha error of 0.05 and a beta error of 0.2 were calculated to arrive at a total of 32 subjects. Group comparisons of baseline demographics were performed using Student's *t*-test for continuous variables and χ^2 test for categorical variables to test imbalance between groups. Likewise, the paired *t*-test was used for comparison between paired variables (pre- and post-training in groups). Finally, the comparison of the absolute increase in strength between groups was performed with Student's *t*-test. The significance level was set at $p < 0.025$ to consider alpha-level adjustments for multiple comparisons.

3. Results

The mean baseline maximum head extension angle in G1 was 39.6 ± 9.9 (25–55) degrees, which significantly increased to 57.7 ± 7.8 (40–70) degrees after 4 weeks. The increase in maximum head extension angle was positively correlated with the increase in tongue strength in the G1 group (Spearman's Rho, r = 0.651, $p = 0.016$)

The average baseline maximum isometric pressures (average ± standard deviation) of G1 and G2 were 40.5 ± 9.2 kPa and 43.5 ± 10.4 kPa, respectively, showing no significant differences between groups ($p = 0.455$). The average baseline peak pressures during swallowing of G1 and G2 were 26.1 ± 12.4 kPa and 31.3 ± 12.6 kPa, respectively, and also there was no significant difference between the groups ($p = 0.297$). After four weeks of exercise, the tongue strength in both isometric and swallowing tasks was increased significantly in both groups (G1, $p < 0.001$, Cohen's d = 2.222 and G2, $p < 0.001$, Cohen's d = 1.469 for isometric pressure; G1, $p = 0.001$, Cohen's d = 0.882 and G2, $p = 0.003$, Cohen's d = 0.763 for pressure during swallowing) (Figure 3). However, no significant difference in strength increment in both tasks was detected between the groups (G1, 17.6 ± 7.5 kPa and G2, 14.0 ± 7.9 kPa, $p = 0.244$ for isometric pressure; G1, 11.9 ± 10.3 kPa and G2, 10.2 ± 10.1 kPa, $p = 0.662$ for pressure during swallowing) (Figure 4).

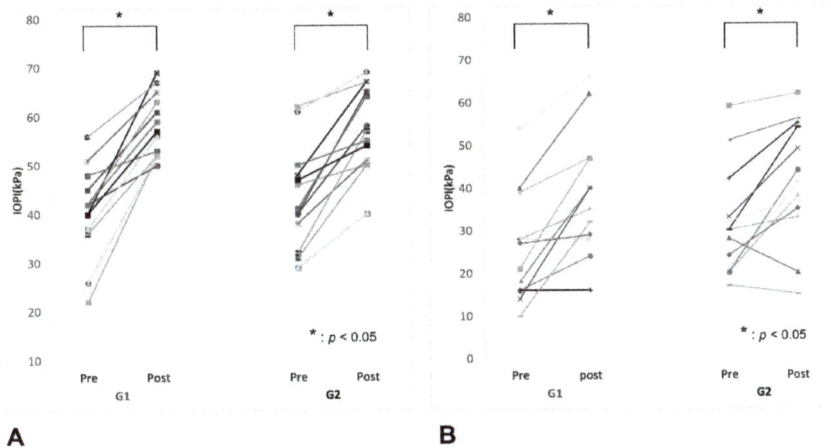

Figure 3. Comparisons of maximal tongue pressure between baseline and post-training sessions in both groups. G1, Tongue progressive resistance exercise group; G2, Tongue isometric exercise group. (**A**) Maximum isometric pressure. Tongue strength was increased significantly in both exercise groups (G1, $p = 0.000$; G2, $p = 0.000$). (**B**) Peak pressure during swallowing. Tongue strength was also increased significantly in both exercise groups (G1, $p = 0.001$; G2, $p = 0.003$).

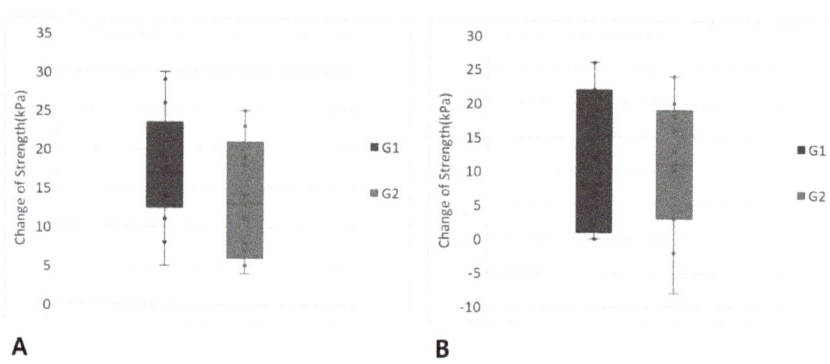

Figure 4. Comparison of the degree of strength increment between the two groups. G1, Tongue progressive resistance exercise group; G2, Tongue isometric exercise group. (**A**) Maximum isometric pressure. There were no significant differences between the groups (G1, 17.6 ± 7.5 kPa and G2, 14.0 ± 7.9 kPa, $p = 0.244$). (**B**) Peak pressure during swallowing. No significant differences were detected between groups. (G1, 11.9 ± 10.3 kPa and G2, 10.2 ± 10.1 kPa, $p = 0.662$). Box: 1st quartile and 3rd quartile; Whisker: minimum and maximum; Line: median; X: average.

4. Discussion

Four weeks of progressive head extension swallowing exercise improved tongue strength in older volunteers. However, this method was not superior to conventional isometric strengthening exercise. Likewise, the head extension swallowing exercise strengthens the tongue and suprahyoid muscles. It was originally a compensatory method administered to inpatients with head and neck cancer who generally present with problems associated with oral food intake [16]. However, the use of head extension as a resistance mechanism to strengthen the tongue was applicable to young and old alike [13,17]. We modified this exercise by additionally increasing the angle of head extension to control the intensity of exercise. Progressive head extension swallow training that meets training specificity criteria and overload principle is expected to be the most effective method to increase lingual strength.

However, lingual strengthening training does not follow standard exercise principles. In fact, the unique physiology of the lingual musculature may defy many types of exercise principles [18]. The tongue is a muscular hydrostat, which generates force via contraction of muscle fibers to generate hydraulic pressure within a limited area. However, the muscles of the human tongue are unique in that they are attached to only a single static support (mandible or styloid process), or to a floating support (hyoid bone). The tongue is a cylindrical structure with a constant volume that adjusts its shape and size by co-activating many of its muscular components. The implication in this case is that because the muscles cannot contract by attaching to a bony support, as in the arm or leg, the hydrostatic pull on the muscles results in a net productive movement. In contrast, skeletal muscles usually contract with joints to create force, and most of the theory underlying exercise physiology is based on skeletal muscle studies. Regardless of the direction, most tongue motions require simultaneous contraction of several tongue muscles to produce hydraulic pressure that alters the functional strength in any untrained tongue movements [10].

Robbins et al. reported that average baseline peak isometric pressure was 41 (36–46) kPa and the pressure increased 7 kPa in older adults after an 8-week program of lingual resistance exercise entailing compression of an air-filled bulb [6]. Van den Steen et al. performed tongue-strengthening exercises for 8 weeks using IOPI in healthy older adults and reported an approximate increase in strength of 26.0 kPa in the anterior maximum isometric pressure (baseline 35.9 ± 6.0 kPa) [14]. Park et al. performed a home-based program for the older adults involving tongue-pressing effortful swallow exercise. Baseline mean tongue pressure was 37.51 ± 15.26 kPa. Four weeks after exercise, the average of the maximum tongue pressure increased by 8.17 kPa [8]. Four weeks of progressive head extension swallowing exercise increased the maximal isometric pressure of 17.6 kPa in this study.

Few studies reported attempts to strengthen the tongue muscles in the form of resistance-swallowing exercise (consistent with exercise principles). Repetitive tongue-holding swallowing exercise was proposed for improving swallowing function in young healthy people, but it showed the same effects as compared to normal swallowing exercise [19]. Park et al. showed that chin-down swallowing exercise improved the lingual strength of healthy young people. However, this exercise was not superior to other tongue-strengthening trainings [20]. The results reinforced our findings in this study.

This study has a few limitations. First, although increasing the degree of head extension requires additional effort during swallowing, evidence is insufficient to show that the resistance increases in proportion to the increasing angle of head extension. However, the maximum head extension angle was increased with exercise. The increment of maximum head extension angle significantly correlated with the increase in the tongue strength, which might support the role of increasing head extension as an appropriate mechanism for achieving overload. Second, we had the participants stare at a point, which was set to maintain the same posture during exercise, but we did not ensure that this direction was perfectly followed in each case. However, we supervised the exercise of all participants to ensure that they followed our instructions correctly. Third, the head extension exercise was conducted with effortful swallows but lingual pressure during swallowing was measured during non-effortful swallows. In terms of training specificity, this limitation might have affected the results of this study.

5. Conclusions

Swallowing exercise with progressive head extension increased tongue strength in the older participants. It was easy to monitor the participants anytime and anywhere without any equipment. However, the benefits of this training intervention were not better than other conventional tongue-strengthening exercise. The results suggest that since lingual musculature exhibits atypical response to strength training and all tongue-strength training interventions yield favorable results regardless of the type, it is best to select an exercise option that is easy and most appropriate for the participant and the specific circumstances.

Author Contributions: Conceptualization, J.-W.P.; methodology, C.-H.O., B.-U.C., H.-J.H. and J.-H.P.; validation, J.-W.P.; formal analysis, T.-Y.K. and Y.-J.C.; investigation, T.-Y.K. and Y.-J.C.; writing—original draft preparation, J.-W.P.; writing—review and editing, J.-W.P.; visualization, J.-W.P.; funding acquisition, J.-W.P. All authors have read and agreed to the published version of the manuscript.

Funding: This research was funded by a grant (NRF-2019R1F1A1043950) of the Basic Science Research Program through the National Research Foundation of Korea (NRF) funded by the Ministry of Science and ICT, Republic of Korea. The funder had no role in the design of the study and collection, analysis, and interpretation of data and in writing the manuscript.

Institutional Review Board Statement: The study was conducted according to the guidelines of the Declaration of Helsinki, and approved by the Dongguk University Ilsan Hospital Institutional Review Board. (Approval No. 2019-07-010-002).

Informed Consent Statement: We obtained from all subjects participating in the study.

Data Availability Statement: Data presented in this study are provided by the corresponding authors upon reasonable request.

Conflicts of Interest: The authors have no conflict of interest.

References

1. Robbins, J.; Hamilton, J.W.; Lof, G.L.; Kempster, G.B. Oropharyngeal swallowing in normal adults of different ages. *Gastroenterology* **1992**, *103*, 823–829. [CrossRef]
2. Rofes, L.; Arreola, V.; Romea, M.; Palomera, E.; Almirall, J.; Cabre, M.; Serra-Prat, M.; Clave, P. Pathophysiology of oropharyngeal dysphagia in the frail elderly. *Neurogastroenterol. Motil.* **2010**, *22*, 851–858.e230. [CrossRef]
3. McConnel, F.M. Analysis of pressure generation and bolus transit during pharyngeal swallowing. *Laryngoscope* **1988**, *98*, 71–78. [CrossRef]
4. Clark, H.M.; Henson, P.A.; Barber, W.D.; Stierwalt, J.A.; Sherrill, M. Relationships among subjective and objective measures of tongue strength and oral phase swallowing impairments. *Am. J. Speech Lang. Pathol.* **2003**, *12*, 40–50. [CrossRef]
5. Stierwalt, J.A.; Youmans, S.R. Tongue measures in individuals with normal and impaired swallowing. *Am. J. Speech Lang. Pathol.* **2007**, *16*, 148–156. [CrossRef]
6. Robbins, J.; Gangnon, R.E.; Theis, S.M.; Kays, S.A.; Hewitt, A.L.; Hind, J.A. The effects of lingual exercise on swallowing in older adults. *J. Am. Geriatr. Soc.* **2005**, *53*, 1483–1489. [CrossRef]
7. Wakabayashi, H.; Matsushima, M.; Momosaki, R.; Yoshida, S.; Mutai, R.; Yodoshi, T.; Murayama, S.; Hayashi, T.; Horiguchi, R.; Ichikawa, H. The effects of resistance training of swallowing muscles on dysphagia in older people: A cluster, randomized, controlled trial. *Nutrition* **2018**, *48*, 111–116. [CrossRef]
8. Park, T.; Kim, Y. Effects of tongue pressing effortful swallow in older healthy individuals. *Arch. Gerontol. Geriatr.* **2016**, *66*, 127–133. [CrossRef]
9. Brukner, P.; Khan, K. *Brukner & Khan's Clinical Sports Medicine*, 3rd ed.; McGraw-Hill: Sydney, Australia; New York, NY, USA, 2010; 117p.
10. Clark, H.M.; O'Brien, K.; Calleja, A.; Corrie, S.N. Effects of directional exercise on lingual strength. *J. Speech Lang. Hear. Res.* **2009**, *52*, 1034–1047. [CrossRef]
11. Yeates, E.M.; Molfenter, S.M.; Steele, C.M. Improvements in tongue strength and pressure-generation precision following a tongue-pressure training protocol in older individuals with dysphagia: Three case reports. *Clin. Interv. Aging* **2008**, *3*, 735–747. [CrossRef]
12. Clark, H.M.; Shelton, N. Training effects of the effortful swallow under three exercise conditions. *Dysphagia* **2014**, *29*, 553–563. [CrossRef]
13. Oh, J.C. Effect of the head extension swallowing exercise on suprahyoid muscle activity in elderly individuals. *Exp. Gerontol.* **2018**, *110*, 133–138. [CrossRef]
14. Van den Steen, L.; Schellen, C.; Verstraelen, K.; Beeckman, A.S.; Vanderwegen, J.; De Bodt, M.; Van Nuffelen, G. Tongue-Strengthening Exercises in Healthy Older Adults: Specificity of Bulb Position and Detraining Effects. *Dysphagia* **2018**, *33*, 337–344. [CrossRef]
15. Robbins, J.; Levine, R.; Wood, J.; Roecker, E.B.; Luschei, E. Age effects on lingual pressure generation as a risk factor for dysphagia. *J. Gerontol. A Biol. Sci. Med. Sci.* **1995**, *50*, M257–M262. [CrossRef]
16. Pauloski, B.R. Rehabilitation of dysphagia following head and neck cancer. *Phys. Med. Rehabil. Clin. N Am.* **2008**, *19*, 889–928. [CrossRef] [PubMed]
17. Oh, J.C. A Pilot Study of the Head Extension Swallowing Exercise: New Method for Strengthening Swallowing-Related Muscle Activity. *Dysphagia* **2016**, *31*, 680–686. [CrossRef]
18. Kier, W.M. Tongues, tentacles and trunks: The biomechanics of movement in muscular-hydrostats. *Zool. J. Linn. Soc.* **1985**, *83*, 30–324. [CrossRef]
19. Oh, J.C.; Park, J.W.; Cha, T.H.; Woo, H.S.; Kim, D.K. Exercise using tongue-holding swallow does not improve swallowing function in normal subjects. *J. Oral Rehabil.* **2012**, *39*, 364–369. [CrossRef]
20. Park, J.W.; Hong, H.J.; Nam, K. Comparison of three exercises on increasing tongue strength in healthy young adults. *Arch. Oral Biol.* **2020**, *111*, 104636. [CrossRef]

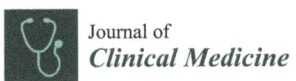

Article

Validation and Classification of the 9-Item Voice Handicap Index (VHI-9i)

Felix Caffier [1,†], Tadeus Nawka [1,†], Konrad Neumann [2], Matthias Seipelt [3] and Philipp P. Caffier [1,*,†]

1. Department of Audiology and Phoniatrics, Charité-Universitätsmedizin Berlin, Charitéplatz 1, D-10117 Berlin, Germany; felix.caffier@charite.de (F.C.); tadeus.nawka@charite.de (T.N.)
2. Institute of Biometry and Clinical Epidemiology, Charité-Universitätsmedizin Berlin, Campus Charité Mitte, Charitéplatz 1, D-10117 Berlin, Germany; konrad.neumann@charite.de
3. Department of Otorhinolaryngology, Ernst von Bergmann Klinikum Potsdam, Charlottenstr. 72, D-14467 Potsdam, Germany; MatthiasSeipelt@web.de
* Correspondence: philipp.caffier@charite.de
† Corporate Member of Freie Universität Berlin and Humboldt-Universität zu Berlin, Campus Charité Mitte.

Abstract: The international nine-item Voice Handicap Index (VHI-9i) is a clinically established short-scale version of the original VHI, quantifying the patients' self-assessed vocal handicap. However, the current vocal impairment classification is based on percentiles. The main goals of this study were to establish test–retest reliability and a sound statistical basis for VHI-9i severity levels. Between 2009 and 2021, 17,660 consecutive cases were documented. A total of 416 test–retest pairs and 3661 unique cases with complete multidimensional voice diagnostics were statistically analyzed. Classification candidates were the overall self-assessed vocal impairment (VHIs) on a four-point Likert scale, the dysphonia severity index (DSI), the vocal extent measure (VEM), and the auditory–perceptual evaluation (GRB scale). The test–retest correlation of VHI-9i total scores was very high (r = 0.919, $p < 0.01$). Reliability was excellent regardless of gender or professional voice use, with negligible dependency on age. The VHIs correlated best with the VHI-9i, whereas statistical calculations proved that DSI, VEM, and GRB are unsuitable classification criteria. Based on ROC analysis, we suggest modifying the former VHI-9i severity categories as follows: 0 (healthy): $0 \leq 7$; 1 (mild): $8 \leq 16$; 2 (moderate): $17 \leq 26$; and 3 (severe): $27 \leq 36$.

Keywords: Voice Handicap Index (VHI-9i); international short scale; VHI-9i severity levels; test–retest reliability; validation of classification ranges; self-assessed vocal impairment (VHIs); hoarseness; dysphonia severity categories; voice diagnostics

Citation: Caffier, F.; Nawka, T.; Neumann, K.; Seipelt, M.; Caffier, P.P. Validation and Classification of the 9-Item Voice Handicap Index (VHI-9i). J. Clin. Med. 2021, 10, 3325. https://doi.org/10.3390/jcm10153325

Academic Editor: Renee Speyer

Received: 31 May 2021
Accepted: 25 July 2021
Published: 28 July 2021

Publisher's Note: MDPI stays neutral with regard to jurisdictional claims in published maps and institutional affiliations.

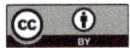

Copyright: © 2021 by the authors. Licensee MDPI, Basel, Switzerland. This article is an open access article distributed under the terms and conditions of the Creative Commons Attribution (CC BY) license (https://creativecommons.org/licenses/by/4.0/).

1. Introduction

A patient's self-assessment of his or her own voice is an important tool for diagnosing voice disorders and vocal treatment outcomes [1,2]. Only the patients themselves can quantify how much a voice disorder impacts their daily lives. For instance, mild hoarseness affects professional voice users such as opera singers in a different way than non-professional voice users such as office workers [3,4].

The Voice Handicap Index (VHI) was developed and validated as a statistically robust method to measure the subjective impact of voice disorders [5]. The original questionnaire consists of 30 items (VHI-30) addressing functional, physical and emotional impairments in the context of dysphonia according to the patient's own experience. Each question is answered on a scale from 0 (never) to 4 (always), resulting in an overall score ranging from 0 to 120. The VHI-30 was translated and validated cross-culturally to form international variants (e.g., [6–11]) which were proven to be equivalent with each other [12,13].

From our own clinical experience, many patients and medical staff perceive the original 30-item questionnaire as rather time-consuming. To increase overall acceptance and practicability, shortened versions with fewer items were developed. A 12-item questionnaire [14,15] was soon followed by another reduction to 10 items [16,17]. Since 2009, the commonly used variant at the Charité-Universitätsmedizin Berlin is the VHI-9i international questionnaire [14]. It consists of only nine items, after item reduction based on the original VHI-30 and European translations. A detailed discussion of the item and scale development can be found in the original VHI-9i publication [14]. In everyday diagnostic practice, the German translation of the VHI-9i is widely used by laryngologists and phoniatricians in German-speaking countries (e.g., [18–22]). Despite its clinical adoption, the reliability and validity of this VHI short scale as well as its classification have not yet been statistically verified. Instead, the current classification scale is based on the 25th, 50th, and 75th percentiles, dividing the scores into four severity classes. Thus far, clinical experience seems to plausibly reflect the self-perceived voice impairment. However, to overcome this arbitrary percentile-based exploration, we looked for a sound statistical basis for VHI-9i severity levels by revising the current cut-off points. In the context of expert opinion, thorough classifications of vocal parameters are essential for the assessment of dysphonia. In addition, a reliable and valid VHI-9i severity classification is needed to improve clinician-rated evaluations of treatment outcomes (e.g., better characterization of the quantified extent of subjective vocal impairment, more comprehensible assessment of individual pre- vs. post-therapeutic comparisons).

This study aims to address these shortcomings. Initially, we investigated whether the VHI-9i produces reliable results independent of age, gender or professional voice use. Next, the questionnaire validity was examined. For this purpose, the relationship between VHI-9i total scores and other established vocal parameters was statistically analyzed to establish cut-off values for healthy voices and mild to severe dysphonia. For external criteria, we intended to use objective acoustic–aerodynamic voice function diagnostics including voice range profile (VRP) measurements, dysphonia severity index (DSI) and vocal extent measure (VEM) calculations, as well as the subjective auditory–perceptual evaluation of voices by experienced examiners (GRB scale). Furthermore, the overall self-assessed vocal impairment (VHIs) served as an internal criterion.

2. Materials and Methods

2.1. Study Design and Patients

This study was conducted in accordance with the Declaration of Helsinki and approved by the local ethical review board. Selection criteria involved informed consent and the completion of the standard phoniatric examination procedures. After taking the medical history, all patients presenting in the Department of Audiology and Phoniatrics, Charité-Universitätsmedizin Berlin, Germany, received a digital videolaryngostroboscopy to assess the laryngeal findings and to establish a medical diagnosis. Subsequently, multi-dimensional voice function diagnostics were carried out as recommended by the European Laryngological Society (ELS) [1], starting with subjective evaluations (GRB, VHI-9i) and followed by objective voice function diagnostics (VRP, DSI, VEM). For subjective vocal self-assessment, patients completed the VHI-9i questionnaire. To estimate the voice use of every study participant, we also asked about their occupation and categorized them according to Koufman and Isaacson [23]: elite vocal performers (Level 1; e.g., actors, singers, voice artists), professional voice users (Level 2; e.g., teachers, politicians, moderators), non-vocal professionals (Level 3; e.g., lawyers, medical personnel, civil service employees), and non-vocal non-professionals (Level 4; e.g., IT staff, office workers, mechanics).

Between May 2009 and March 2021, a total of 17,660 consecutive cases were documented in the clinical database. To analyze the reliability of the VHI-9i, 718 patients were asked to complete the same questionnaire for a second time, without therapeutical intervention. The retest form had to be returned within one week to study the differences between the original answers and the retest. The second VHI-9i questionnaire was returned by 517 patients, corresponding to a response rate of 72%. Some questionnaires containing unanswered items or ambiguous checkmarks (e.g., between items) had to be excluded, resulting in 416 test–retest pairs.

The remaining 16,942 consecutive cases were analyzed to establish the validity of the questionnaire and to calculate statistically valid classification ranges. Since the VHI-9i should be compared with other established vocal parameters, only 7766 cases with complete multi-dimensional diagnostic assessment were considered. Cases with unreliable perturbation measures (jitter > 5%) were excluded, as recommended in the literature [1,24], resulting in a sample size of 6882. After another exclusion of follow-up visits, 3661 complete and unique cases were left for statistical analysis.

2.2. Subjective Examination Instruments

The VHI-9i represents an item-reduced short scale of the established VHI-30 [14], available in several languages (i.e., Dutch, English, French, German, Italian, Portuguese and Swedish). In this study, the German translation of the questionnaire was used (see Appendix A). Study participants were asked to answer all 9 items on a scale from 0 to 4 (0: never, 1: almost never, 2: sometimes, 3: almost always, 4: always), resulting in a total score between 0 and 36. The total score was then assigned to one of four dysphonia severity categories, ranging from 0 (healthy; $0 \leq 5$), 1 (mild; $6 \leq 13$), 2 (moderate; $14 \leq 22$), to 3 (severe; $23 \leq 36$). However, these categories correspond to a classification proposed by Nawka et al., based on the percentiles of a representative investigation of 716 patients [25]. Since these classification ranges have not yet been validated, statistical calculation of potential cut-off values for the VHI-9i classification was a main goal of this study.

Additionally, participants were asked to rate their overall voice impairment at present on a scale from 0 to 3 (0: normal, 1: mild, 2: moderate, 3: severe), the VHI summary assessment (VHIs). This index allows patients to assess how they feel about their voice with only one number. The relationship between VHI-9i and VHIs scores was examined to determine whether patients would rate themselves differently when asked about specific situations in their lives (VHI-9i items) or directly about their overall impairment (VHIs).

Apart from self-assessment, voices were also evaluated by auditory–perceptual assessment using the GRB system [26–28]. Based on the GRBAS scale, our department developed the modified GRB classification [29,30]. Only the first three criteria are used, focusing on the overall grade of hoarseness (G) and both main pathophysiological hoarseness components: roughness (R) and breathiness (B). The assessment of voice quality can be carried out more quickly and easily. Therefore, this system has become established in German-speaking countries and is also recommended in the ELS protocol [1]. Patients were asked to read the standardized text "The north wind and the sun" (German version), while the perceived G, R and B were scored on a scale from 0 to 3. To increase objectivity, each voice recording was rated independently by one experienced phoniatric physician and one senior speech–language therapist. The means were used for further exploration. While the degree of G serves as the overall indicator of dysphonia in the original GRBAS scale, it is regarded as gold standard for hoarseness evaluation in the GRB system presented here [31].

2.3. Objective Acoustic Assessment

For objective external validation criteria, we applied acoustic–aerodynamic voice function diagnostics. Voice recordings of all participants were conducted at the voice lab of our outpatient department, which is a sound-treated room with a background noise <40 dB(A). Study participants were asked to wear a head-mounted microphone with a stable mouth–microphone distance of 30 cm [32]. The equipment used for this purpose was the XION microphone headset (model number 352,009,010; XION GmbH, Berlin, Germany), which enables the realization of speech and singing VRP measurements and voice analyses under reproducible conditions. Technical microphone specifications include a frequency response of 70 Hz–20 kHz and a dynamic range of 40–120 dB(A). The microphone headset incorporates a calibrated audio interface that transmits digitized data to the PC via USB. The built-in electronics ensure the automatic calibration of the microphone connection without additional adjustments. The audio was processed via the DiVAS 2.8 software using the Singing Voice Analysis module (product number 350,020,013) and the Speaking

Voice Analysis module (product number 350,020,024; XION GmbH, Berlin, Germany). VRP measurements were performed to show the functional interactions of different components of voice generation regarding vocal frequency and intensity [33,34]. The detailed procedure of VRP recordings is described in previous publications [35,36].

The established parameter DSI was automatically calculated as a weighted combination of the highest possible fundamental frequency, the lowest phonation intensity, maximum phonation time and jitter [37]. Regarding jitter, the waveform matching method was used for fundamental frequency extraction as it meets the high-precision criterion of being able to extract a 1% frequency change per cycle with a 1% accuracy, as long as the signal-to-noise ratio is greater than about 40 dB and concomitant amplitude modulations are below about 5% [24]. Measurements were conducted in a standing position. Subjects were asked to produce a sustained vowel (/na/ or /a/) for about 3 seconds at comfortable pitch and loudness. The most stable recording out of 3 trials was chosen for DSI calculation. Based on Gonnermann's investigation of 495 subjects [38], the DSI scores were sorted into 4 severity categories, discriminating healthy voices (≥ 4.2) from mildly (<4.2 to ≥ 1.8), moderately (<1.8 to ≥ -1.2), or severely (<-1.2) dysphonic voices. Since the DSI quantifies dysphonia as a negative criterion and involves the risk of imprecise results due to its multidimensional data acquisition, the one-dimensional parameter VEM was recently developed [35].

VEM calculation was performed automatically after VRP recording via the proprietary AVA software [39,40]. The VEM quantifies a subject's dynamic performance and frequency range. It is calculated as a relation of the area and perimeter of the VRP and describes the vocal function by an interval-scaled value without unit, usually between 0 and 120. These limits may be exceeded at both ends by either severely impaired or exceptionally capable voices with a large ambitus and dynamic range. A small vocal capacity is described by a low VEM, a large VRP by a high VEM. The VEM emphasizes the vocal abilities and enables a classification of voice performance as a positive criterion [21,31,41]. Based on Müller's investigation of 994 subjects [36], the resulting VEM scores were divided into percentiles, distinguishing a normal vocal capacity (≥ 108) from mildly reduced (<108 to ≥ 93), moderately (<93 to ≥ 69) and severely reduced (<69) vocal capacities.

Table 1 summarizes the severity classification of different objective and subjective vocal parameters by reference range. In contrast to the ordinally scaled GRB and VHIs, the classifications of metrically scaled parameters (VEM, VHI-30, VHI-9i) are based on the percentiles of the respective study cohorts (Level 0: 100th percentile/4th quartile; Level 1: 75th percentile/3rd quartile; Level 2: 50th percentile/2nd quartile; Level 3: 25th percentile/1st quartile).

Table 1. Severity classification of different vocal parameters, assessed by study participants (VHI-30, VHI-9i, VHIs), experienced clinicians (GRB), and acoustic–aerodynamic analysis (VEM, DSI). Although all parameters share the same classification scale (0–3), equal levels of severity among different parameters do not imply equivalence (* classification ranges based on percentiles).

Level of Severity	VHI-30 *[25]	VHI-9i *[25]	VHIs	Grade (G)	VEM *[36]	DSI [38]
0: healthy	$0 \leq 14$	$0 \leq 5$	0	0	≥ 108	≥ 4.2
1: mild	$15 \leq 28$	$6 \leq 13$	1	1	$93 < 108$	$1.8 < 4.2$
2: moderate	$29 \leq 50$	$14 \leq 22$	2	2	$69 < 93$	$-1.2 < 1.8$
3: severe	$51 \leq 120$	$23 \leq 36$	3	3	<69	<-1.2

3. Data Analysis

Statistical analysis was performed using IBM SPSS version 26.0.0.1. To establish the questionnaire as reliable, the absolute differences in total VHI-9i scores between test and retest were compared. An analysis of the differences of every single item in the questionnaire is individually important, but only the total scores are relevant in diagnostic practice. Paired-sample *t*-tests were used to check for biases, and correlations were established through Pearson's r. To test the dependency of the VHI-9i total score on age, a regression analysis was performed. Gender differences were analyzed through independent sample t-tests. We checked for a dependency on voice use by means of the nonparametric Kruskal–Wallis H-test.

Before the cut-off points for the VHI-9i severity categories could be validated, the correlations between the VHI-9i and the severity classifications for VHIs, DSI, VEM, G, R and B had to be determined using Spearman's rho (ρ), in order to choose which of them was best suited for classification. These vocal parameters had to be balanced in terms of sensitivity (i.e., true positive rate, TPR) and specificity (i.e., true negative rate, TNR) when applied to the VHI-9i scores. Receiver operator characteristic (ROC) curves were used, which plot the TPR against the false positive rate (FPR = 1 − TNR). Since ROC is a binary classifier, the curves had to be plotted three times to establish possible cut-off points for every severity level (0 vs. 1–3, 0–1 vs. 2–3, 0–2 vs. 3). The area under the curve (AUC) was used to rank the performance of every curve to distinguish between two severity classes. Values between 0.8 and 0.9 are considered excellent, 0.7 to 0.8 acceptable, 0.5 to 0.7 poor.

Several methods exist to determine good class boundaries from ROC curves. As a starting point, we used Youden's index (J) [42]. The highest J (Max J) is achieved when sensitivity and specificity are at optimal balance (J = TPR − FPR = TPR + TNR − 1). As a second possible class boundary, we determined the point where the number of correctly classified cases (CCCs) was the highest. The CCC is calculated as follows:

CCC = TPR * (n cases of classifying index above class boundary)
    + TNR * (n cases of classifying index below class boundary)

To find plausible cut-off values or categories of reasonable size, we selected a value between the two suggested class boundaries based on the median between Max J and Max CCC, also taking into account well over a decade of clinical experience with the VHI-9i.

4. Results

4.1. Test–Retest Reliability

After eliminating all incomplete questionnaires, 416 test–retest pairs were left. The mean age (±SD) was 50 (±17), with males skewing generally older at 56 (±16) compared to female patients at 46 (±17) years of age. A total of 26 participants (6.3%) were classified as elite vocal performers, 59 as professional voice users (14.2%), 78 as non-vocal professionals (18.7%) and 253 as non-vocal non-professionals (60.8%). An overview of the test–retest population is given in Figure 1 and Table 2.

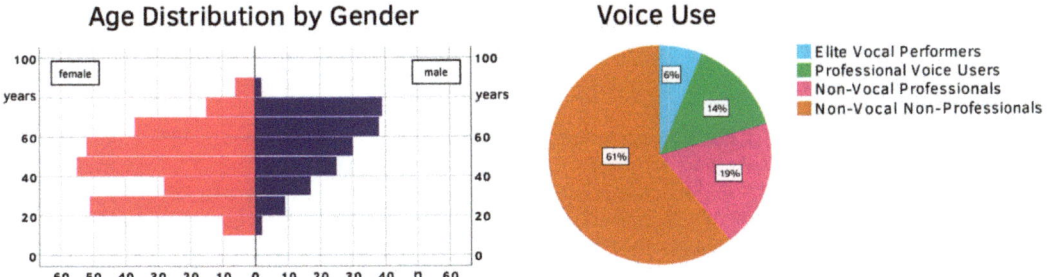

Figure 1. Overview of the test–retest population (age, gender, voice use classification).

Table 2. Study participant distribution and VHI-9i score differences between test and retest.

	Number *n* (%)	Mean Total Score Difference (±SD)
Male	162 (38.9%)	0.38 (±3.68)
Female	254 (61.1%)	0.17 (±3.42)
Voice Use Level 1	26 (6.3%)	0.75 (±3.45)
Voice Use Level 2	59 (14.2%)	0.82 (±3.48)
Voice Use Level 3	78 (18.7%)	0.40 (±2.91)
Voice Use Level 4	253 (60.8%)	0.02 (±3.70)
Age Group 0–24 years	46 (11.1%)	0.41 (±2.17)
Age Group 25–64 years	267 (64.2%)	0.45 (±3.47)
Age Group 65–99 years	103 (24.7%)	−0.33 (±4.06)

The median gap between test and retest was 2 days, with a mean of 3.3 days. The overall mean difference between VHI-9i scores (± SD) was very small at 0.25 (±3.52). Gender, voice use or age showed similarly minor differences (see Figure 2 and Table 2).

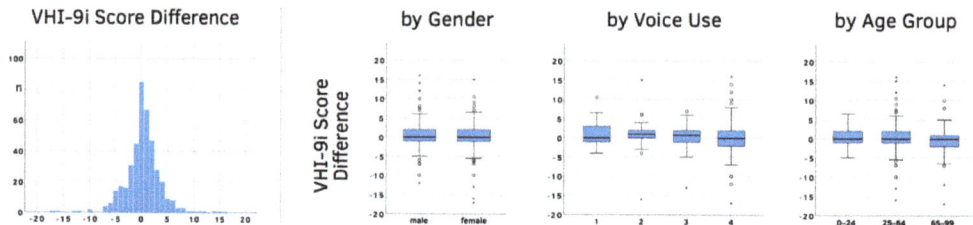

Figure 2. VHI-9i score difference between test and retest (total differences, by gender, by voice use, by age group). Age dependency was analyzed using discrete age values; age groups were only used in the diagram to improve the graphical representation. Circles (○) mark outliers (3rd quartile + 1.5*interquartile range; 1st quartile − 1.5*interquartile range) and asterisks (*) mark far outliers (3rd quartile + 3*interquartile range; 1st quartile − 3*interquartile range).

A paired-sample *t*-test between the VHI-9i total scores showed no significant differences ($p = 0.146$). Test and retest scores also correlated very well ($r = 0.919$, $p < 0.01$), indicating a highly reliable questionnaire. Only 5% of the population had a difference larger than 7 points. Gender had no impact on the reliability of the questionnaire. The independent sample *t*-test for the absolute VHI-9i score difference between males and females was not significant ($p = 0.589$). The level of voice use did also not affect reliability. The Kruskal–Wallis H-test showed no significance between the four voice use classifications ($p = 0.701$). The absolute score differences lightly depended on age. For every year of life, the difference rose by 0.016 points ($p = 0.028$).

4.2. Validation

Of the 3661 participants remaining for VHI-9i validation, 1456 were male (39.8%) and 2205 were female (60.2%). The mean age (±SD) was 48 (±17), with males being on average slightly older at 50 (±18) years compared to females at 47 (±17) years of age. Vocal impairment was caused by functional dysphonia in 40.8% of the study population. Patients with organic dysphonia (50.8%) showed various pathologies: mostly lesions of the lamina propria (e.g., vocal fold nodules, polyps, cysts, Reinke's edema), followed by benign and malignant changes of the epithelium (e.g., leukoplakia, papillomatosis, carcinoma), as well as neurogenic voice disorders (e.g., unilateral paralyses of the recurrent laryngeal nerve, spasmodic dysphonia). The remaining 8.4% were healthy subjects without dysphonia, mainly college applicants who presented to receive a vocal fitness examination, or prior to starting a profession associated with high vocal demands (e.g., teachers, singers, lecturers). The population pyramid and pathology classification are shown in Figure 3.

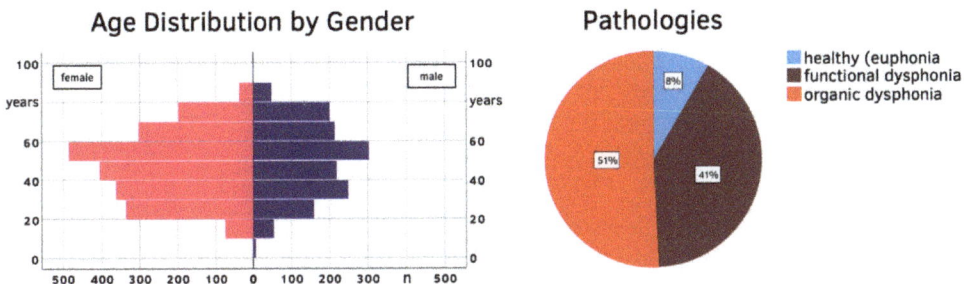

Figure 3. Overview of the validation population (age, gender, pathology classification).

As the test–retest examinations demonstrated, the reliability of VHI-9i scores is not affected by gender or voice use. Although statistically significant, the age dependency is so small that it can be neglected in clinical practice. Therefore, all further observations and calculations were conducted for the entire population of 3661 participants. Using the old VHI-9i classification scale based on percentiles [25], 15.5% of our participants had healthy voices (total score $0 \leq 5$), 25.7% mild dysphonia ($6 \leq 13$), 32.3% moderate ($14 \leq 22$) and 26.5% severe dysphonia ($23 \leq 36$). Applying the same method to the current database, 25% of patients had a score between 0 and 9, 50% up to 16, and 75% up to 22 points. The severity distribution for the other vocal parameters can be found in Table 3. Regarding VHIs, 63 cases had to be excluded (n = 3598 instead of 3661), because these test subjects had marked this question outside or in-between the provided options for the severity levels, rendering them invalid.

Table 3. Collected voice data by vocal parameter, classified according to the associated level of severity as shown in Table 1.

Vocal Parameter		Level of Severity			
		0: Healthy	1: Mild	2: Moderate	3: Severe
VHIs	number (%)	559 (15.5%)	1170 (32.5%)	1425 (39.6%)	444 (12.4%)
	mean VHI-9i score (±SD)	6.6 (±6.8)	12.8 (±7.2)	19.5 (±7.4)	23.9 (±7.8)
DSI	number (%)	879 (24.0%)	1210 (33.0%)	1244 (34.0%)	328 (9.0%)
	mean VHI-9i score (±SD)	11.9 (±8.1)	15.5 (±8.8)	17.7 (±8.9)	21.0 (±8.5)
VEM	number (%)	732 (20.0%)	673 (18.4%)	945 (25.8%)	1311 (35.8%)
	mean VHI-9i score (±SD)	11.1 (±8.0)	13.5 (±8.2)	15.7 (±8.3)	19.9 (±8.8)
G	number (%)	537 (14.7%)	1693 (46.2%)	1169 (31.9%)	262 (7.2%)
	mean VHI-9i score (±SD)	10.4 (±8.3)	14.2 (±8.4)	19.1 (±8.4)	23.3 (±7.8)
R	number (%)	602 (16.4%)	1864 (50.9%)	1031 (28.2%)	164 (4.5%)
	mean VHI-9i score (±SD)	11.7 (±8.9)	15.0 (±8.7)	18.9 (±8.4)	21.8 (±8.2)
B	number (%)	1865 (50.9%)	1205 (32.9%)	446 (12.2%)	145 (4.0%)
	mean VHI-9i score (±SD)	12.8 (±8.4)	17.3 (±8.4)	21.8 (±8.1)	25.6 (±6.7)

The size and mean of each severity category as well as the distribution of scores were notably different between parameters. The VHI-9i histogram shows a centered flat curve (skewness 0.063, kurtosis -0.90), the DSI is still centered but steeper (skewness -0.04, kurtosis 0.48) and the VEM is even steeper and skewed towards lower VEM values (skewness -1.08, kurtosis 1.94), with most patients falling into severity category 3 (Figure 4).

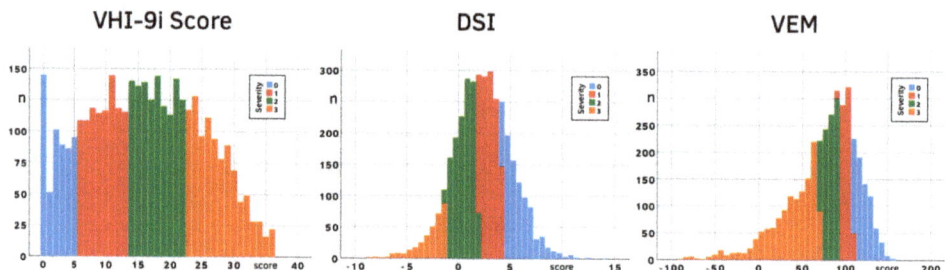

Figure 4. Observed VHI-9i, DSI and VEM scores with their associated severities.

The VHI-9i total scores correlated the most with the VHIs, even though ρ was only moderate (ρ = 0.592; see Table 4). All other parameters correlated notably weaker with the VHI-9i. The objective DSI and VEM were also moderately correlated to each other at ρ = 0.663. The distribution of subjects into G and R severity levels was rather similar, while B showed a different result with over 50% of all cases falling into the "healthy" category. G and R also had the strongest correlation among each other (ρ = 0.871), reinforcing clinical experience that G serves as the gold standard for hoarseness evaluations via the GRB scale.

Table 4. Results of correlation analysis between vocal parameters (Spearman's rho). All correlation coefficients were significant ($p < 0.001$).

	VHIs (0–3)	DSI (0–3)	VEM (0–3)	G (0–3)	R (0–3)	B (0–3)
VHI-9i	0.592	0.292	0.373	0.393	0.299	0.386
VHIs (0–3)		0.229	0.261	0.328	0.263	0.287
DSI (0–3)			0.663	0.525	0.454	0.494
VEM (0–3)				0.494	0.390	0.501
G (0–3)					0.871	0.665
R (0–3)						0.449

Figure 5 shows the distribution of VHI-9i total scores using the classifications for VHIs, DSI, VEM and G. The boxplots reveal a clear tendency: the higher the severity level, the higher the associated median. However, there is also a lot of overlap between the quartiles of different severity levels. This especially applies to DSI and VEM, which makes these parameters less suitable for VHI-9i classification.

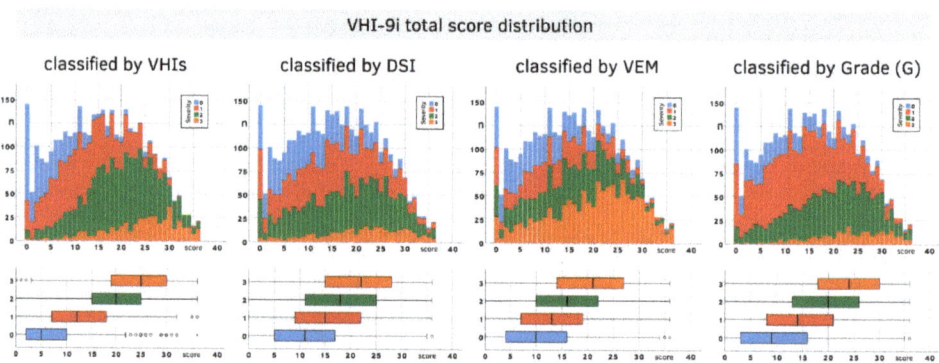

Figure 5. Distribution of VHI-9i total scores classified by VHIs, DSI, VEM and G severity levels. Upper row: stacked bar chart showing the number of subjects with their VHI-9i scores. Lower row: boxplots showing the percentiles of patients' VHI-9i scores by severity level. Circles (○) and asterisks (*) mark outliers and far outliers.

The ROC plots (Figure 6) also favor the VHIs as the best classifying index. DSI, VEM and G are visibly less suitable classifiers, because their curves are closer to the hypothetical diagonal through the ROC plot, signifying weaker discriminating performance.

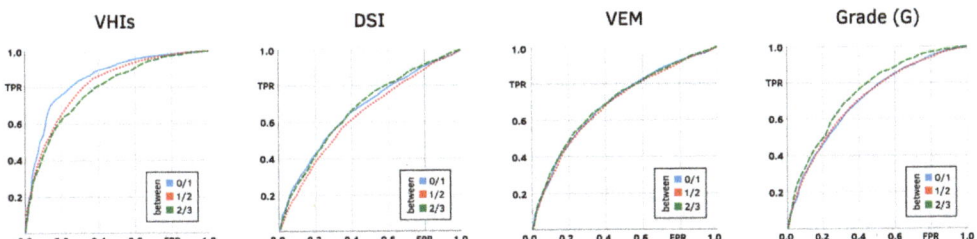

Figure 6. Combined ROC plots to determine cut-off points between severity categories 0 and 1 (blue), 1 and 2 (red), 2 and 3 (green).

The AUC results (Table 5) mirror the correlations of vocal parameters (compare Table 4). The best performance was achieved by the VHIs with excellent AUCs, followed by acceptable values for G. The parameters DSI and VEM turned out to be poor discriminators, with AUCs below 0.7.

As shown by our reliability analysis, severity categories must be at least 7 points in size to account for significant changes and minimize the possibility of retest artifacts. Neither optimizing for sensitivity and specificity (Max J) nor correctly classified cases (Max CCC) alone produced classes that were all wide enough (>7 points). Apart from the VHIs, Max CCC even produced cut-off recommendations that would eliminate the lowest (VEM) or lowest and highest (DSI, G) severity categories (highlighted in Table 5). Since both methods did not produce plausible cut-off values or categories of reasonable size, medians between the Max J and Max CCC measurements had to be calculated.

Table 5. ROC results for potential cut-offs between severity categories (0–1, 1–2, 2–3) using Max J, Max CCC and Median calculations. Yellow cells mark impossible cut-offs. Median calculations for every ROC parameter (TPR, FPR, J, CCC) resulted in slightly different class boundaries, which were specified by the ranges of cut-off values.

		VHIs			G		
		Cut 0–1	Cut 1–2	Cut 2–3	Cut 0–1	Cut 1–2	Cut 2–3
AUC		0.846	0.811	0.783	0.704	0.709	0.748
Max J	TPR	0.737	0.781	0.743	0.633	0.664	0.683
	FPR	0.174	0.298	0.316	0.33	0.352	0.311
	J	0.564	0.483	0.427	0.303	0.311	0.372
	CCC	2702	2674	2486	2336	2394	2521
	cut-off	11.5	14.75	19.5	13.5	16.75	20.5
Max CCC	TPR	0.966	0.818	0.115	1	0.464	0
	FPR	0.651	0.337	0.014	1	0.193	0
	J	0.315	0.481	0.101	0	0.271	0
	CCC	3132	2675	3162	3124	2464	3399
	cut-off	2.5	13.5	32.5	0	21.25	36
J–CCC–Median	TPR	0.86	0.78	0.43	0.83	0.59	0.32
	FPR	0.35	0.3	0.1	0.56	0.28	0.09
	J	0.51	0.48	0.33	0.27	0.31	0.23
	CCC	2988	2674	3026	2813	2443	3182
	cut-off	7–8	14–15	26–27	7–8	19	28

Table 5. Cont.

		DSI			VEM		
		Cut 0–1	Cut 1–2	Cut 2–3	Cut 0–1	Cut 1–2	Cut 2–3
	AUC	0.667	0.64	0.674	0.692	0.689	0.699
Max J	TPR	0.651	0.569	0.683	0.648	0.585	0.639
	FPR	0.39	0.344	0.416	0.35	0.296	0.329
	J	0.26	0.226	0.267	0.298	0.289	0.31
	CCC	2346	2266	2170	2373	2309	2415
	cut-off	13.5	17.25	17.75	13.5	16.75	17.75
Max CCC	TPR	1	0.408	0	1	0.786	0.44
	FPR	1	0.216	0	1	0.537	0.167
	J	0	0.193	0	0	0.25	0.273
	CCC	2782	2280	3333	2929	2425	2535
	cut-off	0	21.75	36	0	10.75	22.5
J–CCC–Median	TPR	0.83	0.48	0.3	0.83	0.66	0.53
	FPR	0.66	0.28	0.13	0.61	0.38	0.23
	J	0.17	0.2	0.17	0.22	0.28	0.3
	CCC	2604	2266	3012	2718	2360	2512
	cut-off	7–8	18–20	26–27	7–8	14	20–21

However, both median calculations did not always return the exact same result, which is why the J–CCC–Median cut-off values are expressed as ranges in Table 5. In general, the difference between both medians was below 0.25 points most of the time and very rarely exceeded 0.5 points. The medians for all vocal parameters agreed on the first boundary (i.e., between severity levels 0 and 1) at 7 or 8. Between "mild" and "moderate" (severity levels 1 and 2), the median recommendations ranged from 14 to 20. Except for the VEM, the medians led to a cut-off point between 26 and 28 for the boundary distinguishing "moderate" from "severe" impairment (i.e., severity levels 2 and 3).

5. Discussion

The VHI-9i short scale has proven to be a valuable diagnostic tool in our clinical practice for well over a decade. The total number of 17,660 consecutively completed questionnaires documented in our database confirms its high acceptance among patients and medical staff. In our test–retest analysis, the VHI-9i questionnaire demonstrated very high reliability independent of gender or voice use. Age had a minor influence, which we do not consider clinically relevant: For every year of life, the absolute score difference between test and retest increased by 0.016. If we applied that difference to the entire age range of our study population, the VHI-9i total score of an adolescent compared to a senior person would differ by about 1. The reliability analysis also showed that the severity classes for the VHI-9i need to be at least 7 points in size (2*SD of paired sample t-test), since only differences of 7 points and above account for significant changes and minimize the possibility of retest artifacts. Our interpretation of the ROC analysis had to consider this requirement. Unfortunately, neither optimizing for Max J nor Max CCC resulted in categories that were all large enough. Calculating the median between them for each cut-off point, however, yielded satisfactory results for clinical use.

All classification ranges are listed in Table 6. The Median J method strikes a good balance between sensitivity, specificity and the minimum class width of 7 points. The new boundary of a score of 7 corresponds directly with the VHIs Median J result for healthy voices (class 0). Finding a reasonable upper boundary for severity level 1 is more difficult: using VHIs Median J (a score of 14) would result in a category that is too small. The median for the expert auditory–perceptual assessment (G) points towards an even higher boundary (a score of 19). Since we were trying to find a mid-point for our severity classes, we decided to use the upper boundary of the 50% quartile (a score of 16). The upper boundary for severity level 2 (moderate impairment) can be taken once again from the VHIs Median J row, placing class 2 between $17 \leq 26$ and class 3 between $27 \leq 36$.

Table 6. Sizes of severity classes based on Max J, Max CCC and Median calculations. Green cells serve as the basis for our proposed new VHI-9i severity classification.

Classifying Method	Level of Severity			
	0: Healthy	1: Mild	2: Moderate	3: Severe
VHIs (Max J)	$0 \leq 12$	$13 \leq 15$	$16 \leq 20$	$21 \leq 36$
VHIs (Max CCC)	$0 \leq 3$	$4 \leq 14$	$15 \leq 33$	$34 \leq 36$
VHIs (Median J)	$0 \leq 7$	$8 \leq 14$	$15 \leq 26$	$27 \leq 36$
VHIs (Median CCC)	$0 \leq 8$	$9 \leq 15$	$16 \leq 27$	$28 \leq 36$
G (Max J)	$0 \leq 14$	$15 \leq 17$	$18 \leq 21$	$22 \leq 36$
G (Max CCC)	-	$0 \leq 21$	$22 \leq 36$	-
G (Median J)	$0 \leq 7$	$8 \leq 19$	$20 \leq 28$	$29 \leq 36$
G (Median CCC)	$0 \leq 8$	$9 \leq 19$	$20 \leq 28$	$29 \leq 36$
DSI (Max J)	$0 \leq 14$	$15 \leq 17$	18	$19 \leq 36$
DSI (Max CCC)	-	$0 \leq 22$	$23 \leq 36$	-
DSI (Median J)	$0 \leq 8$	$9 \leq 20$	$21 \leq 27$	$28 \leq 36$
DSI (Median CCC)	$0 \leq 8$	$9 \leq 18$	$19 \leq 26$	$27 \leq 36$
VEM (Max J)	$0 \leq 14$	$15 \leq 17$	18	$19 \leq 36$
VEM (Max CCC)	-	$0 \leq 11$	$12 \leq 23$	$24 \leq 36$
VEM (Median J)	$0 \leq 8$	$9 \leq 14$	$15 \leq 20$	$21 \leq 36$
VEM (Median CCC)	$0 \leq 7$	$8 \leq 14$	$15 \leq 21$	$22 \leq 36$
VHI-9i quartiles	$0 \leq 9$	$10 \leq 16$	$17 \leq 22$	$23 \leq 36$
Proposed new classification	$0 \leq 7$	$8 \leq 16$	$17 \leq 26$	$27 \leq 36$

Compared to the old VHI-9i classification scale based on percentiles [25], the revised severity ranges classify more patients towards the lower categories. Severity level 3 is reduced by 4 points and is no longer the largest category. Level 1 and 2 start at higher class boundaries due to the size increase in level 0.

The best correlation was observed between VHI-9i and VHIs, making the overall self-assessed vocal impairment the best candidate for the validation process. However, the VHI-9i did not correlate well with the two objective parameters DSI and VEM, and had only slightly higher correlations with GRB. This supports recent studies that all these vocal parameters measure different aspects of a patient's voice and are neither mutually interchangeable nor redundant [31,36,41,43]. Due to the weak correlations, poor discriminating performance and sometimes impossible cut-off points, DSI, VEM and G ultimately had no part in our recommendation for the revised VHI-9i cut-off points. It is important to remember that the VHI-9i does not measure objective voice impairment (DSI) or vocal capacity (VEM), but personal suffering due to a subjectively perceived vocal handicap. None of the parameters allow conclusions to be drawn about the diagnoses or underlying causes of the voice disorder.

Study Limitations

Over 60% of our test–retest population were categorized as non-vocal non-professionals. Ideally, the study would have included more subjects with professional backgrounds in singing, acting or teaching, especially since establishing independence from voice use was one of our goals during the rest-retest analysis. A bigger population of elite vocal performers and professional voice users would have been preferable, but does not represent the actual proportions of our clinic clientele.

Furthermore, males are underrepresented in our study, so there may be participation bias. Despite the limited number of male subjects, we concluded that the VHI-9i was independent of gender, but a more balanced gender involvement would have been more representative. However, our clinical experience shows that women are generally more likely to see a doctor for voice problems.

In addition, signal-to-noise ratio (SNR) analysis and signal typing are considered to be important for valid and reliable perturbation measurements [44–46]. Unfortunately, this functionality is not included in the DiVAS software, which was specified in our study design as the main tool for objective voice analysis. One of the fundamental limitations of the DSI is the inclusion of jitter without sufficient evaluation of the signal type. In general, only type 1 and 2 are considered viable for perturbation analysis. The 5% jitter cut-off applied in our study was established to exclude type 4 signals only [46]. However, the categorization of a small test sample ($n = 40$) revealed signal type 1 and 2 exclusively, even for patients with low DSI and high jitter values. Furthermore, the majority of SNR results were between 42 and 50 dB ("recommended"), with a smaller number between 30 and 42 dB ("acceptable") [45]. Therefore, we believe that our exclusion criteria were sufficient to eliminate voices which are not suitable for perturbation analysis. We recognize that this estimate cannot be taken as proof for the entire dataset and plan to include SNR and signal typing analyses in our future studies from the outset. It should also be noted that jitter was only used for DSI calculation, which proved to be irrelevant for the main goal of our study, i.e., a revised VHI-9i classification. Therefore, our recommendations regarding VHI-9i severity categories should not have been distorted.

Moreover, our initial ROC analysis produced boundary recommendations that were not feasible for diagnostic purposes. The resulting severity categories would have been either too small (<7 points) or would even not exist at all. Calculating the median between Max J and Max CCC is not a commonly used method for solving these problems. However, based on the frequent use of the VHI-9i in clinical investigations [18–22,31,36,41], it appears that the new classification will be a practical option for clinical settings.

In general, the auditory-perceptual assessment of voices via GRB was conducted only by two experienced examiners. Safer larger group judgments were not made. Due to the enormous number of cases ($n = 17,660$) and over a decade of diagnostic voice recordings, a retrospective blinded voice evaluation with 4-5 raters was not an option.

6. Conclusions

The VHI-9i is a reliable questionnaire which is independent of gender and professional voice use. Its dependency on age is negligible. Based on many years of clinical experience, it also has high acceptance among patients and medical staff, making it a valuable diagnostic tool.

The old cut-off values for the VHI-9i severity categories based on percentiles had to be adjusted. We recommend setting class 0 (healthy) between $0 \leq 7$, class 1 (mild impairment) between $8 \leq 16$, class 2 (moderate impairment) between $17 \leq 26$ and class 3 (severe impairment) between $27 \leq 36$.

The subjective VHI-9i does not correlate well with objective vocal parameters (DSI, VEM) or subjective auditory–perceptual assessment (GRB), reinforcing the notion that all these parameters measure different dimensions of a patient's voice and are neither mutually interchangeable nor redundant.

Author Contributions: Conceptualization, T.N., M.S. and P.P.C.; Methodology, F.C., T.N. and P.P.C.; Literature Review, F.C. and P.P.C.; Investigation, T.N., M.S. and P.P.C.; Data Analysis, F.C. and K.N.; Original Draft Writing, F.C. and P.P.C.; Draft Review and Editing, F.C., T.N., K.N. and P.P.C.; Visualization, F.C. and K.N.; Supervision, T.N. All authors have read and agreed to the published version of the manuscript.

Funding: This research received no external funding.

Institutional Review Board Statement: The study was conducted according to the guidelines of the Declaration of Helsinki, and approved by the Ethics Committee of Charité-Universitätsmedizin Berlin, Berlin, Germany (reference number: EA4/140/10).

Informed Consent Statement: Informed consent was obtained from all study participants.

Data Availability Statement: All data of the study are available in the Department of Audiology and Phoniatrics, Charité-Universitätsmedizin Berlin, Berlin, Germany.

Acknowledgments: The authors wish to thank Tatiana Ermakova for the statistical advice.

Conflicts of Interest: The authors declare no conflict of interest.

Appendix A

Table A1. VHI-9i questionnaire items (*German translation*) as used in the study.

Item Text	Score				
My voice makes it difficult for people to hear me. (*Man hört mich wegen meiner Stimme schlecht.*)	0	1	2	3	4
People have difficulty understanding me in a noisy room. (*Anderen fällt es schwer, mich in einem lauten Raum zu verstehen.*)	0	1	2	3	4
The sound of my voice varies throughout the day. (*Der Klang meiner Stimme ändert sich im Laufe des Tages.*)	0	1	2	3	4
My family has difficulty hearing me when I call them throughout the house. (*Meine Familie hört mich kaum, wenn ich zuhause nach ihnen rufe.*)	0	1	2	3	4
My voice difficulties restrict my personal and social life. (*Meine Stimmschwierigkeiten schränken mich in meinem Privatleben ein.*)	0	1	2	3	4
The clarity of my voice is unpredictable. (*Bevor ich spreche, weiß ich nicht, wie klar meine Stimme klingen wird.*)	0	1	2	3	4
My voice is worse in the evening. (*Abends ist meine Stimme schlechter.*)	0	1	2	3	4
I am less outgoing because of my voice problem. (*Ich bin weniger kontaktfreudig wegen meines Stimmproblems.*)	0	1	2	3	4
My voice makes me feel incompetent. (*Wegen meiner Stimme fühle ich mich unfähig.*)	0	1	2	3	4

Scoring: 0 = never (*nie*), 1 = almost never (*selten*), 2 = sometimes (*manchmal*), 3 = almost always (*oft*), 4 = always (*immer*).

Table A2. Global VHIs question added to the study questionnaire.

Question	Score			
How do you rate your voice today? (*Wie schätzen Sie Ihre Stimme heute ein?*)	0	1	2	3

Scoring: 0 = normal (*normal*), 1 = mildly (*leicht*), 2 = moderately (*mittelgradig*), 3 = severely disturbed (*hochgradig gestört*).

References

1. Dejonckere, P.H.; Bradley, P.; Clemente, P.; Cornut, G.; Crevier-Buchman, L.; Friedrich, G.; Van de Heyning, P.; Remacle, M.; Woisard, V. A basic protocol for functional assessment of voice pathology, especially for investigating the efficacy of (phonosurgical) treatments and evaluating new assessment techniques. Guideline elaborated by the Committee on Phoniatrics of the European Laryngological Society (ELS). *Eur. Arch. Oto-Rhino-Laryngol.* **2001**, *258*, 77–82. [CrossRef]
2. Carding, P.N.; Wilson, J.; MacKenzie, K.; Deary, I.J. Measuring voice outcomes: State of the science review. *J. Laryngol. Otol.* **2009**, *123*, 823–829. [CrossRef]
3. Sataloff, R.T. Professional voice users: The evaluation of voice disorders. *Occup. Med.* **2001**, *16*, 633–647.
4. Mori, M.C.; Francis, D.O.; Song, P.C. Identifying Occupations at Risk for Laryngeal Disorders Requiring Specialty Voice Care. *Otolaryngol. Neck Surg.* **2017**, *157*, 670–675. [CrossRef] [PubMed]
5. Jacobson, B.H.; Johnson, A.; Grywalski, C.; Silbergleit, A.; Jacobson, G.; Benninger, M.S.; Newman, C.W. The Voice Handicap Index (VHI): Development and Validation. *Am. J. Speech Lang. Pathol.* **1997**, *6*, 66–70. [CrossRef]
6. Frajkova, Z.; Krizekova, A.; Missikova, V.; Tedla, M. Translation, Cross-Cultural Validation of the Voice Handicap Index (VHI-30) in Slovak Language. *J. Voice* **2020**. [CrossRef]
7. Sakaguchi, Y.; Kanazawa, T.; Okui, A.; Hirosaki, M.; Konomi, U.; Sotome, T.; Tashiro, N.; Kurihara, M.; Omae, T.; Nakayama, Y.; et al. Assessment of Dysphonia Using the Japanese Version of the Voice Handicap Index and Determination of Cutoff Points for Screening. *J. Voice* **2020**. [CrossRef] [PubMed]

8. Sotirović, J.; Grgurević, A.; Mumović, G.; Grgurević, U.; Pavićević, L.; Perić, A.; Erdoglija, M.; Milojević, M. Adaptation and Validation of the Voice Handicap Index (VHI)-30 into Serbian. *J. Voice* **2016**, *30*, 758.e1–758.e6. [CrossRef] [PubMed]
9. Jaruchinda, P.; Suwanwarangkool, T. Cross-Cultural Adaptation and Validation of the Voice Handicap Index into Thai. *J. Med. Assoc. Thail.* **2015**, *98*, 1199–1208.
10. Trinite, B.; Sokolovs, J. Adaptation and Validation of the Voice Handicap Index in Latvian. *J. Voice* **2014**, *28*, 452–457. [CrossRef]
11. Nawka, T.; Wiesmann, U.; Gonnermann, U. Validation of the German version of the Voice Handicap Index (VHI). *Hno* **2003**, *51*, 921–929. [CrossRef] [PubMed]
12. Leeuw, I.V.-D.; Kuik, D.; De Bodt, M.; Guimarães, I.; Holmberg, E.; Nawka, T.; Rosen, C.; Schindler, A.; Whurr, R.; Woisard, V. Validation of the Voice Handicap Index by Assessing Equivalence of European Translations. *Folia Phoniatr. Logop.* **2008**, *60*, 173–178. [CrossRef] [PubMed]
13. Seifpanahi, S.; Jalaie, S.; Nikoo, M.R.; Sobhani-Rad, D. Translated Versions of Voice Handicap Index (VHI)-30 across Languages: A Systematic Review. *Iran. J. Public Health* **2015**, *44*, 458–469.
14. Nawka, T.; Leeuw, I.V.-D.; De Bodt, M.; Guimarães, I.; Holmberg, E.; Rosen, C.; Schindler, A.; Woisard, V.; Whurr, R.; Konerding, U. Item Reduction of the Voice Handicap Index Based on the Original Version and on European Translations. *Folia Phoniatr. Logop.* **2009**, *61*, 37–48. [CrossRef]
15. Hanschmann, H.; Lohmann, A.; Berger, R. Comparison of Subjective Assessment of Voice Disorders and Objective Voice Measurement. *Folia Phoniatr. Logop.* **2011**, *63*, 83–87. [CrossRef]
16. Gilbert, M.R.; Gartner-Schmidt, J.L.; Rosen, C.A. The VHI-10 and VHI Item Reduction Translations—Are we all Speaking the Same Language? *J. Voice* **2017**, *31*, 250.e1–250.e7. [CrossRef] [PubMed]
17. Rosen, C.A.; Lee, A.S.; Osborne, J.; Zullo, T.; Murry, T. Development and validation of the voice handicap index-10. *Laryngoscope* **2004**, *114*, 1549–1556. [CrossRef]
18. Song, W.; Caffier, F.; Nawka, T.; Ermakova, T.; Martin, A.; Mürbe, D.; Caffier, P. T1a Glottic Cancer: Advances in Vocal Outcome Assessment after Transoral CO_2-Laser Microsurgery Using the VEM. *J. Clin. Med.* **2021**, *10*, 1250. [CrossRef]
19. Langenfeld, A.; Bohlender, J.E.; Swanenburg, J.; Brockmann-Bauser, M. Cervical Spine Disability in Correlation with Subjective Voice Handicap in Patients with Voice Disorders: A Retrospective Analysis. *J. Voice* **2020**, *34*, 371–379. [CrossRef] [PubMed]
20. Reetz, S.; Bohlender, J.E.; Brockmann-Bauser, M. Do Standard Instrumental Acoustic, Perceptual, and Subjective Voice Outcomes Indicate Therapy Success in Patients With Functional Dysphonia? *J. Voice* **2019**, *33*, 317–324. [CrossRef]
21. Salmen, T.; Ermakova, T.; Schindler, A.; Ko, S.-R.; Göktas, O.; Gross, M.; Nawka, T.; Caffier, P. Efficacy of microsurgery in Reinke's oedema evaluated by traditional voice assessment integrated with the Vocal Extent Measure (VEM). *Acta Otorhinolaryngol. Ital.* **2018**, *38*, 194–203. [CrossRef]
22. Caffier, P.P.; Salmen, T.; Ermakova, T.; Forbes, E.; Ko, S.-R.; Song, W.; Gross, M.; Nawka, T. Phonomicrosurgery in Vocal Fold Nodules: Quantification of Outcomes in Professional and Non-Professional Voice Users. *Med Probl. Perform. Artist.* **2017**, *32*, 187–194. [CrossRef] [PubMed]
23. Koufman, J.A.; Isaacson, G. The spectrum of vocal dysfunction. *Otolaryngol. Clin. N. Am.* **1991**, *24*, 985–988. [CrossRef]
24. Titze, I.R.; Liang, H. Comparison of F o Extraction Methods for High-Precision Voice Perturbation Measurements. *J. Speech Lang. Heart Res.* **1993**, *36*, 1120–1133. [CrossRef] [PubMed]
25. Nawka, T.; Rosanowski, F.; Gross, M. How to render an expert opinion on dysphonia. *Laryngorhinootologie* **2014**, *93*, 591–598.
26. Hanschmann, H.; Berger, R. Perceptual and acoustic evaluation of hoarseness. *Laryngorhinootologie* **2011**, *90*, 68–70.
27. Ptok, M.; Schwemmle, C.; Iven, C.; Jessen, M.; Nawka, T. On the auditory evaluation of voice quality. *Hno* **2006**, *54*, 793–802. [CrossRef]
28. Schönweiler, R.; Wübbelt, P.; Hess, M.; Ptok, M. Psychoacoustic scaling of acoustic voice parameters by multicenter voice ratings. *Laryngorhinootologie* **2001**, *80*, 117–122. [CrossRef]
29. Wendler, J.; Rauhut, A.; Krüger, H. Classification of voice qualities. *J. Phon.* **1986**, *14*, 483–488. [CrossRef]
30. Anders, L.; Hollien, H.; Hurme, P.; Sonninen, A.; Wendler, J. Perception of Hoarseness by Several Classes of Listeners. *Folia Phoniatr. Logop.* **1988**, *40*, 91–100. [CrossRef] [PubMed]
31. Seipelt, M.; Möller, A.; Nawka, T.; Gonnermann, U.; Caffier, F.; Caffier, P.P. Monitoring the Outcome of Phonosurgery and Vocal Exercises with Established and New Diagnostic Tools. *BioMed Res. Int.* **2020**, *2020*, 4208189. [CrossRef]
32. Schutte, H.; Seidner, W. Recommendation by the Union of European Phoniatricians (UEP): Standardizing Voice Area Measurement/Phonetography. *Folia Phoniatr. Logop.* **1983**, *35*, 286–288. [CrossRef]
33. Ternström, S.; Pabon, P.; Södersten, M.; Peter, P.; Maria, S. The Voice Range Profile: Its Function, Applications, Pitfalls and Potential. *Acta Acust. United Acust.* **2016**, *102*, 268–283. [CrossRef]
34. Printz, T.; Godballe, C.; Grøntved, Å.M. The Dual-Microphone Voice Range Profile Assessment—Interrater Reliability. *J. Voice* **2020**. [CrossRef] [PubMed]
35. Caffier, P.P.; Möller, A.; Forbes, E.; Müller, C.; Freymann, M.-L.; Nawka, T. The Vocal Extent Measure: Development of a Novel Parameter in Voice Diagnostics and Initial Clinical Experience. *BioMed Res. Int.* **2018**, *2018*, 3836714. [CrossRef] [PubMed]
36. Müller, C.; Caffier, F.; Nawka, T.; Müller, M.; Caffier, P.P. Pathology-Related Influences on the VEM: Three Years' Experience since Implementation of a New Parameter in Phoniatric Voice Diagnostics. *BioMed Res. Int.* **2020**, *2020*, 5309508. [CrossRef] [PubMed]

37. Wuyts, F.L.; Bodt, M.S.D.; Molenberghs, G.; Remacle, M.; Heylen, L.; Millet, B.; Lierde, K.V.; Raes, J.; Heyning, P.H.V.D. The dysphonia severity index: An objective measure of vocal quality based on a multiparameter approach. *J. Speech Lang. Heart Res.* **2000**, *43*, 796–809. [CrossRef]
38. Gonnermann, U. *Quantifizierbare Verfahren zur Bewertung von Dysphonien [Quantifiable Techniques for Evaluation of Dysphonia]*; Peter Lang: Frankfurt/Main, Germany, 2007.
39. Möller, A. Vocal Extent Measure as a New Parameter in Instrumental Voice Diagnostics. Unpublished. Bachelor Thesis, Fachhochschule Stralsund—University of Applied Sciences, Stralsund, Germany, 2010.
40. Caffier, P.P.; Möller, A. Das Stimmumfangsmaß SUM als neuer Parameter in der objektiven Stimmdiagnostik. *Sprache · Stimme · Gehör* **2016**, *40*, 183–187. [CrossRef]
41. Salmen, T.; Ermakova, T.; Möller, A.; Seipelt, M.; Weikert, S.; Rummich, J.; Gross, M.; Nawka, T.; Caffier, P.P. The Value of Vocal Extent Measure (VEM) Assessing Phonomicrosurgical Outcomes in Vocal Fold Polyps. *J. Voice* **2017**, *31*, 114.e7–114.e15. [CrossRef]
42. Youden, W.J. Index for rating diagnostic tests. *Cancer* **1950**, *3*, 32–35. [CrossRef]
43. Woisard, V.; Bodin, S.; Yardeni, E.; Puech, M. The Voice Handicap Index: Correlation Between Subjective Patient Response and Quantitative Assessment of Voice. *J. Voice* **2007**, *21*, 623–631. [CrossRef] [PubMed]
44. Titze, I.R. *Workshop on Acoustic Voice Analysis: Summary Statement*; National Center for Voice and Speech: Iowa City, IA, USA, 1995.
45. Deliyski, D.D.; Shaw, H.S.; Evans, M.K. Adverse Effects of Environmental Noise on Acoustic Voice Quality Measurements. *J. Voice* **2005**, *19*, 15–28. [CrossRef] [PubMed]
46. Sprecher, A.; Olszewski, A.; Jiang, J.J.; Zhang, Y. Updating signal typing in voice: Addition of type 4 signals. *J. Acoust. Soc. Am.* **2010**, *127*, 3710–3716. [CrossRef] [PubMed]

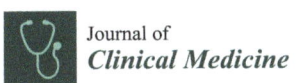 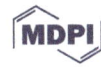

Article

Reliability of Machine and Human Examiners for Detection of Laryngeal Penetration or Aspiration in Videofluoroscopic Swallowing Studies

Yuna Kim [1], Hyun-Il Kim [2], Geun Seok Park [1], Seo Young Kim [1], Sang-Il Choi [2,3,*] and Seong Jae Lee [1,4,*]

1. Department of Rehabilitation Medicine, Dankook University Hospital, Cheonan 31116, Korea; kimyuna727@dkuh.co.kr (Y.K.); geunpark@dkuh.co.kr (G.S.P.); juliet8383@naver.com (S.Y.K.)
2. Department of Computer Science and Engineering, Dankook University, Yongin 16890, Korea; gusdlf93@naver.com
3. Department of Computer Engineering, Dankook University, Yongin 16890, Korea
4. Department of Rehabilitation Medicine, College of Medicine, Dankook University, Cheonan 31116, Korea
* Correspondence: choisi@dankook.ac.kr (S.-I.C.); rmlee@dankook.ac.kr (S.J.L.)

Abstract: Computer-assisted analysis is expected to improve the reliability of videofluoroscopic swallowing studies (VFSSs), but its usefulness is limited. Previously, we proposed a deep learning model that can detect laryngeal penetration or aspiration fully automatically in VFSS video images, but the evidence for its reliability was insufficient. This study aims to compare the intra- and inter-rater reliability of the computer model and human raters. The test dataset consisted of 173 video files from which the existence of laryngeal penetration or aspiration was judged by the computer and three physicians in two sessions separated by a one-month interval. Intra- and inter-rater reliability were calculated using Cohen's kappa coefficient, the positive reliability ratio (PRR) and the negative reliability ratio (NRR). Intrarater reliability was almost perfect for the computer and two experienced physicians. Interrater reliability was moderate to substantial between the model and each human rater and between the human raters. The average PRR and NRR between the model and the human raters were similar to those between the human raters. The results demonstrate that the deep learning model can detect laryngeal penetration or aspiration from VFSS video as reliably as human examiners.

Keywords: dysphagia; swallowing; laryngeal penetration or aspiration; deglutition; reliability; videofluoroscopic swallowing study; deep learning; machine learning

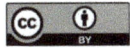

1. Introduction

The videofluoroscopic swallowing study (VFSS) is currently regarded as the gold standard method for evaluating swallowing function because it allows real-time visualization of bolus movement along with the dynamics of anatomical structures associated with the swallowing process [1,2]. A VFSS makes it possible to detect the presence and timing of laryngeal penetration or aspiration and helps to identify its physiological mechanisms [2–4].

The videofluoroscopic images are recorded while the patients swallow boluses mixed with contrast, and physicians or speech–language pathologists analyze the recorded videos [2]. VFSS analysis depends on the subjective visual judgment of the reviewers and is inevitably susceptible to human bias [5–7]. Human examiners usually have the burden of reviewing the images dozens of times for one patient because the swallowing process is repeated 10 to 15 times per test and repeated replay is required due to the fast and complex nature of swallowing. Consequently, it is difficult to avoid human error due to the fatigue that results from high concentration and repetitive examination. Because of this vulnerability to human error, the reported reliability of VFSS analysis is not excellent; wide variation is present in both intra- and inter-rater agreement (intrarater κ = 0.530~1.00, interrater κ = 0.269~0.700) [5–9].

As an alternative to overcome the limitations of human reading, recent studies have attempted to develop computer-assisted analysis [10–15]. Aung et al. suggested that automated reading enables more objective and immediate analysis with a quantifiable level of accuracy, eliminates the need for high levels of training for analysis and reporting, and provides a platform for larger-scale screening of populations with dysphagia [10]. Computer-assisted analysis typically tracks anatomical landmarks automatically after they are demarcated by humans in the first few frames of the videos [10–15]. However, its clinical usefulness has been limited because most of the models use obsolete semi-automated tracking and segmentation algorithms that require manual demarcation of anatomical landmarks.

Recently, deep learning technology has increased the accuracy of image classification to a level exceeding that of human eyes and is expected to reduce error in reading medical images [16–19]. In a previous study, we developed and proposed a model capable of detecting laryngeal penetration or aspiration from VFSS images in a fully automated manner without any human intervention by applying deep learning algorithms [20]. The model showed an overall accuracy of 97.2% in classifying image frames and 93.2% in classifying video files in which laryngeal penetration or aspiration was evident, exceeding the accuracy of previous semiautomated computer-assisted analysis. The results showed the potential value of the model for clinical practice in many respects, but the evidence for its reliability still seems to be insufficient.

This study aims to examine and compare the intra- and inter-rater reliability of our deep learning model and human examiners for the detection of laryngeal penetration or aspiration from VFSS images. We anticipate that the results of this study may provide further evidence to support the clinical application of deep learning technology in VFSS analysis, although dichotomous results of whether penetration/aspiration was detected or not on VFSS does not always represent the degree of pathology in the swallowing mechanism.

2. Materials and Methods

2.1. Dataset

We collected a total of 205 VFSS video files from 49 patients, aiming for an even distribution of attributes including gender, age, viscosity of diet and degree of laryngeal penetration or aspiration. Presence of the penetration or aspiration was determined using the PAS (Penetration/Aspiration Scale) [21] and videos scored as PAS 2 or higher were included. The video files were selected from the database of Dankook University Hospital, which contains the videos of VFSSs conducted between January 2015 and June 2020. The VFSS was performed according to the protocol described by Logemann [22] with minor modifications. Briefly, video images were acquired via lateral projection at a speed of 30 fps (frames per second) while the seated patients swallowed boluses of various consistencies mixed with contrast medium; the videos were stored digitally. The types of boluses swallowed were as follows: 3 mL of thick liquid (water-soluble barium sulfate diluted to 70%); 3 mL of rice porridge; 3 mL of curd-type yogurt; 3 mL of thin liquid (water-soluble barium sulfate diluted to 35%) from a spoon; or 5 mL of thin liquid from a cup. The video files were selected by an investigator who had more than two years of experience in analysis of VFSS. Every effort was made to select videos in which the presence or absence was evident. The video files were edited to contain only one swallowing event. Each swallowing was defined as the process from the backward movement of bolus in oral cavity to the returning of larynx to original position. A little space was also put on the front and back of the swallowing event to include the whole swallowing event. When the bolus was not fully swallowed in first attempt, subsequent swallows were also included until the bolus was completely swallowed. The videos were not included if they showed remaining of the bolus aspirated from previous swallow in the larynx. Among those files, 32 were excluded due to poor image quality. Ultimately, 173 video files from 42 patients were included in the VFSS dataset; the distribution of their attributes is shown in Table 1. The shortest video lasted 4 s, and the longest video lasted 240 s. The depth of penetration/aspiration was categorized as shallow (PAS 2 or 3), deep (PAS 4 or 5) and aspiration (PAS 6 or higher) and their distribution is shown in Table 1. The proportion of presence and depth was set to equal the overall distribution in database of authors' institution.

Table 1. Characteristics of VFSS dataset for test.

Factors		Number of Video Files (Number of Patients)	%
Gender	Male	87 (21)	50
	Female	86 (21)	50
Age (years)	40–49	35 (8)	20
	50–59	31 (7)	18
	60–69	30 (8)	17
	70–79	35 (7)	20
	80+	42 (12)	24
Viscosity of diet	Thick liquid	40	23
	Rice porridge	41	24
	Curd-type yogurt	35	20
	Thin liquid	33	19
	Cup drinking	24	14
Laryngeal penetration or aspiration	Absent	79	46
	PA2 2–3	44	25
	PAS 4–5	29	17
	PAS 6–8	21	12

2.2. Analysis of VFSS

2.2.1. Machine Reading

The video files were examined for the presence of laryngeal penetration or aspiration using the computer model described in a previous study [20]. In summary, the model consisted of three phases: (1) image normalization, (2) dynamic ROI (region of interest) determination, and (3) detection of laryngeal penetration or aspiration (Figure 1). After the input images were normalized using CLAHE (contrast-limited adaptive histogram equalization) [23], an ROI was defined with reference to the cervical spinal column segmented using U-net. The ROI was set to include the larynx, the cervical spine, and adjacent areas. Noise from the movement of head and neck could be minimized by setting the ROI to move dynamically with the cervical spines. Within the ROI, the presence of laryngeal penetration or aspiration was classified by the deep learning network trained with the Xception module [24]. The output was reported and displayed in the form of histograms as shown in Figure 2. The classification and reporting process was conducted in a fully automated manner without any human intervention except for inputting the image data. Display of at least one peak was considered "positive" result.

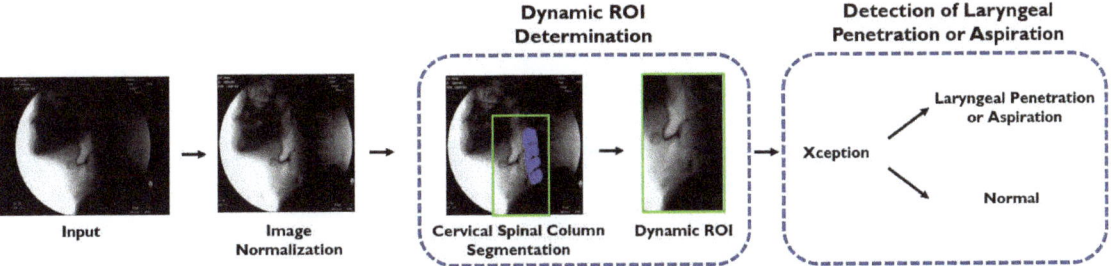

Figure 1. The same deep learning model we proposed in our previous study [20] is used in this study. After normalization of the input images, a dynamic ROI is defined with reference to the cervical spinal column segmented by U-net. The presence of laryngeal penetration or aspiration in the ROI can be identified by the Xception module.

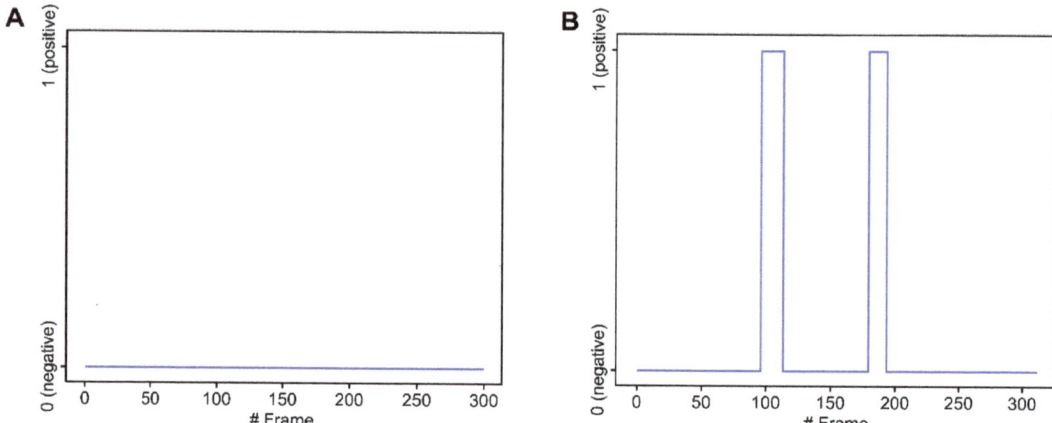

Figure 2. Example output of the deep learning model represented as histograms: (**A**) No laryngeal penetration or aspiration was detected in any frame of the video. (**B**) Laryngeal penetration or aspiration occurred in approximately the 100th to 115th frames and the 180th to 200th frames of the video.

2.2.2. Human Reading

The human raters were three physicians: "Human 1", with more than 20 years of experience in VFSS analysis; "Human 2", with 10 years; and "Human 3", the novice with 1 year. Working in separate locations, the three human examiners judged the existence of laryngeal penetration or aspiration, regardless of severity or depth, in the same video files. When multiple swallowing attempts were included in the video clip, the result was rated as "positive" if any one of the attempts shows penetration/aspiration. Discussion was not allowed, and no information about the subjects in the videos (including gender, age, and medical history) or the viscosity of the bolus was given to the raters.

2.3. Analysis of Intra- and Inter-Rater Reliability

2.3.1. Intrarater Reliability

Trials were conducted in two sessions, separated by four weeks, to calculate the intrarater reliability of machine and human reading. In both sessions, the presence or absence of laryngeal penetration or aspiration was judged by three human raters and the deep learning model. In the second session, 173 video files were reordered and randomly assigned to the raters by an investigator who was blinded to the results of the first session. The results were collected from the three human raters and the model in both sessions, and Cohen's kappa coefficient was calculated. However, the meaning of epidemiological statistics derived in this way can be limited because there is no absolute gold standard for VFSS analysis. Therefore, we used the positive reliability ratio (PRR) and negative reliability ratio (NRR), as suggested by Kuhlemeier et al. [8]. In the absence of a gold standard, PRR and NRR can provide statistics about the agreement between session results from the same interpreter [8]. According to the definition of Kuhlemeier et al. [8], we calculated the PRR as the percentage of cases a given rater judged abnormal in the first session that he or she also judged abnormal in the second session. The NRR was calculated in the same way for normal ratings.

Therefore, the PRR and NRR were calculated by the following formulas:

PRR = Abn(1 and 2)/Abn(1), where Abn(1 and 2) = number rated abnormal in both the first and second sessions and Abn(1) = number rated abnormal in the first session.

NRR = Normal(1 and 2)/Normal(1), where Normal(1 and 2) = number rated normal in both the first and second sessions and Normal(1) = number rated normal in the first session.

2.3.2. Interrater Reliability

The interrater reliability was verified in the same way as the intrarater reliability. As with the intrarater reliability, the interrater PRR and NRR were defined according to the definition by Kuhlemeier et al. [8]. PRR and NRR were calculated between each possible combination of human raters and machine, not between sessions. For interrater reliability, PRR denoted the percentage of cases judged abnormal (i.e., having laryngeal penetration or aspiration) by rater "A" that were also judged abnormal by rater "B". In the same way, NRR was calculated based on the cases judged to be normal.

Thus, interrater PRR and NRR were calculated by the following formulas:

PRR = Abn(A and B)/Abn(A), where Abn(A and B) = number rated abnormal by both "A" and "B" and Abn(A) = number rated abnormal by "A".

NRR = Normal(A and B)/Normal(A), where Normal(A and B) = number rated normal by both "A" and "B" and Normal(A) = number rated normal by "A".

All statistical analysis was performed with SPSS for Windows version 26.0, and the whole study protocol was approved by the institutional review board of Dankook University Hospital (approval No. 2020-11-015).

3. Results

3.1. Intrarater Reliability

Intrarater reliability is shown in Table 2. The kappa coefficients of all human raters showed almost perfect agreement except for Human 3 (a novice physician), who had only moderate agreement. The kappa coefficients of the model showed perfect agreement (intrarater kappa = 1.00), as expected. The PRRs of all human raters were above 90%. The NRRs of experienced human raters (Human 1 and Human 2) were above 90%, but Human 3 showed an NRR of only 68%. The PRR and NRR of the model were both 100%.

Table 2. Intrarater reliability represented by kappa coefficients, PRR and NRR.

	Kappa	PRR (%)	NRR (%)
Human 1	0.830	93	91
Human 2	0.930	96	97
Human 3	0.693	98	68
Model	1.000	100	100

3.2. Interrater Reliability

The interrater kappa coefficients are shown in Table 3. All pairs of two human raters showed substantial agreement in both sessions, except that there was only moderate agreement between Human 2 and Human 3 in the second session. The machine and every human rater also showed substantial agreement in both sessions, except that there was only moderate agreement between the machine and Human 3 in the second session.

Table 3. The interrater Cohen's kappa coefficients.

	Session	Human 2	Human 3	Machine
Human 1	1	0.672	0.781	0.660
	2	0.672	0.668	0.705
Human 2	1		0.672	0.732
	2		0.457	0.732
Human 3	1			0.705
	2			0.488

Scale for kappa coefficient: below 0.00 = poor agreement; 0.00–0.20 = slight agreement; 0.21–0.40 = fair agreement; 0.41–0.60 = moderate agreement; 0.61–0.80 = substantial agreement; 0.81–1.00 = almost perfect agreement.

The calculated PRRs and NRRs are shown in Table 4. Overall, the PRR values ranged from 62% to 100%, and the NRR values ranged from 50% to 100%. No particular pattern was found in the distribution of PRR or NRR among the human and machine ratings. The ratios were somewhat variable among the raters and between sessions. In order to delineate the difference in reliability, the PRR and NRR values were averaged and compared. The average PRR was 86.6% when measured between each pair of human raters and 85.5% when measured between the machine and each human rater. The average NRRs were 82.4%, and 81.3%, respectively. PRR and NRR values were not significantly different regardless of whether they were between human raters or between machine and human raters (Figure 3).

Table 4. PRR and NRR values calculated between each human rater and the machine.

		PRR [1] (%)				NRR [2] (%)			
	Session	Human 1	Human 2	Human 3	Machine	Human 1	Human 2	Human 3	Machine
Human 1	1		73	91	73		100	88	99
	2		73	97	75		99	66	100
Human 2	1	100		99	86	70		70	87
	2	99		99	86	70		50	50
Human 3	1	92	73		75	85	99		100
	2	82	62		63	94	98		100
Machine	1	99	85	100		69	88	72	
	2	100	85	100		72	88	51	

[1] positive reliability ratio = Abn(A and B)/Abn(A), [2] negative reliability ratio = Normal(A and B)/Normal(A).: A changes according to rows into Human 1, Human 2, Huma 3, Model, and B changes according to columns into Human 1, Human 2, Human 3, Model. See the method Section 2.3 for further details.

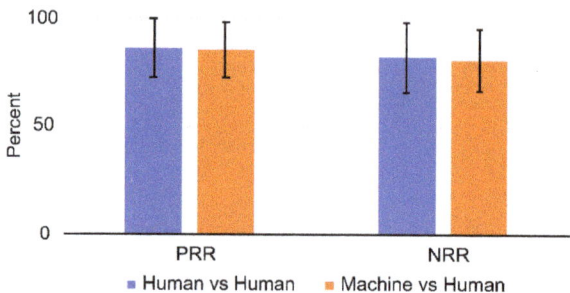

Figure 3. PRR and NRR values averaged between human raters and between machine and human raters.

4. Discussion

One of the major limitations of VFSS is unsatisfactory interrater reliability. Its poor reliability may originate from the rapidity and complexity of the swallowing process and resultant difficulties in its analysis [25], as well as incomplete standardization of the definitions and judgment criteria of parameters [9]. Several methods have been used to improve the reliability of VFSS, including training and education [26], group discussion [25], directed search [27], frame-by-frame observation [5] and computer-assisted automated analysis [10–15]. Most previously proposed computer-assisted analyses use semiautomated algorithms that require human manual demarcation of salient anatomical structures [10–15]. To our knowledge, the deep learning model we proposed in our previous study was the first fully automated model capable of detecting laryngeal penetration or aspiration in VFSS images [20]. The model showed more than 90% accuracy, but its reliability has not been tested sufficiently. The reliability of computer-assisted analysis, whether with semiautomated or deep learning models, has never been compared with that of human examination. This is the first study designed to compare the reliability of machine and human examiners for VFSS analysis and demonstrate the reliability of VFSS analysis using a deep learning model.

Since there is not yet an absolute gold standard for the analysis of VFSS results, the significance of classical epidemiologic statistics, such as the kappa coefficient, intraclass correlation coefficient or positive and negative predictive values, may be limited for assessing the reliability or validity of VFSS analysis. Kuhlemeier et al. [8] proposed that the PRR and NRR, modified from the positive and negative predictive values, can be useful for verifying the reliability or agreement among raters in the absence of a gold standard. They used the PRR to denote the probability that a condition that has been judged to be abnormal by a rater will also be judged the same by a separate rater or in a second rating by the same rater [8]. Similarly, the NRR was used to denote the probability that a rating of "normal" would be followed by a second rating of "normal" either by a different rater or by the same rater at a different time [8]. In this study, we used the PRR and NRR in addition to the kappa coefficient to increase statistical strength.

The results of reliability analysis for VFSS data can be influenced by test videos because VFSS data frequently shows diverse findings according to the severity and type of dysphagia. If the test videos contain only mild or vague laryngeal penetrations and aspirations, raters may have difficulties in judgment, and the reliability will be lowered. If the videos contain only severe laryngeal penetrations and aspirations, agreement between the raters may appear excessively high because judgment of definite laryngeal penetration or aspiration might be easy for all raters. We made our best effort to include test videos with a balanced distribution of characteristics, including the gender and age of patients and the viscosity of the diet. Efforts were also made to include patients with diverse degrees of penetration and aspiration in the test dataset. In this way, we believe that selection bias was minimized in the measurement of reliability.

The experience of the raters may also affect the results of reliability analysis. [25]. Experienced raters usually have highly accurate standards of judgment, while less experienced raters can have confusion or difficulty in making decisions. We invited and compared three human raters with different levels of experience to minimize the effect of experience. The raters comprised one with more than 20 years of experience, one with approximately 10 years and one with approximately one year. We believe that the bias caused by different degrees of experience was minimized by comparing human raters with different experience levels. In addition to experiences, more extensive training also affected the difference between experienced and less experienced examiners because it had been recommended for precise use of the Penetration/Aspiration Scale [26].

As expected, the intrarater reliability was excellent for human and machine reading except in the novice physician (Human 3). Regarding interrater reliability, the kappa coefficients between the deep learning model and each human rater showed moderate to substantial agreement, except for Human 2 vs Human 3 and the machine vs Human 3 in the second session. Human 3 showed the lowest agreement with other human raters and machines as well as the lowest intrarater reliability, suggesting that experience may play an important role in the analysis of VFSS results by humans. It is reasonable to speculate that our deep learning model might be more reliable than an inexperienced human reader for VFSS analysis.

The PRRs showed inconsistent results both between human raters and between the machine and human raters, but the values were generally above 70%, except for Human 3 in the second session. It can be speculated that the agreement between experienced human raters and the deep learning model is high for positive results (the presence of penetration or aspiration). The lower PRR values between Human 3 and the other human raters as well as the machine may again suggest that interrater agreement may be affected by the raters' experience level. The PRRs of the machine to the human raters showed almost perfect agreement (above 80%), although the PRRs of the human raters to the machine showed much lower values. The meaning of the difference between "machine-to-human" and "human-to-machine" PRRs is unclear. The NRRs, meaning the agreement for negative results (the absence of laryngeal penetration or aspiration), were generally lower, but not by a wide margin. To compare the agreement between the human raters and the agreement between the machine and human raters, we averaged and compared the PRRs and NRRs. The differences were not significant, suggesting that the overall agreement between the machine and human raters was noninferior to that between the human raters for both positive and negative results.

These results indicate that computer-assisted analysis using a deep learning model is a reliable method for detecting laryngeal penetration or aspiration through a VFSS. Considering its consistency and efficiency, deep learning computer analysis could provide good assistance to human examiners, who are vulnerable to fatigue and variability. It is anticipated that machine reading with a deep learning model will be able to improve the reliability and accuracy of VFSS analysis by reducing the time and effort required of human observers. The concept of computer-assisted detection of penetration or aspiration is of great clinical value for many reasons such as the potential for lower cost screening for aspiration or the facilitation of telehealth.

This study has several limitations. In the present study, human raters and the machine judged the existence of laryngeal penetration or aspiration only, although most VFSS examiners evaluate the depth and amount of laryngeal penetration or aspiration as well as its presence. The ultimate purpose of VFSS is not only to detect penetration or aspiration, but also to evaluate the pathophysiology and mechanism of swallowing. However, variables other than laryngeal penetration and aspiration were not considered in the analysis because the deep learning model was designed and trained only for the detection of laryngeal penetration or aspiration. Therefore, the machine described in this study is at best a prototype that proves that penetration/aspiration can be detected by computers, but in no way resembles human interpretation of VFSS at least for now. There was no distinction between penetration and aspiration in this study, although they have different clinical meanings [28]. Dynamics of continuous eating was not verified in this study because the analysis was limited to the video containing only one swallowing event. Additionally, the meaning and usefulness of the reliability results might be limited by the absence of a gold standard for comparison. For the same reason, selection bias could not be eliminated completely in choice of video files although we made every effort to avoid it. Despite these limitations, we believe that machine reading by a deep learning algorithm can assist human observers, helping to minimize the variability and improve the efficiency of VFSS analysis. Further studies are required to develop more sophisticated models that can assess VFSS images more comprehensively. The results presented in this study are only descriptive statistics. This study did not aim to determine the superiority or inferiority of machine reading, only to demonstrate its usefulness.

5. Conclusions

Computer analysis using a deep learning model can provide a reliable method for detecting the existence of laryngeal penetration or aspiration in VFSS images. This deep learning model has promising prospects for use in VFSS analysis although further research will be required to increase its reliability and accuracy.

Author Contributions: Conceptualization, S.J.L. and Y.K.; methodology, S.-I.C., H.-I.K., S.J.L. and Y.K.; software, H.-I.K. and S.-I.C.; validation, S.J.L. and S.-I.C.; formal analysis, S.J.L. and Y.K.; investigation, Y.K., S.J.L., G.S.P. and S.Y.K.; resources, S.J.L. and Y.K.; data curation, Y.K. and S.J.L.; writing—original draft preparation, Y.K.; writing—review and editing, S.J.L., S.Y.K. and S.-I.C.; visualization, Y.K. and H.-I.K.; supervision, S.J.L. and S.-I.C.; project administration, S.J.L.; funding acquisition, S.J.L. and S.-I.C. All authors have read and agreed to the published version of the manuscript.

Funding: This work was supported in part by the National Research Foundation of Korea through the Korean Government (MSIT) under 2021R1A2B5B01001412 and in part by the Basic Science Research Program through the National Research Foundation of Korea (NRF) funded by the Ministry of Education (Grant Number 2018R1D1A3B07049300).

Institutional Review Board Statement: The study was conducted according to the guidelines of the Declaration of Helsinki and approved by the Institutional Review Board of Dankook University Hospital (IRB No. 2020-11-015).

Informed Consent Statement: Not applicable.

Data Availability Statement: The data presented in this study are available from the corresponding author upon reasonable request.

Conflicts of Interest: The authors declare no conflict of interest.

References

1. Martin-Harris, B.; Logemann, J.A.; McMahon, S.; Schleicher, M.; Sandidge, J. Clinical utility of the modified barium swallow. *Dysphagia* **2000**, *15*, 136–141. [CrossRef] [PubMed]
2. Martin-Harris, B.; Jones, B. The videofluorographic swallowing study. *Phys. Med. Rehabil. Clin. N. Am.* **2008**, *19*, 769–785. [CrossRef] [PubMed]
3. Logemann, J.A. Behavioral management for oropharyngeal dysphagia. *Folia Phoniatr. Et Logop.* **1999**, *51*, 199–212. [CrossRef]
4. Robbins, J.; Coyle, J.; Rosenbek, J.; Roecker, E.; Wood, J. Differentiation of normal and abnormal airway protection during swallowing using the penetration–aspiration scale. *Dysphagia* **1999**, *14*, 228–232. [CrossRef] [PubMed]
5. Baijens, L.; Barikroo, A.; Pilz, W. Intrarater and interrater reliability for measurements in videofluoroscopy of swallowing. *Eur. J. Radiol.* **2013**, *82*, 1683–1695. [CrossRef] [PubMed]
6. Kim, D.H.; Choi, K.H.; Kim, H.M.; Koo, J.H.; Kim, B.R.; Kim, T.W.; Ryu, J.S.; Im, S.; Choi, I.S.; Pyun, S.B. Inter-rater reliability of videofluoroscopic dysphagia scale. *Ann. Rehabil. Med.* **2012**, *36*, 791. [CrossRef]
7. McCullough, G.H.; Wertz, R.T.; Rosenbek, J.C.; Mills, R.H.; Webb, W.G.; Ross, K.B. Inter-and intrajudge reliability for videofluoroscopic swallowing evaluation measures. *Dysphagia* **2001**, *16*, 110–118. [CrossRef]
8. Kuhlemeier, K.; Yates, P.; Palmer, J. Intra-and interrater variation in the evaluation of videofluorographic swallowing studies. *Dysphagia* **1998**, *13*, 142–147. [CrossRef]
9. Stoeckli, S.J.; Huisman, T.A.; Seifert, B.A.; Martin–Harris, B.J. Interrater reliability of videofluoroscopic swallow evaluation. *Dysphagia* **2003**, *18*, 53–57. [CrossRef]
10. Aung, M.S.; Goulermas, J.Y.; Hamdy, S.; Power, M. Spatiotemporal visualizations for the measurement of oropharyngeal transit time from videofluoroscopy. *IEEE Trans. Biomed. Eng.* **2009**, *57*, 432–441. [CrossRef]
11. Aung, M.; Goulermas, J.; Stanschus, S.; Hamdy, S.; Power, M. Automated anatomical demarcation using an active shape model for videofluoroscopic analysis in swallowing. *Med. Eng. Phys.* **2010**, *32*, 1170–1179. [CrossRef] [PubMed]
12. Chang, M.W.; Lin, E.; Hwang, J.-N. Contour tracking using a knowledge-based snake algorithm to construct three-dimensional pharyngeal bolus movement. *Dysphagia* **1999**, *14*, 219–227. [CrossRef] [PubMed]
13. Hossain, I.; Roberts-South, A.; Jog, M.; El-Sakka, M.R. Semi-automatic assessment of hyoid bone motion in digital videofluoroscopic images. *Comput. Methods Biomech. Biomed. Eng. Imaging Vis.* **2014**, *2*, 25–37. [CrossRef]
14. Lee, W.H.; Chun, C.; Seo, H.G.; Lee, S.H.; Oh, B.-M. STAMPS: Development and verification of swallowing kinematic analysis software. *BioMed. Eng. OnLine* **2017**, *16*, 1–12. [CrossRef]
15. Natarajan, R.; Stavness, I.; Pearson, W., Jr. Semi-automatic tracking of hyolaryngeal coordinates in videofluoroscopic swallowing studies. *Comput. Methods Biomech. Biomed. Eng. Imaging Vis.* **2017**, *5*, 379–389. [CrossRef]
16. Dong, Y.; Pan, Y.; Zhang, J.; Xu, W. Learning to read chest X-ray images from 16000+ examples using CNN. In Proceedings of the 2017 IEEE/ACM International Conference on Connected Health: Applications, Systems and Engineering Technologies (CHASE), Philadelphia, PA, USA, 17–19 July 2017; pp. 51–57.
17. Le, M.H.; Chen, J.; Wang, L.; Wang, Z.; Liu, W.; Cheng, K.-T.T.; Yang, X. Automated diagnosis of prostate cancer in multi-parametric MRI based on multimodal convolutional neural networks. *Phys. Med. Biol.* **2017**, *62*, 6497. [CrossRef] [PubMed]
18. Lundervold, A.S.; Lundervold, A. An overview of deep learning in medical imaging focusing on MRI. *Z. Für Med. Phys.* **2019**, *29*, 102–127. [CrossRef]
19. Song, Q.; Zhao, L.; Luo, X.; Dou, X. Using deep learning for classification of lung nodules on computed tomography images. *J. Healthc. Eng.* **2017**, *2017*. [CrossRef] [PubMed]
20. Lee, S.J.; Ko, J.Y.; Kim, H.I.; Choi, S.-I. Automatic Detection of Airway Invasion from Videofluoroscopy via Deep Learning Technology. *Appl. Sci.* **2020**, *10*, 6179. [CrossRef]
21. Rosenbek, J.C.; Robbins, J.A.; Roecker, E.B.; Coyle, J.L.; Wood, J.L. A penetration-aspiration scale. *Dysphagia* **1996**, *11*, 93–98. [CrossRef] [PubMed]
22. Logemann, J.A. Evaluation and treatment of swallowing disorders. *Am. J. Speech-Lang. Pathol.* **1994**, *3*, 41–44. [CrossRef]
23. Zuiderveld, K. Contrast limited adaptive histogram equalization. In *Graphics Gems IV*; Academic Press Professional Inc.: Cambridge, MA, USA, 1994; pp. 474–485.
24. Chollet, F. Xception: Deep Learning with Depthwise Separable Convolutions. In Proceedings of the 2017 IEEE Conference on Computer Vision and Pattern Recognition (CVPR), Honolulu, HI, USA, 21–26 July 2017; pp. 1800–1807.

25. Scott, A.; Perry, A.; Bench, J. A study of interrater reliability when using videofluoroscopy as an assessment of swallowing. *Dysphagia* **1998**, *13*, 223–227. [CrossRef]
26. Hind, J.A.; Gensler, G.; Brandt, D.K.; Gardner, P.J.M.; Blumenthal, L.; Gramigna, G.D.; Kosek, S.; Lundy, D.; McGarvey-Toler, S.; Rockafellow, S. Comparison of trained clinician ratings with expert ratings of aspiration on videofluoroscopic images from a randomized clinical trial. *Dysphagia* **2009**, *24*, 211. [CrossRef]
27. Bryant, K.N.; Finnegan, E.; Berbaum, K. VFS interjudge reliability using a free and directed search. *Dysphagia* **2012**, *27*, 53–63. [CrossRef] [PubMed]
28. Allen, J.E.; White, C.J.; Leonard, R.J.; Belafsky, P.C. Prevalence of penetration and aspiration on videofluoroscopy in normal individuals without dysphagia. *Otolaryngol. Head Neck Surg.* **2010**, *142*, 208–213. [CrossRef] [PubMed]

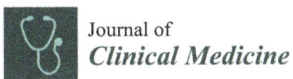

Article

The Effectiveness of Rehabilitation of Occupational Voice Disorders in a Health Resort Hospital Environment

Anna Sinkiewicz [1,*], Agnieszka Garstecka [1], Hanna Mackiewicz-Nartowicz [1], Lidia Nawrocka [1], Wioletta Wojciechowska [2] and Agata Szkiełkowska [3]

1. Department of Otolaryngology, Audiology and Phoniatrics, University Hospital No. 2, Collegium Medicum, Nicolaus Copernicus University in Toruń, Ujejskiego 75 Street, 85-168 Bydgoszcz, Poland; agnieszka@laryngolog.org (A.G.); hamack@cm.umk.pl (H.M.-N.); lidia.nawrocka@cm.umk.pl (L.N.)
2. Health Resort Hospital in Ciechocinek, Institute of Medical Sciences, Cuiavian University in Włocławek, PlacWolności 1 Street, 87-800 Włocławek, Poland; w.wojciechowska@ksuc.pl
3. Department of Audiology and Phoniatrics, Institute of Pathology and Physiology of Hearing, Maurycego Mochnackiego 10 Street, 02-042 Warszawa, Poland; a.szkielkowska@ifps.org.pl
* Correspondence: manuscriptsubmission02.21@gmail.com

Citation: Sinkiewicz, A.; Garstecka, A.; Mackiewicz-Nartowicz, H.; Nawrocka, L.; Wojciechowska, W.; Szkiełkowska, A. The Effectiveness of Rehabilitation of Occupational Voice Disorders in a Health Resort Hospital Environment. *J. Clin. Med.* **2021**, *10*, 2581. https://doi.org/10.3390/jcm10122581

Academic Editor: Renee Speyer

Received: 8 April 2021
Accepted: 8 June 2021
Published: 11 June 2021

Publisher's Note: MDPI stays neutral with regard to jurisdictional claims in published maps and institutional affiliations.

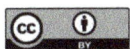

Copyright: © 2021 by the authors. Licensee MDPI, Basel, Switzerland. This article is an open access article distributed under the terms and conditions of the Creative Commons Attribution (CC BY) license (https://creativecommons.org/licenses/by/4.0/).

Abstract: Background: The aim of this study was to present a rehabilitation program of occupational voice disorders for teachers, conducted in the form of health resort stays, and evaluate its effectiveness depending on job seniority. Methods: The study included 420 teachers who participated in a complex vocal prophylactic and rehabilitation program carried out during a 24-day stay at a health resort hospital. Employment time varied from 4 to 45 years (mean 28.3 years). The participants were divided into three groups: employment time < 21 years (57 teachers), 21–30 years (182 teachers) and > 30 years (181 teachers). All of the subjects underwent maximum phonation time assessment as well as jitter, shimmer and NHR (noise to harmonic ratio) parameters assessment before and after the program; they also underwent perceptual evaluation using the GRBAS scale and voice self-assessment using the VHI-30 scale. Results: The perceptual evaluation using the GRBAS scale and self-report measures of voice function assessed using the VHI scale revealed improvement ($p < 0.001$). The parameters of jitter, shimmer and NHR improved significantly: jitter $p < 0.001$, shimmer $p < 0.001$ and NHR $p < 0.003$. Maximum phonation time increased slightly but significantly ($p < 0.001$). For all of the studied groups regardless of their employment time, maximum phonation time increased ($p < 0.001$). Initially, the lowest values of maximum phonation time were observed in teachers with longer job seniority, which improved after the rehabilitation but remained <15 s. Conclusions: Voice care for teachers is crucial regardless of their job seniority. Early prophylaxis for voice disorders is effective, as the results of rehabilitation are better in teachers with a shorter employment time.

Keywords: occupational voice disorders; prevention; prophylaxis; teachers; occupational health; voice training; balneotherapy

1. Introduction

For teachers, the ability to tolerate strain on their vocal organ is essential for safe and comfortable work. Vocal hygiene and stress resistance also play an important role. School teaching is considered to be a profession at a higher risk for developing voice disorders [1,2]. The percentage of teachers with voice problems ranges from 13% [3] to 94% [4]. Lack of sufficient preparation of some teachers for frequent use of their voice at work [5–7], difficult working conditions such as noise, working long hours without rest and poor climatic conditions in classrooms result in a higher prevalence of voice disorders than in the general population [8]. The influence of other significant factors on the occurrence of voice disorders, such as age and gender, is also important [9]. Long periods of treatment, surgical interventions and sick leave are associated with high financial costs [2]. This is a widespread social problem involving not only health but also economical aspects [10,11]. It is therefore important to search for effective methods of prevention and rehabilitation programs for occupational voice disorders.

The effectiveness of complex voice rehabilitation programs in ambulatory care has been assessed by many authors [12–15]. It was observed that vocal hygiene training significantly improves voice quality and reduces disorder symptoms [16,17]. Multicenter efforts to improve quality of care for persons professionally and strenuously using their voice resulted in the development of an interdisciplinary 24-day vocal prophylactic and rehabilitation program conducted in health resort hospitals [18].

The aim of this study was to evaluate the effectiveness of the prevention and rehabilitation program for voice disorders in teachers conducted in a health resort hospital, with analyses of the factors affecting the outcomes.

2. Materials and Methods

The study was completed in accordance with the ethical standards of the institutional research committee and principles of the World Medical Association Declaration of Helsinki Ethical Principles for Medical Research involving Human Subjects. Ethical approval for this study was obtained from the Ethics Committee of the Collegium Medicum, Nicolaus Copernicus University. Written informed consent was obtained from patients before the study.

This program has been implemented in 5 health resort hospitals in Poland, localized in places with a mild climate favorable to the treatment of respiratory diseases. A total of 3685 participants, 3440 female (93.3%) and 245 male (6.7%) participated in a complex rehabilitation program conducted in one health resort hospital between the years 2015–2019.

The study included teachers who had participated in a 24-day vocal prophylactic and rehabilitation program in 2019. The study group consisted of 420 participants aged 28–64 years (mean 51.4 years) with employment time that varied from 4 years to 45 years (mean 28.3 years). As the teaching profession in Poland is female dominated, all participants included in the study were females who were diagnosed with hyperfunctional dysphonia. Dysphonia had been diagnosed by a referring physician, and the diagnosis was confirmed by an initial phoniatric examination. In order to unify the assessment of voice rehabilitation results and the evaluation of voice acoustic parameters, the study group excluded males and females diagnosed with other diseases, such as glottic insufficiency or chronic hypertrophic laryngitis, which are often permanent voice disorders. Male teachers experience voice disorders less frequently and they constituted only 6.7% of the respondents.

Depending on their employment time, the participants were divided into three groups (Table 1).

Table 1. Employment time.

Employment Time (Years)	Number of Patients	Mean Employment Time (Years)
<21	57	15.3
21–30	182	26.8
>30	181	34.0
Total	420	28.3

All of the study participants were subjected to the following initial medical examination: family history taking, laryngological and phoniatric examination. Maximum phonation time (MPT) was obtained as the maximum value of three subsequent trials for each participant to sustain the vowel /a/ for as long as possible using a comfortable pitch and volume [19]:

Perceptual voice evaluation of voice disorders were evaluated using the GRBAS scale: overall grade (G), the degree of hoarse throat intensity; roughness (R), rough voice; breathiness (B), puffing character of voice; asthenia (A), weak voice; and strain (S), voice

tension. Each parameter was evaluated on a 4-point scale: 0 (normal), 1 (mild), 2 (moderate), 3 (severe), (Figure 1). The following were also evaluated:
- Videostroboscopy;
- Voice self-assessment: Voice Handicap Index 30 (VHI 30);
- Acoustic analysis of voice;
- Assessment of vocal effort;
- Speech therapists examination;
- Pure tone audiometry.

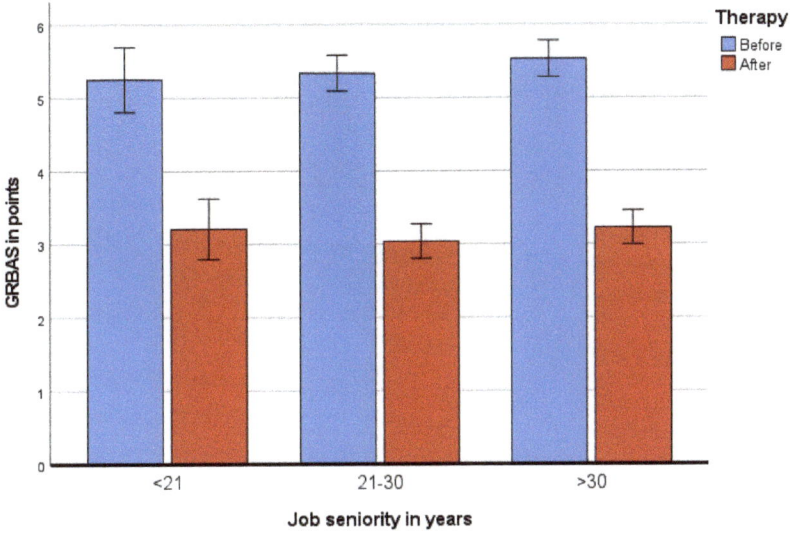

Figure 1. Changes in perceptual voice assessment on the GRBAS scale after the rehabilitation program in groups by their job seniority (the range for the GRBAS scale was 0–15 points).

The assessments were made during the initial examination by a phoniatrist and a speech therapist. The VHI voice self-assessment scale proposed by Jacobson et al. [20] in 1997, the Polish version of which was developed by Pruszewicz et al. in 2004 [21], comprises ten voice disorder variables in three domains: emotional, physical and functional. Patients are requested to note their frequency of each variable on a five-point scale (never, almost never, sometimes, almost ways, always). The score ranges from 30 (unaffected) to 120 (severely affected), (Figure 2) [20,21].

Analysis of voice acoustic parameters (Jitter, Schimmer, NHR) was performed using the DiagnoScope Specialist software [22], before and after the treatment.

The vocal prophylactic and rehabilitation program included educational lectures, voice therapy, physiotherapy and psychotherapy. Educational lectures consisted of vocal hygiene, voice emission mechanisms, voice control, proper voice emission and vocal effort, as well as disorders and laryngeal problems caused by voice abuse, misuse or overuse. The lectures were conducted by a phoniatrist and a speech therapist 5 times per week with durations of 45 min.

Voice rehabilitation consisted of individual and group classes, including relaxation techniques, proper breathing technique, posture, voice emission, articulation and activation of resonators. The aim of the exercises was to eliminate improper breathing, speech and articulation habits, and develop correct habits. Particular attention was paid to voice stabilization and the extension of the phonation time [23]. The exercises were conducted to gain and consolidate the ability to produce a soft voice attack, as well as to enhance the upper vocal tract resonance. A speech therapist conducted individual exercises once a day for 20 min 5 days a week and 30-min group meetings twice a week.

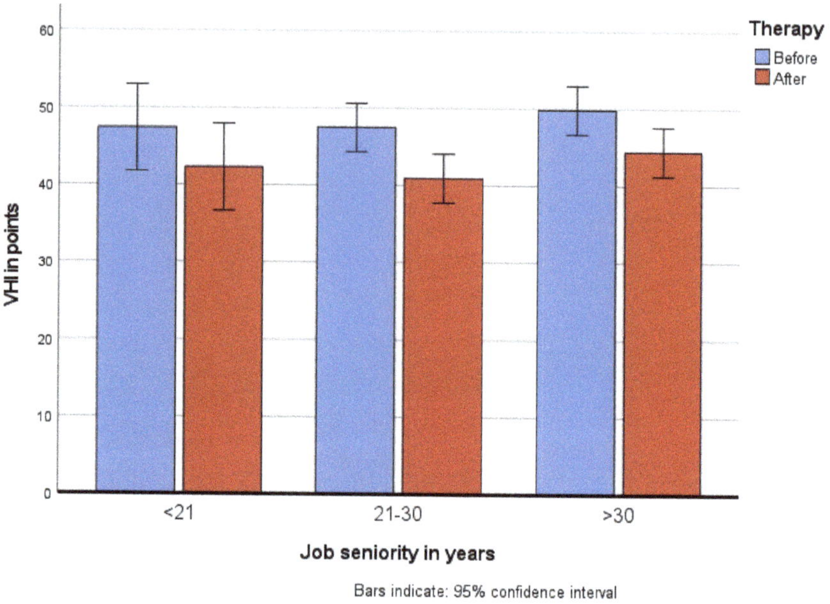

Figure 2. Changes in voice self-assessment on VHI scale after the rehabilitation program in groups by their job seniority.

Physiotherapy included manual therapy, calcium iontophoresis and inhalations. Individual and group psychotherapy was an important part of the program, and focused on stress therapy and stress management techniques. Phoniatric assessment was carried out twice during the program.

All participants were taken care of by the same team of 2 phoniatrists, 3 speech therapists, 3 physiotherapists and 1 psychologist.

The data were statistically analyzed using the IBM SPSS 25.0.0.1 Toruń, Poland. Analysis of variance was conducted (the therapy effects were tested with the repeated measures; 3 groups depending on their employment time were compared using between group factor in analyses of variance). The Greenhouse–Geisser correction was used when the assumption of sphericity was violated.

3. Results

In the perceptual voice evaluation using the GRBAS scale, a statistically significant improvement after therapy ($F_{(1417)} = 730.33$; $p < 0.001$, $\eta_p^2 = 0.64$) was achieved in all voice qualities.

Voice self-assessment on VHI scale improved by more than 6 points after therapy in all the subjects, with a statistical significance of ($F_{(1417)} = 35.96$; $p < 0.001$, $\eta_p^2 = 0.08$).

In all groups, regardless of the employment time, MPT prolongation was observed ($F_{(1417)} = 39.48$; $p < 0.001$, $\eta_p^2 = 0.09$). The initial MPT was the shortest in the group with the longest job seniority. After the rehabilitation, MPT improved, as in the other groups, but remained <15 s. Job seniority had the main effect ($F_{(1417)} = 3.67$; $p = 0.026$, $\eta_p^2 = 0.02$). Group comparison showed that MPT in the group with job seniority of up to 20 years differed significantly ($p = 0.038$) from MPT in the patient group with job seniority of over 30 years (Figure 3).

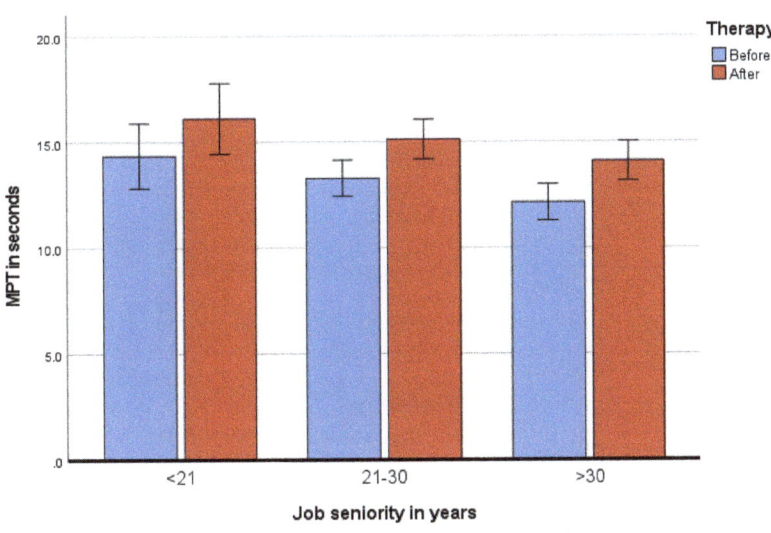

Figure 3. Changes in MPT after the rehabilitation program in groups by their job seniority.

In the presented studies, the perceptual voice evaluation using the GRBAS scale, in all features combined, showed a statistically significant improvement and was consistent with both the results of voice self-assessment (VHI questionnaire) and the objective acoustic analyses of the jitter ($F_{(1417)} = 28.27; p < 0.001, \eta_p^2 = 0.06$), shimmer ($F_{(1417)} = 10.26; p = 0.001, \eta_p^2 = 0.02$) and NHR parameters ($F_{(1417)} = 9.12; p = 0.003, \eta_p^2 = 0.02$), (Figure 4).

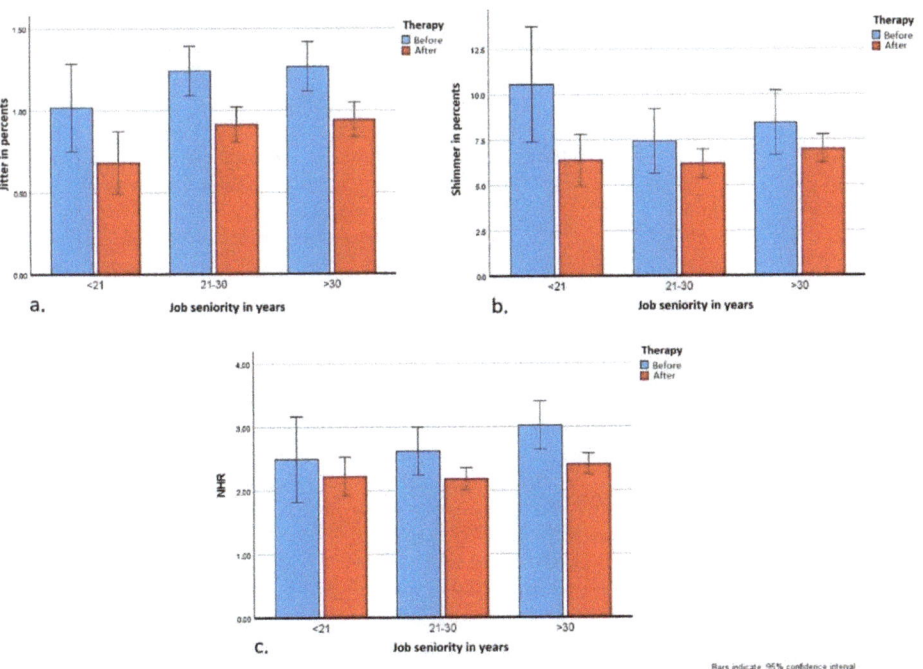

Figure 4. Changes in acoustic parameters after the rehabilitation program in groups by their job seniority: (**a**) jitter; (**b**) shimmer; (**c**) NHR.

4. Discussion

Complex voice rehabilitation in the form of stationary health resort treatments sets up conditions for focusing solely on this activity for 24 days, and gives the opportunity to combine systematic exercises, simultaneous physiotherapy and mental relaxation. It is important that the therapy does not cause any voice strain. A break from work without active voice rehabilitation is just a rest, and returning to work means a return to abnormal voice emission patterns and the recurrence of symptoms. Harmful habits, such as an uneconomical breathing pattern practiced for years, lack of control over the laryngeal muscles, speaking too loudly or clearing the throat by grunting, cannot be changed by a one-time recommendation from a physician.

The main problem of rehabilitation psychology is to stimulate the motivation to implement a rehabilitation program [24]. Health resort treatments give the opportunity to start and maintain a healthy lifestyle. This is facilitated by a comfortable sense of well-being related to rest and relaxation, as well as climatic conditions beneficial to the respiratory tract. An important part of the primary and secondary prevention of voice disorders is physical activity, which is often neglected by teachers. A survey by Rosłaniec et al. showed that over 40% of the respondents did not practice physical activity on a regular basis [25]. Other studies have revealed a relationship between the prevalence of voice disorders and a lack of physical activity. Teachers who did not practice physical activity were diagnosed with dysphonia more often than those who exercised three or more times a week [26]. The rehabilitation program offers daily breathing and relaxation exercises. Moreover, participants receive individual recommendations on how to continue exercising at home.

The conditions of health resort-based treatments are particularly conducive to health education, because highly qualified professionals have extensive experience in conducting lectures, talks or interactive workshops. The patients have also free time during their stay, and therefore are positive about participating in educational activities. An educated patient is more independent, has a better quality of life, understands medical recommendations better and turns to specialists for advice less frequently [27].

Data presented on the basis of extensive meta-analyses show that occupational voice disorders are not only caused by the excessive use of voice but are also related to working environments and general health, as well as psychological and sociodemographic factors [9,13,28]. The presented study did not show any worse results from the health resort treatment in patients with comorbidities according to the MPT, jitter, shimmer and NHR acoustic parameters and the GRBAS perceptual evaluation. On the other hand, better initial MPT values were found in teachers with the shortest job seniority, which made their phonation time the longest after the therapy, with a similar improvement in all study groups. The results of the study showed that voice rehabilitation is important in each group, regardless of the employment time; however, the initial breathing capacity and laryngeal muscles are better in younger patients.

A study by Vaca et al., showed that an age above 50 is associated with an increased risk of voice disorders [29]. Weaker tension of the respiratory and laryngeal muscles can have a negative impact on vocal endurance and voice quality, especially when both deficits occur concomitantly. Voice changes usually refer to difficulties in maintaining the fundamental frequency and shorter phonation time [30]. Patients with the longest work experience are less likely to achieve the desired outcomes of voice rehabilitation, which may not result only from the physiological changes related to age. The study by Rosłaniec et al., showed that teachers over 50 years of age complied with the rules of voice emission and hygiene to a much lesser extent than younger teachers. The VHI voice self-assessment questionnaire is a recognized and useful tool for assessing the progress of voice therapy [31–33]. Teachers' high sensitivity and expectations regarding their own voice make the VHI scale particularly useful in this professional group. However, it is not the numerical value of the VHI test itself that is important but the degree of improvement after treatment [34]. In the study group, after the health resort stay, the voice self-assessment based on the VHI scale improved in all respondents by more than six points ($p < 0.001$).

An improvement in voice parameters after 24 days of an intensive complex rehabilitation program is an expected result. Many authors demonstrated an improvement in the voice of teachers undergoing outpatient rehabilitation [14,35,36].

Therefore, does the presented rehabilitation program allow the intended aim to be achieved more effectively?

Launching a preventive and rehabilitative program based on a health resort hospital environment requires the initial organization of a diagnostic and rehabilitation base with a team of specialists, and the development of a code of conduct. It is also important to adopt uniform criteria to qualify participants. According to the program assumptions, people with the greatest chance of improving their vocal endurance and voice quality should qualify for the program, which will then enable them to continue their professional career.

Based on over 5 years of experience with complex health resort-based rehabilitation and the meta-analysis by Byeon, it can be concluded that the essential preconditions for the effectiveness and durability of the treatment are: the condition of the vocal apparatus without permanent disorders, comorbidities that affect the vocal function of the larynx and active participation in all conducted activities [32].

Given the benefits of this type of therapy, but also limitations such as a 24-day absence from work and considerable costs of the stay and treatment, it is necessary to develop the optimal, possible frequency of participation in such a rehabilitation program. Repetition of health resort treatments offers a chance to consolidate acquired skills and habits, especially in patients with shorter job seniority.

5. Conclusions

In the search for effective methods of prevention and therapy of voice disorders in teachers, it should be recognized that health resort rehabilitation is an attractive form of treatment, as it combines vocal rest with active rehabilitation and health education. An additional advantage of such rehabilitation is climate therapy. Various studies confirmed the purposefulness of voice care at every career stage; however, from the perspective of health and labor economics, early prevention is more appropriate because there is a better chance for voice regeneration for people with shorter work experience.

The co-financing of such rehabilitation is also of great importance, as its multidisciplinarity is associated with considerable costs. In the end, however, the benefits outweigh the otherwise possible expenses related to illness treatment, sick leave and other problems related to the continuation of participants' professional careers.

Author Contributions: Conceptualization, A.G. and A.S. (Anna Sinkiewicz); Methodology, A.S. (Anna Sinkiewicz), A.G., H.M.-N. and L.N.; Literature Review, A.S. (Anna Sinkiewicz), A.G. and H.M.-N.; Data Analysis, A.S. (Anna Sinkiewicz), A.G. and H.M-N.; Original Draft Preparation, A.S. (Anna Sinkiewicz), L.N. and W.W.; Review and Editing: A.S. (Anna Sinkiewicz), A.G. and A.S. (Agata Szkiełkowska); Visualization, L.N. and W.W.; Validation, A.S. (Anna Sinkiewicz), A.G., W.W. and A.S. (Agata Szkiełkowska); Data Auration, H.M.-N. and W.W.; Supervision A.S. (Anna Sinkiewicz); Project Administration, L.N. and A.S. (Agata Szkiełkowska). All authors have read and agreed to the published version of the manuscript.

Institutional Review Board Statement: The study was completed in accordance with the ethical standards of the institutional research committee and principles of the World Medical Association Declaration of Helsinki Ethical Principles for Medical Research involving Human Subjects. Ethical approval for this study was obtained from Ethics Committee of the Collegium Medicum, Nicolaus Copernicus University.

Informed Consent Statement: Informed consent was obtained from all subjects involved in the study.

Data Availability Statement: All data used to support the finding of this study are available from the corresponding author upon request.

Acknowledgments: In this section, you can acknowledge any support given which is not covered by the author contribution or funding sections. This may include administrative and technical support, or donations in kind (e.g., materials used for experiments).

Conflicts of Interest: The authors declare no conflict of interest.

References

1. Thibeault, S.L.; Merrill, R.M.; Roy, N.; Gray, S.D.; Smith, E.M. Occupational risk factors associated with voice disorders among teachers. *Ann. Epidemiol.* **2004**, *14*, 786–792. [CrossRef]
2. Thomas, G.; De Jong, F.I.; Kooijman, P.G.; Donders, A.R.; Cremers, C.W. Voice complaints, risk factors for voice problems and history of voice problems in relation to puberty in female student teachers. *Folia Phoniatr. Logop.* **2006**, *58*, 305–322. [CrossRef]
3. Jónsdottir, V.I.; Boyle, B.E.; Martin, P.J.; Sigurdardottir, G. A comparison of the occurrence and nature of vocal symptoms in two groups of Icelandic teachers. *Logop. Phoniatr. Vocology* **2002**, *27*, 98–105. [CrossRef]
4. Nelson, R.; Merrill, R.M.; Thibeault, S.; Gray, S.D.; Smith, E.M. Voice disorders in teachers and the general population: Effects on work performance, attendance, and future career choices. *J. Speech Lang. Hear. Res.* **2004**, *47*, 542–551. [CrossRef]
5. Leppanen, K.; Ilomaki, I.; Laukkanen, A.M. One-year followup study of self-evaluated effects of voice massage, voice training, and voice hygiene lecture in female teachers. *Logop. Phoniatr. Vocol.* **2010**, *35*, 13–18. [CrossRef] [PubMed]
6. Niebudek-Bogusz, E.; Śliwińska-Kowalska, M. An overview of occupational voice disorders in Poland. *Int. J. Occup. Med. Environ. Health* **2013**, *26*, 659–669. [CrossRef] [PubMed]
7. Sinkiewicz, A.; Niebudek-Bogusz, E.; Szkiełkowska, A. A proposal for optimisation of the prophylaxis system and treatment of occupational voice disorders. *Otorynolaryngologia* **2018**, *17*, 15–19.
8. Ilomäki, I.; Leppänen, K.; Kleemola, L.; Tyrmi, J.; Laukkanen, A.M.; Vilkman, E. Relationships between self-evaluations of voice and working conditions, background factors, and phoniatric findings in female teachers. *Logop. Phoniatr. Vocol.* **2009**, *34*, 20–31. [CrossRef] [PubMed]
9. Chen, S.H.; Chiang, S.C.; Chung, Y.M.; Hsiao, L.C.; Hsiao, T.Y. Risk factors and effects of voice problems for teachers. *J. Voice* **2010**, *24*, 183–192. [CrossRef] [PubMed]
10. Verdolini, K.; Ramig, L. Review: Occupational risks for voice problems. *Logop. Phoniatr. Vocol.* **2001**, *26*, 37–46. [CrossRef]
11. Jałowska, M.; Wośkowiak, G.; Wiskirska-Woźnica, B. Evaluation of the results of the prevention program "Protect your voice" implemented by The Greater Poland Center of Occupational Medicine of Poznan. *Med. Pr.* **2017**, *68*, 593–603. [CrossRef]
12. Sezin, R.K.; Özcebe, E.; Aydinli, F.E.; Köse, A.; Günaydin, R.Ö. Investigation of the Effectiveness of a Holistic Vocal Training Program Designed to Preserve Theatre Students' Vocal Health and Increase their vocal Performances; A Prospective Research Study. *J. Voice* **2018**, *34*, 302.e21. [CrossRef]
13. Da Rocha, L.M.; de Lima Bach, S.; do Amaral, P.L.; Behlau, M.; de Mattos Souza, L.D. Risk factors for the incidence of perceived voice disorders in elementary and middle school teachers. *J. Voice* **2017**, *31*, 258.e7–258.e12. [CrossRef]
14. Van Houtte, E.; Claeys, S.; Wuyts, F.; Van Lierde, K. The Impact of Voice Disorders among Teachers: Vocal Complaints, Treatment-Seeking Behavior, Knowledge of Vocal Care, and Voice-Related Absenteeism. *J. Voice* **2010**. [CrossRef] [PubMed]
15. Niebudek-Bogusz, E.; Sznurowska-Przygocka, B.; Fiszer, M.; Kotyło, P.; Sinkiewicz, A.; Modrzewska, M.; Sliwinska-Kowalska, M. The effectiveness of voice therapy for teachers with dysphonia. *Folia Phoniatr. Logop.* **2008**, *60*, 134–141. [CrossRef] [PubMed]
16. Meerschman, I.; Van Lierde, K.; Peeters, K.; Meersman, E.; Claeys, S.; D'haeseleer, E. Short-Term Effect of Two Semi-Occluded Vocal Tract Training Programs on the Vocal Quality of Future Occupational Voice Users: "Resonant Voice Training Using Nasal Consonants" Versus "Straw Phonation". *J. Speech Lang. Hear. Res.* **2017**, *60*, 2519–2536. [CrossRef]
17. Barkmeier-Kraemer, J.M.; Patel, R.R. The Next 10 Years in Voice Evaluation and Treatment. *Semin. Speech Lang.* **2016**, *37*, 158–165. [CrossRef]
18. Niebudek-Bogusz, E.; Marszałek, S.; Woźnicka, E.; Minkiewicz, Z.; Hima, J.; Śliwińska-Kowalska, M. Extensive treatment of teacher's voice disorders in health spa. *Med. Pr.* **2010**, *61*, 685–691. [PubMed]
19. Dejonckere, P.H.; Bradley, P.; Clemente, P.; Cornut, G.; Crevier-Buchman, L.; Friedrich, G.; Van De Heyning, P.; Remacle, M.; Woisard, V. Committee on Phoniatrics of the European Laryngological Society (ELS). A basic protocol for functional assessment of voice pathology, especially for investigating the efficacy of (phonosurgical) treatments and evaluating new assessment techniques. Guideline elaborated by the Committee on Phoniatrics of the European Laryngological Society (ELS). *Eur. Arch. Otorhinolaryngol.* **2001**, *258*, 77–82. [CrossRef]
20. Jacobson, B.H.; Johnson, A.; Grywalski, C.; Silbergleit, A.; Jacobson, G.; Benninger, M.S.; Newman, C.W. The voice handicap index (VHI): Development and validation. *Am. J. Speech Lang. Pathol.* **1997**, *6*, 66–70. [CrossRef]
21. Pruszewicz, A.; Obrebowski, A.; Wiskirska-Woźnica, B.; Wojnowski, W. Complex voice assessment–Polish version of the Voice Handicap Index (VHI). *Otolaryngolo. Pol.* **2004**, *58*, 547–549.
22. Diagnova Technologies. Available online: https://www.diagnova.pl/pages/oferta.html#oprogramowanie (accessed on 15 May 2021).
23. Sataloff, R. T. *Treatment of Voice Disorders*; Plural Publishing: San Diego, CA, USA, 2005.
24. Łuszczyńska, A. It's time for effectiveness-implementation hybrid research on behaviour change. *Health Psychol. Rev.* **2020**, *14*, 188–192. [CrossRef]

25. Rosłaniec, A.; Sielska-Badurek, E.; Niemczyk, K. Evaluation of compliance of the principles of voice hygiene and voice production among teachers. *Pol. Otorhino. Rev.* **2019**, *8*, 18–24. [CrossRef]
26. Assunção, A.A.; de Medeiros, A.M.; Barreto, S.M.; Gama, A.C. Does regular practice of physical activity reduce the risk of dysphonia? *Prev. Med.* **2009**, *49*, 487–489. [CrossRef] [PubMed]
27. Bender, T.; Bálint, G.; Prohászka, Z.; Géher, P.; Tefner, I.K. Evidence-based hydro- and balneotherapy in Hungary–a systematic review and meta-analysis. *Int. J. Biometeorol.* **2014**, *58*, 311–323. [CrossRef] [PubMed]
28. Byeon, H. The Risk Factors Related to Voice Disorder in Teachers: A Systematic Review and Meta-Analysis. *Int. J. Environ. Res. Public Health* **2019**, *16*, 3675. [CrossRef] [PubMed]
29. Vaca, M.; Mora, E.; Cobeta, I. The Aging Voice: Influence of Respiratory and Laryngeal Changes. *Otolaryngol. Head Neck Surg.* **2015**, *153*, 409–413. [CrossRef] [PubMed]
30. Hodge, F.S.; Colton, R.H.; Kelley, R.T. Vocal intensity characteristics in normal and elderly speakers. *J. Voice* **2001**, *15*, 503–511. [CrossRef]
31. Behlau, M.; Madazio, G.; Moreti, F.; Oliveira, G.; de Moraes Alves Dos Santos, L.; Paulinelli, B.R.; de Barros Couto, E., Jr. Efficiency and cutoff values of self-assessment instruments on the impact of a voice problem. *J. Voice* **2016**, *30*, 506.e9–506.e18. [CrossRef] [PubMed]
32. Frajkova, Z.; Krizekova, A.; Missikova, V.; Tedla, M. Translation, Cross-Cultural Validation of the Voice Handicap Index (VHI-30) in Slovak Language. *J. Voice* **2020**, S0892-1997(20)30129-6. [CrossRef]
33. Karlsen, T.; Heimdal, J.-H.; Grieg, A.R.H.; Aarstad, H.J. The Norwegian Voice Handicap Index (VHI-N) patient scores are dependent on voice-related disease group. *Eur. Arch. Otorhinolaryngol.* **2015**, *272*, 2897–2905. [CrossRef] [PubMed]
34. Rosen, C.A.; Murry, T.; Zinn, A.; Zullo, T.; Sonbolian, M. Voice handicap index change following treatment of voice disorders. *J. Voice* **2000**, *14*, 619–623. [CrossRef]
35. Ziegler, A.; Gillespie, A.I.; Abbott, K.V. Behavioral treatment of voice disorders in teachers. *Folia Phoniatr. Logop.* **2010**, *62*, 9–23. [CrossRef] [PubMed]
36. Cantor Cutiva, L.C.; Fajardo, A.; Burdorf, A. Associations between self-perceived voice disorders in teachers, perceptual assessment by speech-language pathologists, and instrumental analysis. *Int. J. Speech Lang. Pathol.* **2016**, *18*, 550–559. [CrossRef] [PubMed]

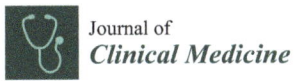

Article

T1a Glottic Cancer: Advances in Vocal Outcome Assessment after Transoral CO_2-Laser Microsurgery Using the VEM

Wen Song [1], Felix Caffier [1], Tadeus Nawka [1], Tatiana Ermakova [2], Alexios Martin [3], Dirk Mürbe [1] and Philipp P. Caffier [1,*]

1. Department of Audiology and Phoniatrics, Charité–Universitätsmedizin Berlin, Corporate Member of Freie Universität Berlin and Humboldt-Universität zu Berlin, Campus Charité Mitte, Charitéplatz 1, D-10117 Berlin, Germany; wensonwen@hotmail.com (W.S.); felix.caffier@charite.de (F.C.); tadeus.nawka@charite.de (T.N.); dirk.muerbe@charite.de (D.M.)
2. Fraunhofer Institute for Open Communication Systems, Kaiserin-Augusta-Allee 31, D-10589 Berlin, Germany; tatiana.ermakova@fokus.fraunhofer.de
3. Klinikum Mutterhaus der Borromäerinnen, Academic Teaching Hospital of Johannes Gutenberg-Universität Mainz, Feldstraße 16, D-54290 Trier, Germany; alexios.martin@mutterhaus.de
* Correspondence: philipp.caffier@charite.de

Abstract: Patients with unilateral vocal fold cancer (T1a) have a favorable prognosis. In addition to the oncological results of CO_2 transoral laser microsurgery (TOLMS), voice function is among the outcome measures. Previous early glottic cancer studies have reported voice function in patients grouped into combined T stages (Tis, T1, T2) and merged cordectomy types (lesser- vs. larger-extent cordectomies). Some authors have questioned the value of objective vocal parameters. Therefore, the purpose of this exploratory prospective study was to investigate TOLMS-associated oncological and vocal outcomes in 60 T1a patients, applying the ELS protocols for cordectomy classification and voice assessment. Pre- and postoperative voice function analysis included: Vocal Extent Measure (VEM), Dysphonia Severity Index (DSI), auditory-perceptual assessment (GRB), and 9-item Voice Handicap Index (VHI-9i). Altogether, 51 subjects (43 male, eight female, mean age 65 years) completed the study. The 5-year recurrence-free, overall, and disease-specific survival rates (Kaplan–Meier method) were 71.4%, 94.4%, and 100.0%. Voice function was preserved; the objective parameter VEM (64 ± 33 vs. 83 ± 31; mean ± SD) and subjective vocal measures (G: 1.9 ± 0.7 vs. 1.3 ± 0.7; VHI-9i: 18 ± 8 vs. 9 ± 9) even improved significantly ($p < 0.001$). The VEM best reflected self-perceived voice impairment. It represents a sensitive measure of voice function for quantification of vocal performance.

Keywords: T1a glottic carcinoma; transoral laser microsurgery; treatment outcome; vocal function; objective voice diagnostics; vocal extent measure (VEM)

Citation: Song, W.; Caffier, F.; Nawka, T.; Ermakova, T.; Martin, A.; Mürbe, D.; Caffier, P.P. T1a Glottic Cancer: Advances in Vocal Outcome Assessment after Transoral CO_2-Laser Microsurgery Using the VEM. *J. Clin. Med.* **2021**, *10*, 1250. https://doi.org/10.3390/jcm10061250

Academic Editor: Renee Speyer

Received: 15 February 2021
Accepted: 15 March 2021
Published: 17 March 2021

Publisher's Note: MDPI stays neutral with regard to jurisdictional claims in published maps and institutional affiliations.

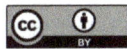

Copyright: © 2021 by the authors. Licensee MDPI, Basel, Switzerland. This article is an open access article distributed under the terms and conditions of the Creative Commons Attribution (CC BY) license (https://creativecommons.org/licenses/by/4.0/).

1. Introduction

Laryngeal cancer is the most frequent malignant tumor in the head and neck area and one of the most common tumors of the respiratory tract [1–3]. GLOBOCAN estimates that more than 177,000 people worldwide developed laryngeal cancer in 2018, with men being affected significantly more often than women (155,000 vs. 22,000) [4]. The prognosis depends mainly on the localization, the TNM classification and the R-status, but also the differentiation and the presence of lymphangiosis carcinomatosa are relevant predictors [5–7]. In the glottis, squamous cell carcinomas are the most frequent type (60 to 80%) compared to other tumor sites within the larynx [8–10]. In early glottic cancer, carcinoma in situ (Tis) must be differentiated from T1 and T2 laryngeal cancer. Invasive T1 glottic cancer is limited to one (T1a) or both (T1b) vocal folds (VF) with normal respiratory but impaired phonatory VF mobility.

T1 and early T2 glottic carcinomas have a very good prognosis due to the early symptom of hoarseness, which usually leads to a quick diagnosis and prompt initiation of therapy. In addition, metastasis rates are low [11–13]. In the literature, the 5-year overall survival after therapy of early glottic cancer is reported to be in the 74–100% range [14,15]. Involvement of the anterior commissure is more likely to have higher local recurrence, lower laryngeal preservation, but no statistical difference in 5-year overall survival [16,17]. In Steiner's landmark study of 240 patients with laryngeal cancer, early-stage carcinomas had an overall 5-year survival rate of 86.5% (disease-specific 100%), 6% local recurrences, with 99.4% larynx preservation [18]. Ledda and Puxeddu evaluated the oncologic efficacy in 103 patients with early glottic carcinoma, reporting for T1 a 5-year recurrence-free rate of 96% (local control 98%, larynx preservation 100%) [19]. Canis et al. showed in 404 pT1a patients the following 5-year Kaplan-Meier estimates: local control 86.8%, overall survival 87.8%, disease-specific survival 98.0%, recurrence-free survival 76.1%, and larynx preservation 97.3% [20]. Batra et al. presented in 53 patients with Tis and T1 comparable results: local control 86.7%, ultimate local control (with CO_2-laser alone) 90.5%, 3-year overall survival 92.4%, 3-year disease-specific survival and larynx preservation 98.1% [21]. An analysis of 2436 transorally treated T1/T2 carcinomas showed a 5-year overall survival of 82% [22]. For disease-specific survival after T1 and T2 transoral resection, 5-year survival rates of 89–100% are reported in the literature [23]. Meta-analyses on laryngeal preservation after transoral laser resection of T1 and T2 report rates of 83–100% [24].

Early detection of laryngeal cancer can minimize surgical trauma, improve therapeutic outcome and reduce mortality [25]. It is a general consensus that the larynx should be examined laryngoscopically in all patients with hoarseness lasting more than 3 to 4 weeks [26,27]. Videolaryngostroboscopy (VLS) can indicate invasive tissue growth by eliminated mucosal wave propagation and reduced or absent phonatory VF mobility [28,29]. Electronic chromoendoscopy can improve the recognition of tumor margins [30]. A recording of connected speech to document the impaired vocal function is considered a minimum requirement for functional assessment [31]. Small glottal findings suspected of malignancy such as precursor lesions, Tis, and T1a carcinomas, can be completely removed during diagnostic microlaryngoscopy to confirm the diagnosis by excision biopsy [32,33]. Apart from the health status, the quality of life in patients with T1 glottic cancer depends mainly on the voice quality and thus on the extent of the resected VF tissue [34–36]. Surgical therapy is preferred [37,38]; primary radiotherapy, however, can also be used as a conservative VF preserving procedure [39,40].

Transoral CO_2-laser microsurgery (TOLMS) was introduced by Strong and Jako for the therapy of early laryngeal cancer in the 1970s [41], and Steiner gave further impetus in the propagation of this technique [18,42]. Today, TOLMS is established for the treatment of early glottic carcinoma with highly satisfying oncological and functional outcomes (e.g., [20,43,44]). However, many studies predominately focus on oncological results and not on functional outcomes. As the vocal outcome depends on the amount of removed tissue, the consistent classification of endoscopic cordectomies of the European Laryngological Society (ELS) allows interpretation of postoperative results with regard to the surgical strategy and comparison between different surgical centers [45]. The main objective of this exploratory study was to examine in detail the vocal outcome in patients with T1a glottic cancer. The hypothesis was that voice function can be preserved after TOLMS. Therefore, we planned to explore the pre- and postoperative vocal function using specific subjective and objective parameters including the vocal extent measure (VEM) based on the voice range profile (VRP) [46].

2. Materials and Methods

2.1. Study Design and Patients

Patients diagnosed with suspected T1a glottic carcinoma underwent direct microlaryngoscopy in general anaesthesia with TOLMS in a prospective study. Clinical examination and data acquisition took place at the initial pre-therapeutic visit, during operation, and at regular follow-ups postoperatively. The voice was examined the day before TOLMS and 3 months after in-sano resection and completed wound healing. Study participants were patients presenting with hoarseness at the Department of Audiology and Phoniatrics, Charité–University Medicine Berlin, Germany. Altogether, 60 consecutive patients were recruited between June 2009 and October 2019. Selection criteria comprised histologically confirmed pT1a cN0 cM0 glottic carcinoma, complete treatment documentation, and informed consent. Patients with Tis, T1b and T2 glottic cancer were not included in this investigation.

2.2. Surgical Procedure and Postoperative Regimen

Microlaryngoscopy was conducted via the operating microscope type OPMI Sensera (Zeiss, Jena, Germany) and the Kleinsasser laryngoscope suspension system (Storz, Tuttlingen, Germany). TOLMS was performed with the AcuPulse 30W/40 ST CO_2-laser system (Lumenis, Yokneam, Israel) using the following parameters: output power 2 to 5 watt, super pulse mode, continuous wave, spot size 200 µm, focal length 400 mm. Conventional intraoperative safety precautions were respected (patient covering with moist cloths, safety goggles, laser-resistant endotracheal tube, ventilation with oxygen concentration below 40%). After inspection and palpation under the microscope, saline containing epinephrine (1 mg/mL; 10 gtt. in 10 mL NaCl) was injected into the VF. As a result, stretching the epithelium allowed to assess the fixation of the lesion to deeper structures. The saline also protected the healthy surrounding VF tissue from thermal damage. Laser incisions were made at the site where the suspicious lesions could be distinguished from normal epithelium, considering a safety margin of at least 1 mm. Depending on the pre- and intraoperative findings, cordectomy was conducted. After having removed the suspicious cancerous tissue, the surgeon classified the resection type according to the cordectomy types of the ELS [45]. Lesions within the epithelial level without fixation or signs of infiltration were superficially removed en bloc. Marginal resections were taken if the complete tumor removal was uncertain. All excision biopsies were sent for histopathological examination. The guidelines of the American Joint Committee on Cancer (AJCC) were used for tumor staging [47]. Patients with histopathologically confirmed R1 status were rescheduled for follow-up resection. All TOLMS operations were performed by 5 experienced laryngologists. After surgery, patients were monitored on the ward for 1–2 nights. Before discharge, all treated patients received vocal hygiene counseling. In the event of recurring voice impairment, they were asked to present again between regular follow-up intervals. Postoperative voice rest was not recommended.

2.3. Examination Instruments and Criteria

The analysis of treatment outcome was based on postoperative histopathological findings, pre- and postoperative VLS, and voice function diagnostics. Digital 2D or 3D VLS was carried out via rigid transoral or flexible transnasal endoscopes with integrated microphones (XION GmbH, Berlin, Germany) [28,48]. According to the ELS protocol, voice function diagnostics consisted of established subjective (i.e., auditory-perceptual assessment, self-evaluation of voice) and objective procedures (i.e., VRP measurement, acoustic-aerodynamic analysis) [49–51]. Objective procedures quantify the investigated aspects of vocal function in an apparatus-based and neutral manner. Subjective tests describe the individual self-perceived vocal impairment from the examined person's point of view as well as auditory-perceptual assessments from the examiner's viewpoint.

Auditory-perceptual assessment of the recorded voice samples was conducted using the GRB system [31]. The perceived overall grade of hoarseness (G), roughness (R), and breathiness (B) were independently rated on a scale from 0 to 3 (0 = not existing, 1 = mild, 2 = moderate, 3 = severe) by two senior phoniatricians. From each audio recording the mean score of both GRB evaluations served for further analysis.

Subjective self-assessment of voice was obtained using the 9-item Voice Handicap Index (VHI-9i) including 9 questions rated on a scale from 0 to 4 (0 = never, 1 = almost never, 2 = sometimes, 3 = almost always, 4 = always) [52]. The VHI-9i reflects the functional, physical and emotional impact of the voice disorder on the patient's quality of life. Additionally, an estimation of the self-perceived overall vocal impairment (VHIs) at the time of questioning was scored between 0 and 3 (0 = normal, 1 = mild, 2 = moderate, 3 = severe).

VRP measurements and acoustic-aerodynamic analyses were performed with the DiVAS software (XION GmbH) to obtain objective quantitative data of the speaking and singing voice. The following parameters were collected: soft phonation threshold, highest and lowest pitch, maximum phonation time (MPT), jitter, dysphonia severity index (DSI) [53], and VEM [46]. The VEM is the logarithmised product of the area of the VRP (A_{VRP}) and the quotient of the circumference of a circle with the same area and the actual VRP circumference (P_{VRP}), supplemented by the addition of a coefficient (50) and an offset (−200). The mathematical formula is:

$$VEM = 50 \ln \left(A_{VRP} \frac{2\pi \sqrt{\frac{A_{VRP}}{\pi}}}{P_{VRP}} \right) - 200 \quad (1)$$

The VEM quantifies the patient's dynamic performance and the frequency range as documented in the VRP. It expresses the vocal capacity as an interval-scaled value, mostly between 0 and 120. A high vocal capacity is characterized by a high VEM; conversely, a small VRP results in a small VEM.

3. Data Analysis

Descriptive statistics were used to describe the quantitative features of all pre- and postoperative parameters and their changes. As graphical techniques to display the data, we chose histograms and violin plots, i.e., box plots with kernel density plots rotated and surrounding them on each side. Being suitable for both continuous and ordinal variables, Spearman's rank-order correlation (r_s) was used to investigate the strength and direction of association between the pre- und postoperatively measured characteristics and their differences. Wilcoxon signed-rank test was used to test whether vocal function parameters significantly improved as the result of TOLMS. Mean values and 95% confidence intervals for these changes were calculated. The impact of patient-related, tumor-related, and treatment-related factors on disease control and survival was analyzed using the Kaplan–Meier method. All statistical tests and graphics were done using R version 4.0.1 (GNU project, Free Software Foundation, Boston, MA, USA). The level of significance was set at α = 0.05. Due to the exploratory nature of the study no adjustment for multiple testing was performed. To show different significance levels, the following abbreviations were used: * = 5%; ** = 1%; *** = 0.1%.

4. Results

4.1. Sample Description and Preoperative Assessment

From 60 patients initially recruited with histopathologically confirmed diagnosis of pT1a, six subjects (10.0%) were lost to follow-up and three subjects (5.0%) had to be excluded due to incomplete treatment documentation. In the remaining 51 patients, all diagnostic tests and therapeutic procedures were carried out as planned. The total sample consisted of 43 men and 8 woman, with a mean age of 65 years (range 31–84). At the time of intervention, women were on average 16 years younger than men (52 ± 14 vs. 68 ± 10, mean ± SD, p < 0.01). Regarding medical history, 39 subjects (76.5%) gave information about current or past tobacco abuse, with 12 subjects (23.5%) having smoked rarely or not at all. While 15.7% of the patients (8/51) never drank alcohol, 62.7% (32/51) reported regular and 21.6% (11/51) daily consumption of alcohol. Relevant preoperative patient characteristics within the examined cohort are shown in Table 1 (left side).

VLS revealed an almost equal distribution of tumor growth on both VF (28 right, 23 left). The lesions appeared flat and hyperkeratotic in 20/51 (39.2%), exophytic in 29/51 (56.9%), and ulcerating in 2/51 (3.9%) subjects. Concerning macroscopic assessment of tumor size at initial presentation, 51.0% of the patients (26/51) showed involvement of the entire VF, while in 27.4% (14/51) two-thirds and in 21.6% (11/51) one-third of the VF were affected. During phonation, phonatory VF mobility was reduced or absent on the affected tumor side in all subjects. Additionally, patients with bulged VF due to exophytic tissue growth displayed highly impaired glottal closure.

Subjective auditory-perceptual evaluation of patient's voices was categorized preoperatively with a mean of G2 R2 B1 (range 0–3). The VHI-9i had an average score of 18 ± 8, corresponding to moderate self-assessed patient complaints. The objective acoustic and aerodynamic parameters also indicated moderate impairment (e.g., VEM 64 ± 33; DSI 1.2 ± 2.4; MPT 13 ± 6 s). Correlation analysis performed on preoperative values showed that both VEM and DSI correlated with VHI-9i ($r_s = -0.62^{***}$ and $r_s = -0.29^*$, respectively), G ($r_s = -0.42^{**}$ and $r_s = -0.34^*$), R ($r_s = -0.41^{**}$ and $r_s = -0.37^{**}$), B ($r_s = -0.47^{***}$ and $r_s = -0.30^*$), and with each other ($r_s = 0.51^{***}$).

Table 1. Patient characteristics ($n = 51$) before TOLMS (left) and after TOLMS (right). Unless otherwise specified, data expressed as number of patients and percentage of group.

	Number	%		Number	%
Gender			Initial cordectomy (via TOLMS)		
male	43	84.3%	type I (subepithelial)	24	47.1%
female	8	15.7%	type II (subligamental)	18	35.3%
			type III (transmuscular)	9	17.6%
Age			Grading of pT1a		
(in years; mean $\pm$ SD)	65 ± 12	-	G1 (well differentiated)	15	29.4%
			G2 (moderately differentiated)	34	66.7%
			G3 (poorly differentiated)	2	3.9%
Occurrence of pT1a			Follow-up	45 ± 26	-
left vocal fold	23	45.1%	(in months; mean $\pm$ SD)		
right vocal fold	28	54.9%			
Vocal fold involvement			Treatment response		
anterior third	3	5.9%	local disease control	41	80.4%
middle third	7	13.7%	local disease recurrence	10	19.6%
posterior third	1	2.0%	contralateral secondary pT1a	2	3.9%
anterior and middle third	7	13.7%	ultimate local disease control	49	96.1%
middle and posterior third	7	13.7%	with TOLMS alone)		
entire length	26	51.0%	larynx preservation	50	98.0%
Appearance of pT1a			Survival		
hyperkeratotic	20	39.2%	disease-specific	51	100.0%
exophytic	29	56.9%	overall	49	96.1%
ulcerating	2	3.9%	recurrence-free	39	76.5%

4.2. Postoperative Assessment

Via TOLMS, 24 patients received subepithelial cordectomy (type I; 47.1%), 18 patients subligamental cordectomy (type II; 35.3%), and nine patients transmuscular cordectomy (type III; 17.6%). According to histopathology, the diagnosis confirmed in all subjects squamous cell carcinoma limited to one VF (pT1a). The grading classification revealed in most patients moderately differentiated tissue (G2; 66.7%), less frequent well differentiated (G1; 29.4%) and seldom poorly differentiated tissue (G3; 3.9%). Through primary operation, the pT1a was completely excised (R0 status) in 29 patients (56.9%). Following the piecemeal strategy, a second excision was necessary in 22 subjects (43.1%), as a residuum could not be ruled out (close tumor margin vs. R1 status). Of these 22 subjects with suspicious findings, 17 patients (77.3%) had no visual or histopathological malignant residue in the scheduled control TOLMS. Among the remaining five patients, the follow-up resections revealed residual invasive tumor in three patients (13.7%), Tis in one patient (4.5%), and a precursor lesion (squamous intraepithelial neoplasia SIN III) in the other patient (4.5%). All these lesions were completely excised during the second TOLMS.

The operative procedures were conducted without complications. Postoperatively, no patient complained about swallowing dysfunction. VLS check-ups showed fibrin formation on the wound surfaces followed by formation of scar tissue during healing. While extensive tumor growth was associated with larger glottal defects after removal, in smaller superficial findings treated via type I cordectomy a stable epithelium regenerated on the preserved lamina propria without relevant defects or scarring. In some patients, the scarred VF developed after about 6 months a restored phonatory mobility. Figure 1 gives an impression of pre- and postoperative VLS findings with videostrobokymographic illustration of VF oscillations.

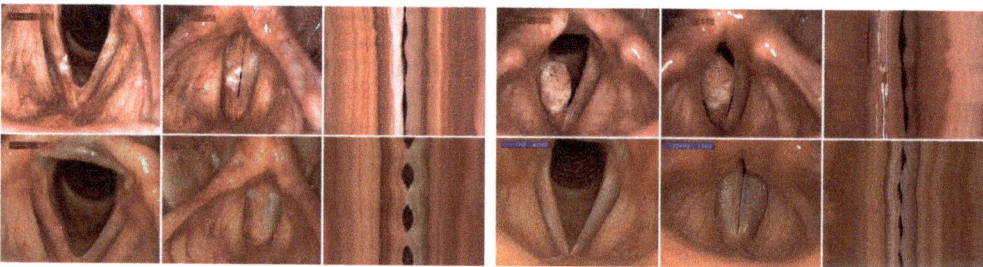

Figure 1. Videolaryngostroboscopic pictures and videostrobokymographic illustration of vocal fold anatomy and function, preoperative (**upper row**) vs. postoperative (**lower row**). Example A (**left side**): 45-year-old male professional theater actor with a flat hyperkeratotic lesion of the right vocal fold. Example B (**right side**): 32-year-old female medical doctor with an exophytic tumor of the right vocal fold. Findings three months postoperatively show: pT1a completely removed, healing process finished, vocal folds with straight margin, complete glottal closure, and restored phonatory mobility (A: normalized, regular and symmetric oscillations; B: oscillations with scarring-related reduced amplitude and phase shift).

Within the mean postoperative observation period of 45 ± 26 months (median: 41 months), 10 patients (19.6%) suffered from a local recurrence (1× Tis, 7× rpT1a, 1× rpT1b, 1× cT3) with an average tumor-free interval of 15 months (median 10 months). Eight of these subjects had only one recurrence within the follow-up period. Among the remaining two, further recurrences occurred: one patient with the initial diagnosis of pT1a (G3) suffered from two recurrences of rpT1a after 17 and 80 months. The other subject with the initial diagnosis of pT1a (G2) had altogether four recurrences; after 13 (rpT1a), 27 (rpT2), 44 (rT3), and 92 months (rpT4a). During follow-up, a secondary glottic pT1a on the contralateral VF was detected in two patients after an interval of 1 and 3 years after removal of the primary tumor, respectively. All recurrent and secondary laryngeal carcinomas were successfully treated: Tis, T1 and T2 via secondary TOLMS, both T3 recurrences via radio-chemotherapy, and the T4 recurrence via total laryngectomy. One subject died due to a secondary pancreas carcinoma, another one died intercurrently. The 5-year recurrence-free, overall, and disease-specific survival rates (Kaplan–Meier method) were 71.4%, 94.4%, and 100.0% (Figure 2). Relevant postoperative and oncological patient characteristics are shown in Table 1 (right side).

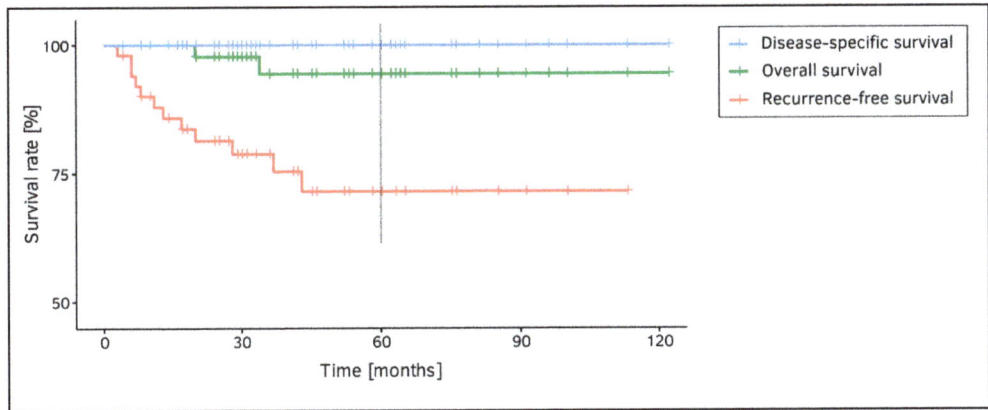

Figure 2. Five-year Kaplan–Meier estimates for recurrence-free survival, overall survival, and disease-specific survival.

Three months after TOLMS, vocal function improved considerably compared to the preoperative measurements (Table 2). With respect to auditory-perceptual GRB evaluation, the pre- vs. post-therapeutical comparison revealed that the voices were less hoarse (1.9 ± 0.7 vs. 1.3 ± 0.7), rough (1.8 ± 0.7 vs. 1.2 ± 0.7), and breathy (1.0 ± 0.6 vs. 0.6 ± 0.6). The subjective vocal self-assessment via VHI-9i questionnaire demonstrated a mean reduction from 18 ± 8 to 9 ± 9 points. The VHIs criterion indicated a change from moderately (2 ± 1) to mildly disturbed voices (1 ± 1). The improvements regarding all these subjective parameters were found significant at the 0.1% level ($p < 0.001$). The subjective vocal parameters both pre- and postoperatively are displayed by histograms in Figure 3.

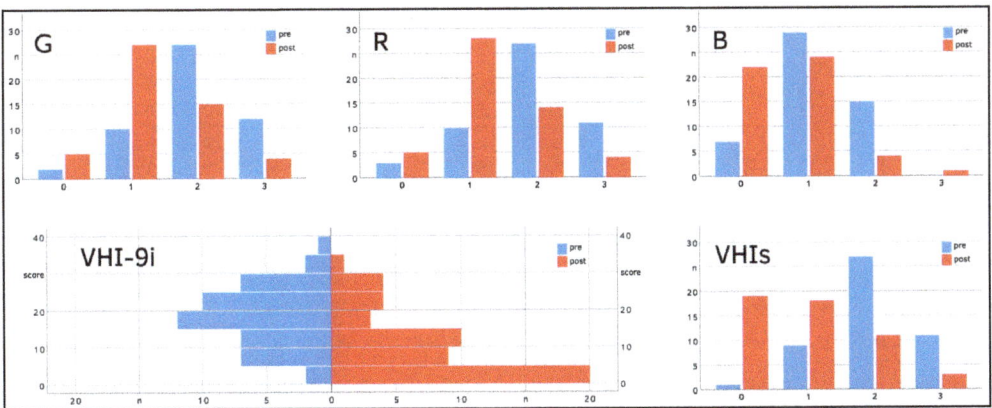

Figure 3. Subjective vocal parameters before and after pT1a removal. Upper row: Comparison of pre- and postoperative voice parameters according to the GRB-classification. Lower row: Comparison of pre- and postoperative VHI-9i and VHIs scores.

Table 2. Pre- and posttherapeutic parameters of vocal function in all patients and all cordectomy types (mean ± SD), their mean therapeutic differences (Diff) and 95% confidence intervals (CI) for changes in vocal measures three months after pT1a removal.

Vocal Measure		Total Group ($n = 51$)	Type I Cordectomy ($n = 24$)	Type II Cordectomy ($n = 18$)	Type III Cordectomy ($n = 9$)
VEM	Pre	64.4 ± 32.7	65.4 ± 36.9	70.3 ± 31.7	51.0 ± 18.4
	Post	82.8 ± 30.5	86.7 ± 33.5	81.9 ± 25.4	74.1 ± 33.2
	Diff (CI)	18.4 (9.0; 29.8) ***	21.3 (5.1; 37.6) *	11.6 (−3.2; 32.6) *	23.1 (−5.7; 52.0) *
DSI	Pre	1.2 ± 2.4	1.5 ± 2.4	1.4 ± 2.3	−0.2 ± 2.6
	Post	1.5 ± 2.3	1.8 ± 2.6	1.0 ± 2.1	1.8 ± 1.8
	Diff (CI)	0.3 (−0.2; 1.3)	0.3 (−0.5; 1.9)	−0.4 (−1.4; 0.6)	2.0 (0.1; 3.9) *
Jitter (%)	Pre	0.9 ± 1.1	0.8 ± 1.1	0.7 ± 0.9	1.5 ± 1.6
	Post	0.6 ± 0.4	0.6 ± 0.3	0.6 ± 0.5	0.5 ± 0.3
	Diff (CI)	−0.3 (−0.7; −0.02)	−0.2 (−0.7; 0.2)	−0.1 (−0.7; 0.3)	−1.0 (−2.0; 0.1) *
MPT (s)	Pre	13.3 ± 5.6	14.1 ± 5.2	12.3 ± 6.6	13.3 ± 4.5
	Post	13.3 ± 6.0	14.7 ± 6.3	10.9 ± 5.7	14.6 ± 4.5
	Diff (CI)	−0.01 (−1.9; 1.9)	0.6 (−2.4; 3.6)	−1.4 (−4.6; 1.7)	1.3 (−3.6; 6.0)
VHI−9i	Pre	17.7 ± 8.1	16.6 ± 8.3	17.1 ± 7.1	22.1 ± 9.1
	Post	9.3 ± 8.8	10.5 ± 9.0	7.7 ± 8.7	9.2 ± 8.8
	Diff (CI)	−8.4 (−10.9; −5.6) ***	−6.1 (−10.5; −2.1) **	−9.4 (−13.1; −4.9) **	−12.9 (−20.4; −4.3) *
VHIs	Pre	2.0 ± 0.7	1.9 ± 0.9	1.9 ± 0.6	2.4 ± 0.5
	Post	1.0 ± 0.9	1.0 ± 1.0	0.8 ± 0.9	1.0 ± 0.9
	Diff (CI)	−1.0 (−1.4; −0.8) ***	−0.9 (−1.3; −0.6) ***	−1.1 (−1.7; −0.7) ***	−1.4 (−2.2; −0.6) *
G	Pre	1.9 ± 0.7	1.5 ± 0.8	2.2 ± 0.4	2.2 ± 0.7
	Post	1.3 ± 0.7	1.0 ± 0.8	1.5 ± 0.6	1.4 ± 0.6
	Diff (CI)	−0.6 (−0.8; −0.4) ***	−0.5 (−0.8; −0.2) **	−0.7 (−0.9; −0.4) **	−0.8 (−1.2; −0.2) *
R	Pre	1.8 ± 0.7	1.5 ± 0.8	2.1 ± 0.5	2.0 ± 0.8
	Post	1.2 ± 0.7	1.0 ± 0.8	1.5 ± 0.6	1.3 ± 0.6
	Diff (CI)	−0.6 (−0.8; −0.4) ***	−0.5 (−0.8; −0.2) **	−0.6 (−0.9; −0.3) **	−0.7 (−1.2; −0.1) *
B	Pre	1.0 ± 0.6	0.8 ± 0.7	1.2 ± 0.4	1.4 ± 0.4
	Post	0.6 ± 0.6	0.4 ± 0.6	0.9 ± 0.5	0.9 ± 0.7
	Diff (CI)	−0.4 (−0.6; −0.2) ***	−0.4 (−0.7; −0.1) **	−0.3 (−0.6; −0.1) **	−0.5 (−1.1; 0.1) *

B: breathiness; DSI: dysphonia severity index; G: (overall) grade of hoarseness; MPT: maximum phonation time; R: roughness; VEM: vocal extent measure; VHI-9i: 9-item voice handicap index, VHIs: self-perceived overall vocal impairment. The level of significance is indicated as follows: * significant at $p < 0.05$; ** significant at $p < 0.01$; *** significant at $p < 0.001$ (Wilcoxon signed-rank test).

Regarding objective measures, the VEM improved significantly in the total cohort (from 64 ± 33 to 83 ± 31; $p < 0.001$), in both genders (males $p < 0.01$; females $p < 0.05$) and all cordectomy types ($p < 0.05$). In contrast, the decrease of jitter (0.9 ± 1.1 to 0.6 ± 0.4) and the increase of DSI (1.2 ± 2.4 to 1.5 ± 2.3) did not reach the level of significance in the total group, only in females ($p < 0.05$) and cordectomy type III ($p < 0.05$). VEM and DSI correlated significantly with each other also postoperatively ($r_s = 0.62$***). The VEM showed a significant negative correlation with VHI-9i ($r_s = −0.29$*) but not with age ($r_s = −0.18$), while the DSI correlated significantly with age ($r_s = −0.39$**) but not with VHI−9i ($r_s = −0.11$). Selected objective parameters before and after pT1a removal are graphically displayed via boxplots in Figure 4 with regard to the total cohort and cordectomy type.

To provide insights into the magnitude of changes induced by TOLMS, Table 2 also presents the mean differences (and 95% confidence intervals) between pre- and posttherapeutic values. As a result, the numeric outcome of all subjective and objective parameters was larger in women compared to men. Similarly, the improvement of these parameters in cordectomy type III was higher compared to the other cordectomy types.

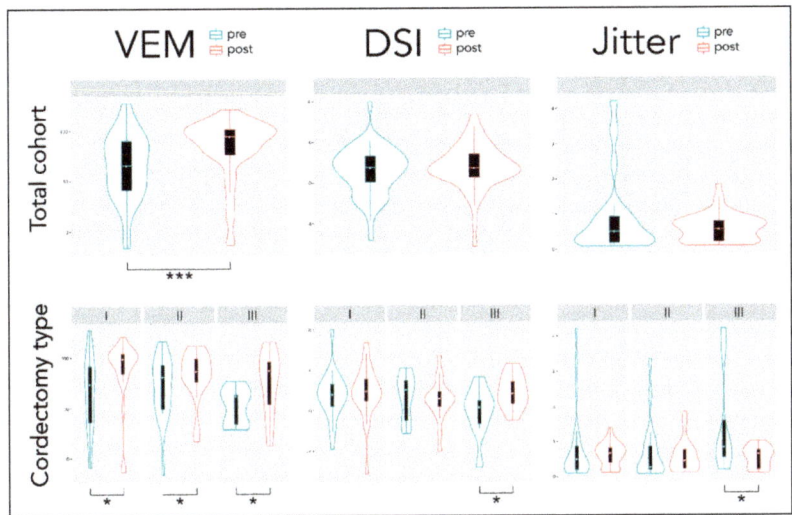

Figure 4. Objective acoustic parameters VEM, DSI, and jitter before and after pT1a removal concerning the total cohort and cordectomy types. Data are compared pre- vs. postoperatively via violin plots, i.e., box plots with kernel density plots rotated and surrounding them on each side. The boxplots display the median, quartiles, and the range of values covered by the data. The density curves display the full distribution of the data including any outliers. The level of significance is indicated as follows: * significant at $p < 0.05$; ** significant at $p < 0.01$; *** significant at $p < 0.001$ (Wilcoxon signed-rank test).

5. Discussion

Given the established favorable oncological results of CO_2-TOLMS in T1a glottic carcinoma, functional aspects should be another treatment objective. We successfully examined the oncological and functional outcomes after TOLMS in pT1a patients, focusing on the evaluation of voice with subjective and objective parameters. Our T1a cohort is consistent with the literature in terms of patient characteristics, treatment methods, and oncological results (see Table 1, Figure 2). Therefore, a closer look at our vocal outcomes is warranted compared to the results of previous investigations.

Many studies were conducted to compare TOLMS with radiotherapy in patients with early glottic cancer [54–56]. The vocal outcomes were either superior in radiotherapy [57,58] or in TOLMS [59,60], or they did not show relevant differences between both treatment groups [61–64]. In general, pre-therapeutic voice data was often not collected [57–59,61,63–69]. In these investigations, it is impossible to relate the postoperative voice function to the pretherapeutic baseline. Some studies evaluated vocal function before and after TOLMS according to the cordectomy type [70–74]. Mainly, voice quality differed depending on the amount of tissue resected: vocal outcomes after lesser-extent cordectomies (ELS type I, II) were superior compared to larger-extent cordectomies. However, a multidimensional, detailed pre- and post-therapeutic documentation and evaluation of voice was only carried out in a few studies [62,70,71,74,75]. To compare the vocal outcomes after TOLMS, Table 3 summarizes the main results of previous investigations including the number of T1a patients treated and the parameters used for evaluation.

Table 3. Published vocal outcomes for T1a glottic cancer treated with TOLMS, taken from representative studies (last 14 years, $n > 10$ T1a patients operated via TOLMS).

Study	Numbers	Clinician-Rated Assessment (Subjective)	Patient's Self-Assessment (Subjective)	Acoustic-Aerodynamic Evaluation (Objective)	Vocal Outcome after Transoral Lasermicrosurgery (TOLMS)
Hamzany et al. (2021) [70]	27 T1a	GRB	VHI	F0, jitter, shimmer, NHR, MPT	significant subjective improvement, no objective improvement
Strieth et al. (2019) [76]	14 T1a	-	VHI	-	improved voice preservation by KTP-TOLMS (lower VHI scores) compared to CO_2-TOLMS (higher VHI scores)
Gandhi et al. (2018) [59]	40 T1a + b (N/S)	GRBAS	VHI	F0, jitter, shimmer, SPL, NHR	excellent vocal outcome (G 0.63, VHI 13); no pretherapeutic data
Hong et al. (2018) [61]	14 T1a + b (N/S)	GRBAS	-	F0, jitter, shimmer, NHR	GRB with mild dysphonia, jitter 2.37%; no pretherapeutic data
Lee et al. (2016) [71]	50 T1a	GRBAS	VHI	F0, jitter, shimmer, NHR, voice intensity, MPT	G significantly improved; voice quality improved over time in limited ELS resections (I-II) but not in extended cordectomies (III-V)
Fink et al. (2016) [72]	38 T1a	VAS (0–100)	VHI	-	similar or improved voice in limited ELS resections (I-III), VHI improved significantly (VAS n.s.); poorer outcomes in extended resections
Kono et al. (2016) [62]	64 T1a	GRBAS	VHI, V-RQOL	F0, jitter, shimmer, NHR, MPT	mild to moderate impairment (GRB, VHI, jitter), better improvement over time in focused excision compared to defocused vaporization
Berania et al. (2015) [65]	18 T1a	PSS-H&N	VHI-10	-	favorable functional outcomes (40% mild voice handicap, VHI-10 > 11); no pretherapeutic data
Bertino et al. (2015) [66]	135 T1a	degree of dysphonia (acc. Ricci Maccarini)	-	F0, HNR	mild to slight dysphonia in limited ELS resections (I-II), moderate to severe dysphonia in extended resections (III-V); no pretherapeutic data
Laoufi et al. (2014) [57]	44 T1a	-	VHI, EORTC QLQ-HN35	-	VHI score mild to moderate impaired (mean 29); no pretherapeutic data
Friedman et al. (2013) [77]	57 T1a	-	V-RQOL	F0, jitter, shimmer, NHR, max. SPL range, max. F0 range, SPL divided by subglottic pressure	significant improvement of subjective (V-RQOL) and most objective (acoustic, aerodynamic) measures
Tomifuji et al. (2013) [73]	33 T1a	GRBAS	VHI	jitter, shimmer, HNR, MPT, MFR	voice quality differs according to the type of cordectomy; no pretherapeutic data
van Gogh et al. (2012) [60]	67 T1a	-	-	F0, jitter, shimmer, NNE	quick voice outcome recovery apart from F0 (remains higher pitched), no significant long-term voice changes
Bajaj et al. (2011) [67]	14 T1a + b (N/S)	GRBAS	VoiSS, UW-QoL	F0, F0 irregularity, CQ range, CQ irregularity	preservation of acceptable vocal function (GRB mild to moderate impaired, low VoiSS score); no pretherapeutic data
Keilmann et al. (2011) [68]	11 T1a	RBH	VHI-12	F0, jitter, shimmer, MPT, GHD, VRP	discrepancy over time (VHI deteriorated; RBH and objective measures improved); no pretherapeutic data

Table 3. Cont.

Study	Numbers	Parameters for Evaluation of Vocal Function			Vocal Outcome after Transoral Lasermicrosurgery (TOLMS)
		Clinician-Rated Assessment (Subjective)	Patient's Self-Assessment (Subjective)	Acoustic-Aerodynamic Evaluation (Objective)	
Lester et al. (2011) [78]	19 T1a + b (N/S)	—	ordinal scale (1–5)	F0, jitter, shimmer, MPT	objective acoustic measures showed no significant changes; deterioration of MPT (13s to 12s) and subjective rating score (3 to 2)
Motta et al. (2008) [69]	49 T1a	—	—	MPT, HNR, average voice intensity	outcomes vary in relation to the main site of the pseudo-glottis, vocal compensation without normal voice quality; no pretherapeutic data
Núñez Batalla et al. (2008) [63]	19 T1a	GRBAS	VHI	F0, jitter, shimmer, NNE, MPT	mild to moderate impairment (GRBAS, VHI); no pretherapeutic data
Sjögren et al. (2008) [64]	18 T1a	GRBAS	VHI	F0, jitter, shimmer, intensity, MPT, VC, phonation quotient	mild to moderate voice dysfunction (G, B, VHI) in ca. half of patients; no pretherapeutic data
Vilaseca et al. (2008) [79]	35 T1a	GRBAS	ordinal scale (1–3)	F0, jitter, shimmer, NHR, vocal range, MPT	self-assessed improvement; compared with healthy controls: increase of F0, jitter, shimmer (MPT decrease in extended resections); no pretherapeutic data
Roh et al. (2007) [75]	50 T1a	GRBAS	VHI, EORTC QLQ-HN35	F0, jitter, shimmer, HNR, MPT, average airflow	improved vocal outcomes, significant in type I and II cordectomies (VHI, G, jitter, shimmer, HNR)

Legend: CQ—closed quotient, EORTC QLQ-HN35—European Organization for Research and Treatment of Cancer Head and Neck Quality of Life questionnaire; F0—fundamental frequency; GHD—Goettinger Hoarseness Diagram; GRBAS—overall Grade, Roughness, Breathyness, Asthenia, Strain; NHR—harmonics-to-noise ratio; KTP—Potassium titanyl phosphate; MFR—mean flow rate; MPT—maximum phonation time; NHR—noise-to-harmonic ratio; NNE—normalized noise energy; N/S—not specified; PSS-H&N—performance status scale for head & neck cancer patients; RBH—Roughness, Breathyness, (overall grade of) Hoarseness; SNR—signal-to-noise ratio; SPL—soft phonation index; SPL—sound pressure level; UW-QoL—University of Washington Quality of Life questionnaire; VAS—visual analogue scale; VC—vital capacity; VHI—voice handicap index; VHI-10—10-item VHI; VHI-12—12-item VHI; VoiSS—voice symptom scale; VRP—voice range profile; V-RQOL—Voice-Related Quality-of-Life survey.

The comparability of published studies is limited due to the lack of standardization regarding (1) vocal outcome assessment (different parameters, follow up), (2) patient selection (e.g., all early glottic cancer patients, low number of T1a), as well as (3) inclusion and treatment criteria (e.g., combined T stages and cordectomy types).

The usefulness of objective acoustic measures has been questioned. Some studies indicated that TOLMS results in an increase of F0, jitter, shimmer, and a moderate decrease of MPT in extended cordectomies when compared with healthy controls (e.g., [79]). Other studies found either a TOLMS-associated improvement [74,75,77], or no relevant changes throughout the postoperative course [70,78]. In our investigation, the patients revealed in all objective and subjective parameters postoperative changes. Similar to the literature, subjective parameters improved significantly [71,72,77,79]: GRB, VHI-9i and VHIs substantially improved in our total cohort, both genders, and in each cordectomy group. Among objective measures, the MPT showed non-specific, undirected changes without any significance. This is in concordance with the results of Hamzany et al., confirming that aerodynamic parameters seem to be less suitable for outcome assessment in T1a glottic carcinoma [70]. Regarding acoustic parameters, VEM seems to be very well suited to assess the resulting voice function after T1a excision compared to other objective acoustic parameters, as only this measure responded significantly in the total cohort and in all subgroups. Among cordectomy types, the larger the resections, the greater the postoperative subjective numerical benefit (Table 2). Similarly, the improvement of acoustic parameters in cordectomy type III was bigger compared to the other cordectomy types. This is related to the fact that larger tumors are associated with more severe voice impairment preoperatively. In contrast, better voice function in smaller tumors results in less postoperative numerical benefit, even if the final voice outcome is better. The relevant differences in the cordectomy groups (types I–III) suggest that pooling these types, as in previous studies of the literature, does not seem appropriate. Although all subjective and objective improvements were larger in women than men, we cannot draw general conclusions due to our limited number of female patients.

While the VEM is not yet widely applied in voice diagnostics, the multidimensional DSI represents an established parameter of instrumental voice evaluation based on a weighted combination of highest possible frequency, lowest intensity, MPT and jitter [53]. Former investigations showed that the DSI might be influenced by using different registration programs, as well as by age or gender [80,81]. These age and gender effects were also confirmed in our study. The DSI appears susceptible to extreme measures (e.g., highest frequency, lowest intensity), which are likely to be influenced by age or gender. In contrast, the VEM, calculated from area and shape of the VRP, is less affected by the above-mentioned extreme measures. Since VEM correlated highly significantly with DSI, both measurements can be seen as related and comparable parameters. Part of their shared variance could be accountable to age, although the linear relationship with age is considerably weaker for the VEM compared to the DSI. However, the VEM as a positive criterion characterizes the vocal abilities and enables a classification of voice performance, while the DSI as a negative criterion particularly describes the severity of dysphonia [80,82]. Among both parameters, the VEM better reflected the subjective vocal impairments. However, DSI, VEM, VHI, and GRB represent different aspects of the voice: They are complementary in objective and subjective evaluation of voice quality, vocal performance, or perceived vocal handicap.

Depending on preoperative T1a tumor characteristics, individual postoperative voice function might be better, similar, or slightly reduced. In general, objective and subjective voice quality improved during long-term postoperative follow-up. This is in line with the results of previous investigations [70,83]. Although voice diagnostics according to ELS protocol is more time-consuming, we consider this effort justified for evidence-based therapy and necessary for documentation of voice preservation. To preserve voice function, the intraoperative laser power should be selected as low as possible to avoid thermal damage in the surrounding healthy tissue. In addition, focused excision achieves better vocal outcomes than defocused vaporization [62]. The application of the KTP laser may be able to offer improved voice preservation with similar oncological control compared to CO_2-TOLMS [76,77]. The focus on voice preservation may increase the number of interventions in cases with histologically questionable tumor margins [84,85]. Our experience confirms the literature, that re-operation can sometimes be avoided by close monitoring of local control using VLS [44,66].

Study Strengths and Limitations

Our study is characterized by the application of multidimensional voice evaluation, extended by the objective VEM. Further strengths comprise cohort homogeneity restricted to T1a instead of all early glottic cancer patients, and evaluation of specific cordectomy types in a sufficient number of patients rather than generalization or grouping into lesser- vs. larger-extent cordectomies. Applying the ELS protocols both for cordectomy classification and multidimensional voice evaluation enables a systematic comparison of our results with the outcomes of future studies.

Some limitations must be considered before drawing general conclusions. First, our results are investigations of a mono-centre study. To prevent centre bias, multicentre trials with a larger number of subjects are needed. Second, females are underrepresented in our study; thus, there may be participation bias. With a limited number of female patients, general gender-specific conclusions cannot be drawn. Our study sample reflects the well-known prevalence of laryngeal cancer in male patients, though. Third, a more precise preoperative assessment of the exact extent of the pathology would be useful. The importance of tumor size and shape should not be underestimated regarding voice function. The histopathologically determined tumor extent does not replace this information, because resections via TOLMS are not always performed en bloc and may lead to thermal tissue artefacts (e.g., shrinkage, coagulation, vaporization). Fourth, there were differences regarding the individual amount of interventions as well as rehabilitation strategies. Voice therapy could influence the vocal outcome in operated patients. Having neglected this may also result in a performance bias. Lastly, some factors influencing the VRP registration have to be considered. One limitation is the fact that in aphonic patients no perimeter of the VRP can be measured. However, in our study no T1a patient suffered from aphonia. Other factors comprise the routine of the examiner, motivation of the patients, and varying quantities of registered tones. Most of these influential factors are of minor importance in our investigation because all VRPs were recorded by one experienced examiner under practically equal conditions. Since precise VEM calculation is based on the actual VRP shape and circumference, future multicenter studies should be standardized by defining the number of registered tones per interval.

6. Conclusions

TOLMS has been proven to be an established and safe standard oncologic therapy for T1a glottic carcinoma with satisfactory preservation of vocal function both subjectively and objectively. Among objective voice parameters, the VEM seems to best reflect self-perceived subjective voice impairment showing significant changes after T1a treatment that incorporates phonosurgical principles. It represents a sensitive, positive measure of voice function, as well as an understandable and easy-to-use parameter for quantifying vocal performance as documented in the VRP. Therefore, it is reasonable to include the VEM as a diagnostic addition to the established voice measures of the ELS protocol.

Author Contributions: Conceptualization, T.N. and P.P.C.; Methodology, W.S., A.M. and P.P.C.; Literature Review, W.S., T.N. and P.P.C.; Investigation, T.N., A.M. and P.P.C.; Data Analysis, W.S. and T.E.; Original Draft Writing, W.S., F.C. and P.P.C.; Draft Review & Editing, W.S., T.N., D.M. and P.P.C.; Visualization, F.C. and T.E.; Supervision, D.M. All authors have read and agreed to the published version of the manuscript.

Funding: This research received no external funding.

Institutional Review Board Statement: The study was conducted according to the guidelines of the Declaration of Helsinki, and approved by the Ethics Committee of Charité–Universitätsmedizin Berlin, Berlin, Germany (reference number: EA4/140/10).

Informed Consent Statement: Informed consent was obtained from all study participants.

Data Availability Statement: All data of the study are available in the Department of Audiology and Phoniatrics, Charité–Universitätsmedizin Berlin, Berlin, Germany.

Conflicts of Interest: The authors declare no conflict of interest.

References

1. Siegel, R.L.; Miller, K.D.; Jemal, A. Cancer Statistics, 2020. *CA Cancer J. Clin.* **2020**, *70*, 7–30. [CrossRef]
2. Nocini, R.; Molteni, G.; Mattiuzzi, C.; Lippi, G. Updates on Larynx Cancer Epidemiology. *Chin. J. Cancer Res.* **2020**, *32*, 18–25. [CrossRef]
3. Steuer, C.E.; El-Deiry, M.; Parks, J.R.; Higgins, K.A.; Saba, N.F. An Update on Larynx Cancer. *CA Cancer J. Clin.* **2017**, *67*, 31–50. [CrossRef]
4. Ferlay, J.; Colombet, M.; Soerjomataram, I.; Mathers, C.; Parkin, D.M.; Pineros, M.; Znaor, A.; Bray, F. Estimating the Global Cancer Incidence and Mortality in 2018: GLOBOCAN Sources and Methods. *Int. J. Cancer* **2019**, *144*, 1941–1953. [CrossRef]
5. El-Naggar, A.K.; Chan, J.K.C.; Grandis, J.R.; Takata, T.; Slootweg, P.J. *WHO Classification of Head and Neck Tumours*, 4th ed.; WHO: Lyon, France, 2017.
6. Brierley, J.D.; Gospodarowicz, M.K.; Wittekind, C. *TNM Classification of Malignant Tumours*, 8th ed.; Wiley: Chichester, UK, 2016.
7. Agaimy, A.; Weichert, W. Grading of Head and Neck Neoplasms. *Pathologe* **2016**, *37*, 285–292. [CrossRef]
8. Williamson, A.J.; Bondje, S. *Glottic Cancer*; StatPearls Publishing: Treasure Island, FL, USA, 2021.
9. Markou, K.; Christoforidou, A.; Karasmanis, I.; Tsiropoulos, G.; Triaridis, S.; Constantinidis, I.; Vital, V.; Nikolaou, A. Laryngeal Cancer: Epidemiological Data from Nuorthern Greece and Review of the Literature. *Hippokratia* **2013**, *17*, 313–318. [PubMed]
10. Pantel, M.; Guntinas-Lichius, O. Laryngeal Carcinoma: Epidemiology, Risk Factors and Survival. *HNO* **2012**, *60*, 32–40. [CrossRef]
11. Nahavandipour, A.; Jakobsen, K.K.; Gronhoj, C.; Hebbelstrup Jensen, D.; Kim Schmidt Karnov, K.; Klitmoller Agander, T.; Specht, L.; von Buchwald, C. Incidence and Survival of Laryngeal Cancer in Denmark: A Nation-wide Study from 1980 to 2014. *Acta Oncol.* **2019**, *58*, 977–982. [CrossRef] [PubMed]
12. Brandstorp-Boesen, J.; Sorum Falk, R.; Boysen, M.; Brondbo, K. Impact of Stage, Management and Recurrence on Survival Rates in Laryngeal Cancer. *PLoS ONE* **2017**, *12*, e0179371. [CrossRef] [PubMed]
13. Wiegand, S. Evidence-Based Review of Laryngeal Cancer Surgery. *Laryngorhinootologie* **2016**, *95* (Suppl. 1), S192–S216. [CrossRef]
14. Forner, D.; Rigby, M.H.; Corsten, M.; Trites, J.R.; Pyne, J.; Taylor, S.M. Oncological and Functional Outcomes after Repeat Transoral Laser Microsurgery for the Treatment of Recurrent Early Glottic Cancer. *J. Laryngol. Otol.* **2020**, 1–5. [CrossRef]
15. Luscher, M.S.; Pedersen, U.; Johansen, L.V. Treatment Outcome after Laser Excision of Early Glottic Squamous Cell Carcinoma–A Literature Survey. *Acta Oncol.* **2001**, *40*, 796–800. [CrossRef]
16. Zhou, J.; Wen, Q.; Wang, H.; Li, B.; Liu, J.; Hu, J.; Liu, S.; Zou, J. Prognostic Comparison of Transoral Laser Microsurgery for Early Glottic Cancer with or without Anterior Commissure Involvement: A Meta-analysis. *Am. J. Otolaryngol.* **2021**, *42*, 102787. [CrossRef] [PubMed]
17. Hendriksma, M.; Sjogren, E.V. Involvement of the Anterior Commissure in Early Glottic Cancer (Tis-T2): A Review of the Literature. *Cancers* **2019**, *11*, 1234. [CrossRef] [PubMed]
18. Steiner, W. Results of Curative Laser Microsurgery of Laryngeal Carcinomas. *Am. J. Otolaryngol.* **1993**, *14*, 116–121. [CrossRef]
19. Ledda, G.P.; Puxeddu, R. Carbon Dioxide Laser Microsurgery for Early Glottic Carcinoma. *Otolaryngol. Head Neck Surg.* **2006**, *134*, 911–915. [CrossRef]
20. Canis, M.; Ihler, F.; Martin, A.; Matthias, C.; Steiner, W. Transoral Laser Microsurgery for T1a Glottic Cancer: Review of 404 Cases. *Head Neck* **2015**, *37*, 889–895. [CrossRef] [PubMed]
21. Batra, A.; Goyal, A.; Goyal, M.; Goel, S. Oncological Outcomes Following Transoral CO2 Laser Microsurgery for T1 Glottic Cancer. *Indian J. Otolaryngol. Head Neck Surg.* **2019**, *71* (Suppl. 1), 542–547. [CrossRef] [PubMed]
22. Arens, C. Transoral Treatment Strategies for Head and Neck Tumors. *GMS Curr. Top. Otorhinolaryngol. Head Neck Surg.* **2012**, *11*. [CrossRef]
23. Wiegand, S. Evidence and Evidence Gaps of Laryngeal Cancer Surgery. *GMS Curr. Top. Otorhinolaryngol. Head Neck Surg.* **2016**, *15*. [CrossRef]
24. Ambrosch, P.; Fazel, A. Functional Organ Preservation in Laryngeal and Hypopharyngeal Cancer. *GMS Curr. Top. Otorhinolaryngol. Head Neck Surg.* **2011**, *10*. [CrossRef]
25. Chatenoud, L.; Garavello, W.; Pagan, E.; Bertuccio, P.; Gallus, S.; La Vecchia, C.; Negri, E.; Bosetti, C. Laryngeal Cancer Mortality Trends in European Countries. *Int. J. Cancer* **2016**, *138*, 833–842. [CrossRef]
26. Stachler, R.J.; Francis, D.O.; Schwartz, S.R.; Damask, C.C.; Digoy, G.P.; Krouse, H.J.; McCoy, S.J.; Ouellette, D.R.; Patel, R.R.; Reavis, C.C.W.; et al. Clinical Practice Guideline: Hoarseness (Dysphonia) (Update). *Otolaryngol. Head Neck Surg.* **2018**, *158* (Suppl. 1), S1–S42. [CrossRef] [PubMed]

27. Tikka, T.; Pracy, P.; Paleri, V. Refining the Head and Neck Cancer Referral Guidelines: A Two Centre Analysis of 4715 Referrals. *Br. J. Oral Maxillofac. Surg.* **2016**, *54*, 141–150. [CrossRef]
28. Caffier, P.P.; Schmidt, B.; Gross, M.; Karnetzky, K.; Nawka, T.; Rotter, A.; Seipelt, M.; Sedlmaier, B. A Comparison of White Light Laryngostroboscopy versus Autofluorescence Endoscopy in the Evaluation of Vocal Fold Pathology. *Laryngoscope* **2013**, *123*, 1729–1734. [CrossRef] [PubMed]
29. Whited, C.W.; Dailey, S.H. Evaluation of the Dysphonic Patient (in: Function Preservation in Laryngeal Cancer). *Otolaryngol. Clin. N. Am.* **2015**, *48*, 547–564. [CrossRef] [PubMed]
30. Piazza, C.; Cocco, D.; De Benedetto, L.; Del Bon, F.; Nicolai, P.; Peretti, G. Narrow Band Imaging and High Definition Television in the Assessment of Laryngeal Cancer: A Prospective Study on 279 Patients. *Eur. Arch. Otorhinolaryngol.* **2010**, *267*, 409–414. [CrossRef] [PubMed]
31. Ptok, M.; Schwemmle, C.; Iven, C.; Jessen, M.; Nawka, T. On the Auditory Evaluation of Voice Quality. *HNO* **2006**, *54*, 793–802. [CrossRef] [PubMed]
32. Ali, S.A.; Smith, J.D.; Hogikyan, N.D. The White Lesion, Hyperkeratosis, and Dysplasia. *Otolaryngol. Clin N. Am.* **2019**, *52*, 703–712. [CrossRef] [PubMed]
33. Nawka, T.; Martin, A.; Caffier, P.P. Microlaryngoscopy and Phonomicrosurgery. *HNO* **2013**, *61*, 108–116. [CrossRef] [PubMed]
34. Hartl, D.M.; Laoufi, S.; Brasnu, D.F. Voice Outcomes of Transoral Laser Microsurgery of the Larynx. *Otolaryngol. Clin. N. Am.* **2015**, *48*, 627–637. [CrossRef] [PubMed]
35. Mau, T.; Palaparthi, A.; Riede, T.; Titze, I.R. Effect of Resection Depth of Early Glottic Cancer on Vocal Outcome: An Optimized Finite Element Simulation. *Laryngoscope* **2015**, *125*, 1892–1899. [CrossRef] [PubMed]
36. Peeters, A.J.; van Gogh, C.D.; Goor, K.M.; Verdonck-de Leeuw, I.M.; Langendijk, J.A.; Mahieu, H.F. Health Status and Voice Outcome after Treatment for T1a Glottic Carcinoma. *Eur. Arch. Otorhinolaryngol.* **2004**, *261*, 534–540. [CrossRef] [PubMed]
37. Bozec, A.; Culie, D.; Poissonnet, G.; Dassonville, O. Current Role of Primary Surgical Treatment in Patients with Head and Neck Squamous Cell Carcinoma. *Curr. Opin. Oncol.* **2019**, *31*, 138–145. [CrossRef]
38. Hartl, D.M.; Brasnu, D.F. Contemporary Surgical Management of Early Glottic Cancer. *Otolaryngol. Clin. N. Am.* **2015**, *48*, 611–625. [CrossRef] [PubMed]
39. Baird, B.J.; Sung, C.K.; Beadle, B.M.; Divi, V. Treatment of Early-stage Laryngeal Cancer: A Comparison of Treatment Options. *Oral Oncol.* **2018**, *87*, 8–16. [CrossRef]
40. Huang, G.; Luo, M.; Zhang, J.; Liu, H. Laser Surgery versus Radiotherapy for T1a Glottic Carcinoma: A Meta-analysis of Oncologic Outcomes. *Acta Otolaryngol.* **2017**, *137*, 1204–1209. [CrossRef]
41. Strong, M.S.; Jako, G.J. Laser Surgery in the Larynx. Early Clinical Experience with Continuous CO_2 Laser. *Ann. Otol. Rhinol. Laryngol.* **1972**, *81*, 791–798. [CrossRef]
42. Harris, A.T.; Tanyi, A.; Hart, R.D.; Trites, J.; Rigby, M.H.; Lancaster, J.; Nicolaides, A.; Taylor, S.M. Transoral Laser Surgery for Laryngeal Carcinoma: Has Steiner Achieved a Genuine Paradigm Shift in Oncological Surgery? *Ann. R. Coll. Surg. Engl.* **2018**, *100*, 2–5. [CrossRef]
43. Sjogren, E.V. Transoral Laser Microsurgery in Early Glottic Lesions. *Curr. Otorhinolaryngol. Rep.* **2017**, *5*, 56–68. [CrossRef]
44. Peretti, G.; Piazza, C.; Cocco, D.; De Benedetto, L.; Del Bon, F.; Redaelli De Zinis, L.O.; Nicolai, P. Transoral CO(2) Laser Treatment for T(is)-T(3) Glottic Cancer: The University of Brescia Experience on 595 Patients. *Head Neck* **2010**, *32*, 977–983. [CrossRef]
45. Remacle, M.; Van Haverbeke, C.; Eckel, H.; Bradley, P.; Chevalier, D.; Djukic, V.; de Vicentiis, M.; Friedrich, G.; Olofsson, J.; Peretti, G.; et al. Proposal for Revision of the European Laryngological Society Classification of Endoscopic Cordectomies. *Eur. Arch. Otorhinolaryngol.* **2007**, *264*, 499–504. [CrossRef] [PubMed]
46. Caffier, P.P.; Moller, A.; Forbes, E.; Muller, C.; Freymann, M.L.; Nawka, T. The Vocal Extent Measure: Development of a Novel Parameter in Voice Diagnostics and Initial Clinical Experience. *BioMed Res. Int.* **2018**, *2018*, 3836714. [CrossRef]
47. Amin, M.B.; Edge, S.; Greene, F.; Byrd, D.R.; Brookland, R.K.; Washington, M.K.; Gershenwald, J.E.; Compton, C.C.; Hess, K.R.; Sullivan, D.C.; et al. *AJCC Cancer Staging Manual*, 8th ed.; Springer: New York, NY, USA, 2017.
48. Caffier, P.P.; Nawka, T.; Ibrahim-Nasr, A.; Thomas, B.; Muller, H.; Ko, S.R.; Song, W.; Gross, M.; Weikert, S. Development of Three-dimensional Laryngostroboscopy for Office-based Laryngeal Diagnostics and Phonosurgical Therapy. *Laryngoscope* **2018**, *128*, 2823–2831. [CrossRef]
49. Patel, R.R.; Awan, S.N.; Barkmeier-Kraemer, J.; Courey, M.; Deliyski, D.; Eadie, T.; Paul, D.; Švec, J.G.; Hillman, R. Recommended Protocols for Instrumental Assessment of Voice: American Speech-Language-Hearing Association Expert Panel to Develop a Protocol for Instrumental Assessment of Vocal Function. *Am. J. Speech Lang. Pathol.* **2018**, *27*, 887–905. [CrossRef] [PubMed]
50. Dejonckere, P.H.; Bradley, P.; Clemente, P.; Cornut, G.; Crevier-Buchman, L.; Friedrich, G.; Van De Heyning, P.; Remacle, M.; Woisard, V.; Committee on Phoniatrics of the European Laryngological Society (ELS). A Basic Protocol for Functional Assessment of Voice Pathology, Especially for Investigating the Efficacy of (Phonosurgical) Treatments and Evaluating New Assessment Techniques. Guideline Elaborated by the Committee on Phoniatrics of the European Laryngological Society (ELS). *Eur. Arch. Otorhinolaryngol.* **2001**, *258*, 77–82. [CrossRef]
51. Ternström, S.; Pabon, P.; Södersten, M. The Voice Range Profile: Its Function, Applications, Pitfalls and Potential. *Acta Acust. United Acust.* **2016**, *102*, 268–283. [CrossRef]

52. Nawka, T.; Verdonck-de Leeuw, I.M.; De Bodt, M.; Guimaraes, I.; Holmberg, E.B.; Rosen, C.A.; Schindler, A.; Woisard, V.; Whurr, R.; Konerding, U. Item reduction of the voice handicap index based on the original version and on European translations. *Folia Phoniatr. Logop.* **2009**, *61*, 37–48. [CrossRef] [PubMed]
53. Wuyts, F.L.; De Bodt, M.S.; Molenberghs, G.; Remacle, M.; Heylen, L.; Millet, B.; Van Lierde, K.; Raes, J.; Van de Heyning, P.H. The Dysphonia Severity Index: An Objective Measure of Vocal Quality Based on a Multiparameter Approach. *J. Speech Lang. Hear Res.* **2000**, *43*, 796–809. [CrossRef]
54. Greulich, M.T.; Parker, N.P.; Lee, P.; Merati, A.L.; Misono, S. Voice Outcomes Following Radiation versus Laser Microsurgery for T1 Glottic Carcinoma: Systematic Review and Meta-analysis. *Otolaryngol. Head Neck Surg.* **2015**, *152*, 811–819. [CrossRef] [PubMed]
55. Spielmann, P.M.; Majumdar, S.; Morton, R.P. Quality of Life and Functional Outcomes in the Management of Early Glottic Carcinoma: A Systematic Review of Studies Comparing Radiotherapy and Transoral Laser Microsurgery. *Clin. Otolaryngol.* **2010**, *35*, 373–382. [CrossRef]
56. Cohen, S.M.; Garrett, C.G.; Dupont, W.D.; Ossoff, R.H.; Courey, M.S. Voice-related Quality of Life in T1 Glottic Cancer: Irradiation versus Endoscopic Excision. *Ann. Otol. Rhinol. Laryngol.* **2006**, *115*, 581–586. [CrossRef]
57. Laoufi, S.; Mirghani, H.; Janot, F.; Hartl, D.M. Voice Quality after Treatment of T1a Glottic Cancer. *Laryngoscope* **2014**, *124*, 1398–1401. [CrossRef]
58. Krengli, M.; Policarpo, M.; Manfredda, I.; Aluffi, P.; Gambaro, G.; Panella, M.; Pia, F. Voice Quality after Treatment for T1a Glottic Carcinoma—Radiotherapy versus Laser Cordectomy. *Acta Oncol.* **2004**, *43*, 284–289. [CrossRef] [PubMed]
59. Gandhi, S.; Gupta, S.; Rajopadhye, G. A Comparison of Phonatory outcome Between Trans-oral CO_2 Laser Cordectomy and Radiotherapy in T1 Glottic Cancer. *Eur. Arch. Otorhinolaryngol.* **2018**, *275*, 2783–2786. [CrossRef]
60. van Gogh, C.D.; Verdonck-de Leeuw, I.M.; Wedler-Peeters, J.; Langendijk, J.A.; Mahieu, H.F. Prospective Evaluation of Voice Outcome during the First Two Years in Male Patients Treated by Radiotherapy or Laser Surgery for T1a Glottic Carcinoma. *Eur. Arch. Otorhinolaryngol.* **2012**, *269*, 1647–1652. [CrossRef] [PubMed]
61. Hong, Y.T.; Park, M.J.; Hong, K.H. Characteristics of Speech Production in Patients with T1 Glottic Cancer who Underwent Laser Cordectomy or Radiotherapy. *Logoped Phoniatr. Vocol.* **2018**, *43*, 120–128. [CrossRef] [PubMed]
62. Kono, T.; Saito, K.; Yabe, H.; Uno, K.; Ogawa, K. Comparative Multidimensional Assessment of Laryngeal Function and Quality of Life after Radiotherapy and Laser Surgery for Early Glottic Cancer. *Head Neck* **2016**, *38*, 1085–1090. [CrossRef] [PubMed]
63. Nunez Batalla, F.; Caminero Cueva, M.J.; Senaris Gonzalez, B.; Llorente Pendas, J.L.; Gorriz Gil, C.; Lopez Llames, A.; Alonso Pantiga, R.; Suárez Nieto, C. Voice Quality after Endoscopic Laser Surgery and Radiotherapy for Early Glottic Cancer: Objective Measurements Emphasizing the Voice Handicap Index. *Eur. Arch. Otorhinolaryngol.* **2008**, *265*, 543–548. [CrossRef]
64. Sjogren, E.V.; van Rossum, M.A.; Langeveld, T.P.; Voerman, M.S.; van de Kamp, V.A.; Friebel, M.O.; Wolterbeek, R.; Baatenburg de Jong, R.J. Voice Outcome in T1a Midcord Glottic Carcinoma: Laser Surgery vs Radiotherapy. *Arch. Otolaryngol. Head Neck Surg.* **2008**, *134*, 965–972. [CrossRef]
65. Berania, I.; Dagenais, C.; Moubayed, S.P.; Ayad, T.; Olivier, M.-J.; Guertin, L.; Bissada, E.; Tabet, J.C.; Christopoulos, A. Voice and Functional Outcomes of Transoral Laser Microsurgery for Early Glottic Cancer: Ventricular Fold Resection as a Surrogate. *J. Clin. Med. Res.* **2015**, *7*, 632–636. [CrossRef]
66. Bertino, G.; Degiorgi, G.; Tinelli, C.; Cacciola, S.; Occhini, A.; Benazzo, M. CO_2 Laser Cordectomy for T1-T2 Glottic Cancer: Oncological and Functional Long-term Results. *Eur. Arch. Otorhinolaryngol.* **2015**, *272*, 2389–2395. [CrossRef]
67. Bajaj, Y.; Uppal, S.; Sharma, R.K.; Grace, A.R.; Howard, D.M.; Nicolaides, A.R.; Coatesworth, A.P. Evaluation of Voice and Quality of Life after Transoral Endoscopic Laser Resection of Early Glottic Carcinoma. *J. Laryngol. Otol.* **2011**, *125*, 706–713. [CrossRef]
68. Keilmann, A.; Napiontek, U.; Engel, C.; Nakarat, T.; Schneider, A.; Mann, W. Long-term Functional Outcome after Unilateral Cordectomy. *ORL J. Otorhinolaryngol. Relat. Spec.* **2011**, *73*, 38–46. [CrossRef]
69. Motta, S.; Cesari, U.; Mesolella, M.; Motta, G. Functional Vocal Results after CO2 Laser Endoscopic Surgery for Glottic Tumours. *J. Laryngol. Otol.* **2008**, *122*, 948–951. [CrossRef]
70. Hamzany, Y.; Crevier-Buchman, L.; Lechien, J.R.; Bachar, G.; Brasnu, D.; Hans, S. Multidimensional Voice Quality Evaluation After Transoral CO2 Laser Cordectomy: A Prospective Study. *Ear Nose Throat J.* **2021**, *100* (Suppl. 1), 27S–32S. [CrossRef] [PubMed]
71. Lee, H.S.; Kim, J.S.; Kim, S.W.; Noh, W.J.; Kim, Y.J.; Oh, D.; Hong, J.C.; Lee, K.D. Voice Outcome According to Surgical Extent of Transoral Laser Microsurgery for T1 Glottic Carcinoma. *Laryngoscope* **2016**, *126*, 2051–2056. [CrossRef]
72. Fink, D.S.; Sibley, H.; Kunduk, M.; Schexnaildre, M.; Kakade, A.; Sutton, C.; McWhorter, A.J. Subjective and Objective Voice Outcomes After Transoral Laser Microsurgery for Early Glottic Cancer. *Laryngoscope* **2016**, *126*, 405–407. [CrossRef]
73. Tomifuji, M.; Araki, K.; Niwa, K.; Miyagawa, Y.; Mizokami, D.; Kitagawa, Y.; Yamashita, T.; Matsunobu, T.; Shiotani, A. Comparison of Voice Quality After Laser Cordectomy with That After Radiotherapy or Chemoradiotherapy for Early Glottic Carcinoma. *ORL J. Otorhinolaryngol. Relat. Spec.* **2013**, *75*, 18–26. [CrossRef] [PubMed]
74. Peretti, G.; Piazza, C.; Balzanelli, C.; Mensi, M.C.; Rossini, M.; Antonelli, A.R. Preoperative and Postoperative Voice in Tis-T1 Glottic Cancer Treated by Endoscopic Cordectomy: An Additional Issue for Patient Counseling. *Ann. Otol. Rhinol. Laryngol.* **2003**, *112*, 759–763. [CrossRef] [PubMed]
75. Roh, J.L.; Kim, D.H.; Kim, S.Y.; Park, C.I. Quality of Life and Voice in Patients After Laser Cordectomy for Tis and T1 Glottic Carcinomas. *Head Neck* **2007**, *29*, 1010–1016. [CrossRef]

76. Strieth, S.; Ernst, B.P.; Both, I.; Hirth, D.; Pfisterer, L.N.; Kunzel, J.; Eder, K. Randomized Controlled Single-blinded Clinical Trial of Functional Voice Outcome after Vascular Targeting KTP laser Microsurgery of Early Laryngeal Cancer. *Head Neck* **2019**, *41*, 899–907. [CrossRef]
77. Friedman, A.D.; Hillman, R.E.; Landau-Zemer, T.; Burns, J.A.; Zeitels, S.M. Voice Outcomes for Photoangiolytic KTP Laser Treatment of Early Glottic Cancer. *Ann. Otol. Rhinol. Laryngol.* **2013**, *122*, 151–158. [CrossRef] [PubMed]
78. Lester, S.E.; Rigby, M.H.; MacLean, M.; Taylor, S.M. 'How Does That sound?': Objective and Subjective Voice Outcomes Following CO(2) Laser Resection for Early Glottic Cancer. *J. Laryngol. Otol.* **2011**, *125*, 1251–1255. [CrossRef] [PubMed]
79. Vilaseca, I.; Huerta, P.; Blanch, J.L.; Fernandez-Planas, A.M.; Jimenez, C.; Bernal-Sprekelsen, M. Voice Quality after CO2 Laser Cordectomy–What Can We Really Expect? *Head Neck* **2008**, *30*, 43–49. [CrossRef]
80. Aichinger, P.; Feichter, F.; Aichstill, B.; Bigenzahn, W.; Schneider-Stickler, B. Inter-device Reliability of DSI Measurement. *Logoped. Phoniatr. Vocol.* **2012**, *37*, 167–173. [CrossRef] [PubMed]
81. Hakkesteegt, M.M.; Brocaar, M.P.; Wieringa, M.H.; Feenstra, L. Influence of Age and Gender on the Dysphonia Severity Index. A Study of Normative Values. *Folia Phoniatr. Logop.* **2006**, *58*, 264–273. [CrossRef]
82. Hakkesteegt, M.M.; Brocaar, M.P.; Wieringa, M.H. The Applicability of the Dysphonia Severity Index and the Voice Handicap Index in Evaluating Effects of Voice Therapy and Phonosurgery. *J. Voice* **2010**, *24*, 199–205. [CrossRef]
83. Chu, P.-Y.; Hsu, Y.-B.; Lee, T.-L.; Fu, S.; Wang, L.-M.; Kao, Y.-C. Longitudinal Analysis of Voice Quality in Patients with Early Glottic Cancer after Transoral Laser Microsurgery. *Head Neck* **2012**, *34*, 1294–1298. [CrossRef] [PubMed]
84. Burns, J.A.; Har-El, G.; Shapshay, S.; Maune, S.; Zeitels, S.M. Endoscopic Laser Resection of Laryngeal Cancer: Is it Oncologically Safe? Position Statement from the American Broncho-Esophagological Association. *Ann. Otol. Rhinol. Laryngol.* **2009**, *118*, 399–404. [CrossRef] [PubMed]
85. Aluffi Valletti, P.; Taranto, F.; Chiesa, A.; Pia, F.; Valente, G. Impact of Resection Margin Status on Oncological Outcomes after CO2 Laser Cordectomy. *Acta Otorhinolaryngol. Ital.* **2018**, *38*, 24–30. [PubMed]

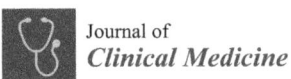

Journal of
Clinical Medicine

Review

Neurostimulation in People with Oropharyngeal Dysphagia: A Systematic Review and Meta-Analyses of Randomised Controlled Trials—Part I: Pharyngeal and Neuromuscular Electrical Stimulation

Renée Speyer [1,2,3,*], Anna-Liisa Sutt [4,5], Liza Bergström [6,7], Shaheen Hamdy [8], Bas Joris Heijnen [3], Lianne Remijn [9], Sarah Wilkes-Gillan [10] and Reinie Cordier [2,11]

1. Department Special Needs Education, Faculty of Educational Sciences, University of Oslo, 0318 Oslo, Norway
2. Curtin School of Allied Health, Faculty of Health Sciences, Curtin University, Perth, WA 6102, Australia
3. Department of Otorhinolaryngology and Head and Neck Surgery, Leiden University Medical Centre, 1233 ZA Leiden, The Netherlands; b.j.Heijnen@lumc.nl
4. Critical Care Research Group, The Prince Charles Hospital, Brisbane, QLD 4032, Australia; annaliisasp@gmail.com
5. School of Medicine, University of Queensland, Brisbane, QLD 4072, Australia
6. Remeo Stockholm, 128 64 Stockholm, Sweden; liza.bergstrom@regionstockholm.se
7. Speech Therapy Clinic, Danderyd University Hospital, 182 88 Stockholm, Sweden
8. GI Sciences, School of Medical Sciences, Faculty of Biology, Medicine and Health, University of Manchester, Manchester M13 9PL, UK; shaheen.hamdy@manchester.ac.uk
9. School of Allied Health, HAN University of Applied Sciences, 6525 EN Nijmegen, The Netherlands; lianne.remijn@han.nl
10. Discipline of Occupational Therapy, Sydney School of Health Sciences, Faculty of Medicine and Health, The University of Sydney, Sydney, NSW 2006, Australia; sarah.wilkes-gillan@sydney.edu.au
11. Department of Social Work, Education and Community Wellbeing, Faculty of Health & Life Sciences, Northumbria University, Newcastle upon Tyne NE7 7XA, UK; reinie.cordier@northumbria.ac.uk
* Correspondence: renee.speyer@isp.uio.no

Abstract: *Objective.* To assess the effects of neurostimulation (i.e., neuromuscular electrical stimulation (NMES) and pharyngeal electrical stimulation (PES)) in people with oropharyngeal dysphagia (OD). *Methods.* Systematic literature searches were conducted to retrieve randomised controlled trials in four electronic databases (CINAHL, Embase, PsycINFO, and PubMed). The methodological quality of included studies was assessed using the Revised Cochrane risk-of-bias tool for randomised trials (RoB 2). *Results.* In total, 42 studies reporting on peripheral neurostimulation were included: 30 studies on NMES, eight studies on PES, and four studies on combined neurostimulation interventions. When conducting meta analyses, significant, large and significant, moderate pre-post treatment effects were found for NMES (11 studies) and PES (five studies), respectively. Between-group analyses showed small effect sizes in favour of NMES, but no significant effects for PES. *Conclusions.* NMES may have more promising effects compared to PES. However, NMES studies showed high heterogeneity in protocols and experimental variables, the presence of potential moderators, and inconsistent reporting of methodology. Therefore, only conservative generalisations and interpretation of meta-analyses could be made. To facilitate comparisons of studies and determine intervention effects, there is a need for more randomised controlled trials with larger population sizes, and greater standardisation of protocols and guidelines for reporting.

Keywords: deglutition; swallowing disorders; RCT; intervention; neuromuscular electrical stimulation; pharyngeal electrical stimulation; PES; NMES

Citation: Speyer, R.; Sutt, A.-L.; Bergström, L.; Hamdy, S.; Heijnen, B.J.; Remijn, L.; Wilkes-Gillan, S.; Cordier, R. Neurostimulation in People with Oropharyngeal Dysphagia: A Systematic Review and Meta-Analyses of Randomised Controlled Trials—Part I: Pharyngeal and Neuromuscular Electrical Stimulation. *J. Clin. Med.* **2022**, *11*, 776. https://doi.org/10.3390/jcm11030776

Academic Editor: Michael Setzen

Received: 7 December 2021
Accepted: 27 January 2022
Published: 31 January 2022

Publisher's Note: MDPI stays neutral with regard to jurisdictional claims in published maps and institutional affiliations.

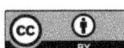

Copyright: © 2022 by the authors. Licensee MDPI, Basel, Switzerland. This article is an open access article distributed under the terms and conditions of the Creative Commons Attribution (CC BY) license (https://creativecommons.org/licenses/by/4.0/).

1. Introduction

The aerodigestive tract facilitates the combined functions of breathing, vocalising, and swallowing. Any dysfunction in this system may lead to oropharyngeal dysphagia (OD)

or swallowing problems [1]. OD can be the result of underlying diseases such as stroke or a progressive neurological disease (e.g., Parkinson's disease, multiple sclerosis) or an adverse effect after head and neck oncological interventions (e.g., radiation or surgery) or intensive care treatment (e.g., intubation and tracheostomy). Prevalence estimates of OD have been reported to be as high as 50% in cerebral palsy [2], 80% in stroke and Parkinson's disease, and over 90% in people with community-acquired pneumonia [3]. OD can have a severe impact on a person's health as it may lead to dehydration, malnutrition, and even death. Research has identified inverse bidirectional relationships between decreased health-related quality of life and increased OD severity [4].

Traditional OD therapy may include physical interventions such as: bolus modification and management (e.g., adjusting the viscosity, volume, temperature and/or acidity of food and drinks); oromotor exercises; body and head postural adjustments; and swallow manoeuvres (e.g., manoeuvres to improve food propulsion into the pharynx and airway protection) [1]. Therapy may also include sensory stimulation, which involves applying techniques like thermal stimulation and chemical stimulation using natural agonists of polymodal sensory receptors (e.g., capsaicin, the spicy component of peppers) [5].

Another type of stimulation considered to be beneficial for promoting rehabilitation of swallowing dysfunction is acupuncture. This practice emerged from traditional Chinese medicine and exerts therapeutic effects by inserting thin needles at strategic places, termed acupuncture points, on the body surface aiming to rebalance the flow of energy or life force ('qi'). Needles are then activated through specific manual movements or electrical stimulation. Although stimulation of acupuncture points seems to be associated with places where nerves, muscles, and connective tissues may be stimulated [6], their intrinsic mechanisms are still part of a continuing scientific debate on acupuncture.

Recently, an increasing number of studies have been published on alternative interventions aiming to enhance neural plasticity by using non-invasive brain stimulation (NIBS) techniques. Repetitive transcranial magnetic stimulation (rTMS) and transcranial direct current stimulation (tDCS) are cortically or centrally applied NIBS techniques. Using electromagnetic induction, rTMS results in depolarisation of post-synaptic connections, whereas tDCS uses direct electrical current to shift the polarity of nerve cells [7]. Alternatively, electrical stimulation techniques like pharyngeal electrical stimulation (PES) and neuromuscular electrical stimulation (NMES) target the peripheral neural pathways [8]. NMES aims to strengthen muscular contractions during swallowing and uses stimulation by electrodes placed on the skin over the anterior neck muscles to activate sensory pathways [9–11]. In contrast, PES has been shown to drive neuroplasticity in the pharyngeal motor cortex through direct stimulation of the pharyngeal mucosa via intraluminal catheters [7].

Over the past decade, several reviews have been published on the effects of neurostimulation in patients with OD. Most of these reviews focused on selected types of neurostimulation: NMES [10,12], rTMS [13,14], tDCS [15], or rTMS and tDCS [16,17]. Only two systematic reviews included both cortical (rTMS and tDCS) and peripheral neurostimulation (PES and NMES) [18,19]. All reviews targeted interventions in post-stroke populations except one review that broadened inclusion criteria to patients with acquired brain injury including stroke [16]. To date, all systematic reviews on neurostimulation as a treatment for OD set boundaries for inclusion based on medical diagnoses.

The aim of this systematic review is to determine the effects of neurostimulation in people with OD without excluding populations based on medical diagnoses. Findings are based on the highest level of evidence only, namely randomised controlled trials (RCTs), and summarised by conducting meta-analyses. The results of this review will be presented in two companion papers. This paper (Part I) reports on pharyngeal and neuromuscular electrical stimulation (PES and NMES) while the second paper (Part II) will report on brain stimulation (i.e., rTMS and tDCS).

2. Methods

The methodology and reporting of this systematic review were based on the Preferred Reporting Items for Systematic Reviews and Meta-Analyses (PRISMA) 2020 statement and checklist (Supplementary Tables S1 and S2) which aim to enhance the essential and transparent reporting of systematic reviews [20,21]. The protocol for this review was registered at PROSPERO, the international prospective register of systematic reviews (registration number: CRD42020179842).

2.1. Information Sources and Search Strategies

Literature searches to identify studies were conducted on 6 March 2021, across four databases: CINAHL, Embase, PsycINFO, and PubMed. Publication dates of coverage ranged from 1937–2021, 1902–2021, 1887–2021, and 1809–2021, respectively. Additional searches, including checking the reference lists of eligible articles, were performed. Two main categories of terms were used in combination: (1) dysphagia and (2) randomised control trials. Search strategies were performed in all four electronic databases using subheadings (e.g., MeSH and Thesaurus terms) and free text terms. The full electronic search strategies for each database are reported in Table 1. To identify other literature beyond that found using these strategies, the reference lists of each eligible article were checked.

Table 1. Search strategies.

Database and Search Terms	Number of Records
Cinahl: ((MH "Deglutition") OR (MH "Deglutition Disorders")) AND (MH "Randomized Controlled Trials")	239
Embase: (swallowing/OR dysphagia/) AND (randomization/or randomized controlled trial/OR "randomized controlled trial (topic)"/OR controlled clinical trial/)	4550
PsycINFO: (swallowing/OR dysphagia/) AND (RCT OR (Randomised AND Controlled AND Trial) OR (Randomized AND Clinical AND Trial) OR (Randomised AND Clinical AND Trial) OR (Controlled AND Clinical AND Trial)).af.	231
PubMed: ("Deglutition"[Mesh] OR "Deglutition Disorders"[Mesh]) AND ("Randomized Controlled Trial" [Publication Type] OR "Randomized Controlled Trials as Topic"[Mesh] OR "Controlled Clinical Trial" [Publication Type] OR "Pragmatic Clinical Trials as Topic"[Mesh])	3039

2.2. Inclusion and Exclusion Criteria

Studies were included in this systematic review if they met the following criteria: (1) participants had a diagnosis of oropharyngeal dysphagia; (2) the study included non-invasive neurostimulation interventions aimed at reducing swallowing or feeding problems; (3) the study included a control group or comparison intervention group; (4) participants were randomly assigned to one of the study arms or groups; and (5) the study was published in the English language.

Interventions such as non-electrical peripheral stimulation (e.g., air-puff or gustatory stimulation), pharmacological interventions and acupuncture, were considered out of the scope of this review, and thus were excluded. Invasive techniques and/or those that did not specifically target OD (i.e., deep-brain stimulation studies after neurosurgical implementation of a neurostimulator) were also excluded. Conference abstracts, doctoral theses, editorials, and reviews were excluded.

Finally, only studies reporting on peripheral neurostimulation (i.e., PES and NMES) were included in this review (Part I). Studies on brain neurostimulation (i.e., rTMS and tDCS) will be reported on in a companion paper (Part II).

3. Systematic Review

3.1. Methodological Quality and Risk of Bias

The methodological quality of the included studies was assessed using the Revised Cochrane risk-of-bias tool for randomised trials (RoB 2) [22]. The RoB 2 tool identifies five domains to consider when assessing where bias may have been introduced into a randomised trial: (1) bias arising from the randomisation process; (2) bias due to deviations from intended interventions; (3) bias due to missing outcome data; (4) bias in measurement of the outcome; and (5) bias in selection of the reported result. The RoB 2 gives a series of signalling questions for each domain whose answers give a judgement (i.e., "low risk of bias," "some concerns," or "high risk of bias"), which can be evaluated to determine a study's overall risk of bias [22].

3.2. Data Collection Process

A data extraction form was created to extract data from the included studies under the following categories: participant diagnosis, inclusion and exclusion criteria, sample size, age, gender, intervention goal, intervention agent/delivery/dosage, outcome measures, and treatment outcome.

3.3. Data, Items and Synthesis of Results

Titles and abstracts of included studies were screened for eligibility by two independent reviewers, after which the eligibility of selected original articles was assessed by these same two reviewers. If agreement could not be reached between the first two reviewers, a third reviewer was consulted to reach consensus. Two independent researchers also assessed the methodological study quality and, where necessary, consensus was reached with involvement of a third reviewer. As none of the reviewers have formal or informal affiliations with any of the authors of the included studies, no evident bias in article selection or methodological study quality rating was present.

Data points across all studies were extracted using comprehensive data extraction forms. Risk of bias per individual study was assessed using the RoB 2 tool [22]. Data were extrapolated and synthesized using the following categories: participant characteristics, inclusion criteria, intervention conditions, outcome measures and intervention outcomes. Effect sizes and significance of findings were the main summary measures for assessing treatment outcome.

4. Meta-Analysis

Data Analysis. Data were extracted from each study to compare the effect sizes for the following: (1) pre-post outcome measures of OD and (2) mean difference between neurostimulation and comparison controls in outcome measures from pre- to post-intervention. Control groups may receive no treatment, sham stimulation and/or traditional dysphagia therapy (DT; e.g., bolus modification, oromotor exercises, body and head postural adjustments, and swallow manoeuvres). Only studies using instrumental assessment (e.g., videofluoroscopic swallow study (VFSS) or fiberoptic endoscopic evaluation of swallowing (FEES)) to confirm OD were included.

Data collected using outcome measures based on visuoperceptual evaluation of instrumental assessment were preferred over clinical non-instrumental assessments. Oral intake measures were only included if no other clinical data were available, whereas screening tools and patient self-report measures were excluded from meta-analyses altogether. When selecting outcome measures for meta-analyses, reducing heterogeneity between studies was a priority. Consequently, measures other than the authors' primary outcomes may have been preferred if these measures contributed to greater homogeneity.

To compare effect sizes, group means, standard deviations, and sample sizes for pre- and post-measurements, data were entered into Comprehensive Meta-Analysis Version 3.3.070 [23]. If only non-parametric data were available (i.e., medians, interquartile ranges), data were converted into parametric data for meta-analytic purposes. Studies with multiple intervention groups were analysed separately for each experimental-control comparison. If studies included the same participants, only one study was included in the meta-analysis. For studies providing insufficient data for meta-analysis, authors were contacted by e-mail to request additional data.

Effect sizes were calculated in Comprehensive Meta-Analysis using a random-effects model since it was unlikely that studies would have similar true effects due to variations in sampling, participant characteristics, intervention approaches, and outcome measurements. Heterogeneity was estimated using the Q statistic to determine the spread of effect sizes about the mean and I^2 was used to estimate the ratio of true variance to total variance. I^2-values of less than 50%, 50% to 74%, and higher than 75% denote low, moderate, and high heterogeneity, respectively [24]. Effect sizes were generated using the Hedges' g formula for standardized mean difference with a confidence interval of 95%. Effects sizes were interpreted using Cohen's d convention as follows: $g \leq 0.2$ as no or negligible effect; $0.2 < g \leq 0.5$ as small effect; $0.5 < g \leq 0.8$ as moderate effect; and $g > 0.8$ as large effect [25].

Forest plots of effect sizes for OD outcome scores were generated for PES and NMES separately: (1) pre-post neurostimulation and (2) neurostimulation interventions versus comparison groups. Subgroup analyses were used to explore effect sizes as a function of various moderators depending on neurostimulation type. For example, outcome measures, medical diagnoses, total treatment duration, total neurostimulation time, and stimulation characteristics (e.g., pulse duration, pulse rate, electrode configuration). To account for the possibility of spontaneous recovery during the intervention period, only between-subgroup meta-analyses were conducted using post-intervention data.

Comprehensive Data Analysis software was utilized to evaluate publication bias. The Begg and Muzumdar's test [26] was used to calculate the rank correlation between the standardised effect size and the ranks of their variances. The Begg and Muzumdar test calculates both a tau and a two tailed p value, with values of close to zero indicating no correlation, while results closer to 1 suggest a correlation. Where asymmetry is the result of publication bias, high standard error values would correspond with larger effect sizes. Where larger effects correspond to low values, tau would be positive (with the inverse also being true). Conversely, when larger effects correspond to high values, tau would be negative.

Publication bias was also evaluated utilising a fail-safe N test. This measure addresses the question of how many omitted studies would be necessary to nullify the effect. It refers to the number of studies where the effect size was zero being included in the meta-analysis prior to the result becoming statistically insignificant [27]. When this value is comparably low, there may be reason to treat the results with caution. When the value is comparably high, however, it can be reasonably concluded that the treatment effect is not nil, although it may be increased due to the omission of some studies.

5. Results

5.1. Study Selection

A total of 8059 studies were identified through subject heading and free text searches from the four databases: CINAHL (n = 239), Embase (n = 4550), PsycINFO (n = 231), and PubMed (n = 3039). Removing duplicate titles and abstracts (n = 1113) left a total of 6946 records. A total of 261 original articles were assessed at a full-text level, with articles grouped based on type of intervention. Four additional studies were found through reference checking of the included articles. At this stage, no studies were excluded based on type of intervention (e.g., behavioural intervention, neurostimulation). Of the reviewed 261 articles, 58 studies on neurostimulation were identified that satisfied the inclusion criteria. As this systematic review reports on PES and NMES interventions only, a final number of 42 studies reporting on peripheral neurostimulation were included in this review. Figure 1 presents the flow diagram of the reviewing process according to PRISMA.

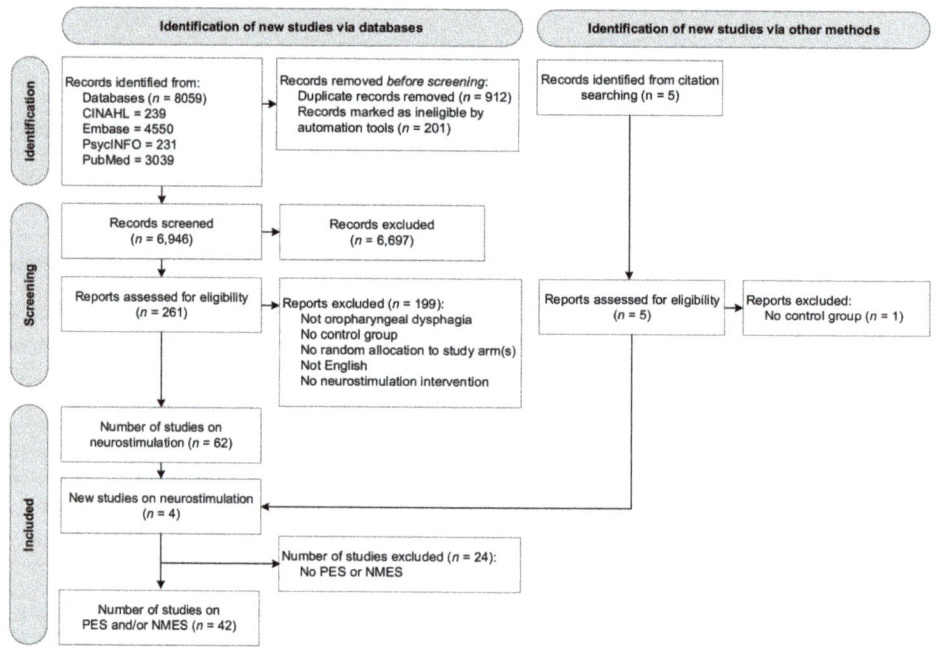

Figure 1. Flow diagram of the reviewing process according to the Preferred Reporting Items for Systematic Reviews and Meta-Analyses (PRISMA).

5.2. Description of Studies

All included studies are described in detail within Tables 2 and 3. Specifically, Table 2 presents data on study characteristics including methodological study quality, inclusion and exclusion criteria, and details on participant groups. The following information is provided for all study groups (control and intervention groups): medical diagnosis, sample size, age and gender. Table 3 reports on intervention goals of included studies, intervention components, outcome measures, intervention outcomes, as well as main conclusions.

Table 2. Study characteristics of studies on NMES and PES interventions for people with oropharyngeal dysphagia.

Study • Country	Inclusion/Exclusion Criteria	Sample (N) • Group	Group Descriptives (Mean ± SD) Age, Gender, Medical Diagnoses
NeuroMuscular Electrical Stimulation (NMES) [a]—n = 30			
Beom, et al. [28] • Country: Korea	OD as per VFSS Inclusion: stroke, traumatic brain injury or brain tumour >1 week ago; hemiplegia caused by hemispheric lesion; able to respond to pain Exclusion: no potential for recovery; severe communication difficulties; contraindications for neuromuscular electrical stimulation (NMES)	n = 132 • Treatment group 1 (66), 50% NMES (Suprahyoid muscle stimulation) + DT [Denoted as 'Beom et al. (2015a)' in Figure 4] • Treatment group 2 (66), 50% NMES (suprahyoid and infrahyoid muscles stimulation) + DT [Denoted as 'Beom et al. (2015b)' in Figure 4]	Treatment group 1: Age 64.4 ± 12.0 50% male Location of lesion: cortex (29), subcortex (20), brainstem (16), cerebellum (1) Treatment group 2: Age 59.8 ± 15.9 66.6% male Location of lesion: cortex (29), subcortex (14), brainstem (19), cerebellum (4) NS difference between groups
Bülow, et al. [29] • Country: Sweden, The Netherlands, France	OD as per VFSS Inclusion: 50–80 years old; hemispheric stroke > 3 months; ability to swallow; ability to communicate Exclusion: brainstem involvement; progressive cerebrovascular disease; other neurologic diseases such as ALS, MS, or Parkinson's disease; patients with tumors of the swallowing apparatus + radiotherapy/surgery to the neck; patients with no pharyngeal swallow; nasogastric tube insitu	n = 25 • Treatment group 1 (13), 52% DT • Treatment group 2 (12), 48% NMES (suprahyoid and infrahyoid muscles stimulation) + Diet modification	Combined treatment groups data: 64% male Treatment group 1: Age 71 (SD not reported) Treatment group 2: Age 70 Statistical difference between groups = NR
El-Tamawy, et al. [30] • Country: Egypt	OD as per bedside screening (confirmed by VFSS once enrolled) Inclusion: acute stroke, severe dysphagia; able to ambulate; normal attention and communication skills; no other neurological disease; able to perform sit to stand test Exclusion: disturbed level of consciousness; dementia; psychiatric disorders; syncope; previous operation or injury to the head and neck area	n = 30 • Treatment group 1 (15), 50% NMES + DT + (Medical treatment) • Control group 2 (15), 50% Medical treatment	Treatment group 1: Age 61.5 ± 7.3 Control group 2: Age 61.3 ± 6.6 No further details on subjects within the groups.
Guillén-Solà, et al. [31] • Country: Spain	OD as per VFSS (PAS ≥ 3) Subacute ischaemic stroke (1–3 weeks) Exclusion: Cognitive impairment (Short portable Mental Status Qnr >3), previous neurological diseases with risk of dysphagia	n = 62 • Treatment group 1 (21), 33.9% DT • Treatment group 2 (20), 32.2% DT + inspiratory and expiratory muscle training • Treatment group 3 (21), 33.9% NMES + DT + sham inspiratory and expiratory muscle training	Treatment 1: Age = 68.9 ± 7 Male = 57.1% Treatment 2: Age = 67.9 ± 10.6 Male = 76.2% Treatment 3: Age = 70.3 ± 8.4 Male = 47.6% NS differences between groups

Table 2. Cont.

Study • Country	Inclusion/Exclusion Criteria	Sample (N) • Group	Group Descriptives (Mean ± SD) Age, Gender, Medical Diagnoses
Heijnen, et al. [32] • Country: The Netherlands	• OD as per clinical assessment by SLT/VFSS • Inclusion: 40–80 year olds with idiopathic Parkinson's disease; stable condition; unaltered antiparkinsonian medication protocol for ≥ 2 months • Exclusion: other neurological disease; severe mental depression or cognitive degeneration (MMSE < 23); deep brain stimulation, malignancies, extensive surgery, radiotherapy to the head&neck region; severe cardiopulmonary disease, epilepsy, carotid sinus syndrome, dermatological diseases in head&neck area; dysphagia treatment in the preceding 6 months	$n = 85$ • Treatment group 1 (28), 32.9% DT • Treatment group 2 (27), 31.8% NMES at motor level + DT • Treatment group 3 (30), 35.3% NMES at sensory level + DT	Treatment group 1: median age 69 78.6% male Treatment group 2: median age 65 74.1% male Treatment group 3: median age 66 76.7% male NS differences between groups
Huang, et al. [33] • Country: Taiwan	• OD as per 100 mL water test + SLT assessment • Inclusion: recent cerebral hemispheric stroke; FOIS ≤ 4 • Exclusion: impaired communication ability; dysphagia caused by other disease; use of an electrically sensitive biomedical device (eg. cardiac pacemaker); pneumonia or acute medical condition	$n = 29$ • Treatment group 1 (11), 37.9% DT • Treatment group 2 (8), 27.6% NMES • Treatment group 3 (10), 34.5% NMES + DT	Treatment group 1: Age 67.0 ± 10.1 54.5% male Infarction (9); haemorrhage (2) Treatment group 2: Age 64.5 ± 14.4 62.5% male Infarction (6); haemorrhage (2) Treatment group 3: Age 68.9 ± 9.8 90% male Infarction (9); haemorrhage (1) NS differences between groups
Huh, et al. [34] • Country: South Korea	• OD as per VFSS • Inclusion: stroke; sufficient cognitive and language skills to perform effortful swallow • Exclusion: other neurological disease; contraindications to electrical stimulation	$n = 31$ • Treatment group 1 (10), 32.3% NMES with horizontal electrodes configuration (supra and infrahyoid muscles stimulation) + DT (effortful swallow) [Denoted as 'Huh et al. (2019a)' in Figure 4] • Treatment group 2 (11), 35.5% NMES with horizontal + vertical electrodes configuration (supra and infrahyoid muscles stimulation) + DT (effortful swallow) [Denoted as 'Huh et al. (2019b)' in Figure 4] • Treatment group 3 (10), 32.3% NMES with vertical electrodes configuration (supra and infrahyoid muscles stimulation) + DT (effortful swallow) [Denoted as 'Huh et al. (2019c)' in Figure 4]	Treatment group 1: Age 64.8 ± 14.1 90% male Infarction 6, haemorrhage 4 Treatment group 2: Age 60.45 ± 16.2 72.7% male Infarction 4, haemorrhage 7 Treatment group 3: Age 62.40 ± 12.7 50% male Infarction 4, haemorrhage 6 NS differences between groups
Jing, et al. [35] • Country: China	• OD as per Rattans dysphagia classification criteria, conducted by a rehabilitation nurse • Inclusion: stroke; dysphagia (grade ≤ 5) within 1–3 days post stroke; no previous rehabilitation training; stable vital signs; signed informed consent • Exclusion: not available	$n = 60$ • Treatment group 1 (30), 50% NMES + DT (+ Medical treatment) • Treatment group 2 (30), 50% DT (+ Medical treatment)	Treatment group 1: Age 67.9 ± 11.4 63.3% male 63% unilateral, 47% bilateral stroke, 70% infarction, 30% haemorrhage Treatment group 2: Age 68.6 ± 12.5 53.3% male 70% unilateral, 30% bilateral stroke, 77% infarction, 23% haemorrhage Statistical difference between groups = NR

Table 2. Cont.

Study • Country	Inclusion/Exclusion Criteria	Sample (N) • Group	Group Descriptives (Mean ± SD) Age, Gender, Medical Diagnoses
Langmore, et al. [36] • Country: USA	OD as per VFSS Inclusion: >21 year old patients ≥ 3 months post a full dose (≥50 Gy) of (chemo)radiotherapy for head&neck cancer, cancer free, severe dysphagia (PAS ≥ 4 on VFSS) Exclusion: dysphagia due to other cause, presence of electrical stimulation, neurologic disease, presence of pacemaker/defibrillator, floor of mouth resection, inability to follow the study protocol	n = 127 • Treatment group 1 (91), 71.7% NMES + DT • Sham/treatment group 2 (36), 28.3% Sham NMES + DT	Treatment group 1: Age 62.1 + 9.2 86.2% male RT site: Oral—9.5%, Nasopharynx—8.6%, Oropharynx—47.4%, Hypopharynx—12.1%, Larynx—11.2%, Other—12.1% Stage: 1—7.4% 2—7.4% 3—21.1% 4—64.2% Sham/Treatment group 2: Age 61.5 ± 10.6 84.6% male RT site: Oral—5.9%, Nasopharynx—13.7%, Oropharynx—45.1%, Hypopharynx—17.6%, Larynx—17.6%, Other—7.8% Stage: 1—0% 2—15.2% 3—13% 4—71.7% NS difference between groups
Lee, et al. [37] • Country: Korea	OD as per VFSS Inclusion: 18–80 years. Supratentorial ischaemic stroke; FOIS of ≤5 as per VFSS within 10days of stroke; Korean Mini-Mental State Examination (K-MMSE) ≥21; stable underlying disease process Exclusion: pre-existing dysphagia; previous stroke; unstable cardiopulmonary status, serious psychological disorder or epilepsy; tumour or radiotherapy of the head&neck region; prior swallowing therapy; unstable medical conditions that may interfere with VFSS	n = 57 • Treatment group 1 (31), 54.4% NMES + DT • Treatment group 2 (26), 45.6% DT	Treatment group 1: Age 63.5 ± 11.4 years 71% male Lesion location: right (13), left (18) Cortical (5), subcortical (26) Treatment group 2: Age: 66.7 ± 9.5 years 77% male Lesion location: right (11), left (15) Cortical (4), subcortical (22) NS difference between groups
Li, et al. [38] • Country: China	OD as per meeting the criteria for diagnosis of dysphagia post stroke. Recruitment through newspaper advertisements and flyers Inclusion: 50–80 year olds > 3 months post hemispheric stroke (first or recurrence); ability to elicit some swallow as per hyoid excursion or pharyngeal constriction on videographic swallow, ability to communicate, Exclusion: brainstem lesion or progressive neurological disease, presence of nasogastric tube, tumour, surgery of radiotherapy to the swallowing apparatus	n = 135 • Treatment group 1 (45), 33.3% NMES + DT • Treatment group 2 (45), 33.3% NMES • Treatment group 3 (45), 33.3% DT 38, 40 and 40 patients in groups 1–3 respectively, completed the treatment. All descriptive data about groups given based on originally enrolled numbers.	Treatment group 1: Age 66.7 ± 14.6 53% male 44% haemorrhage, 56% infarct. Treatment group 2: Age 65.8 ± 13.2 49% male 49% haemorrhage, 51% infarct. Treatment group 3: Age 66.1 ± 13.1 51% male 47% haemorrhage, 53% infarct. NS differences between groups

Table 2. *Cont.*

Study • Country	Inclusion/Exclusion Criteria	Sample (N) • Group	Group Descriptives (Mean ± SD) Age, Gender, Medical Diagnoses
Maeda, et al. [39] • Country: Japan	• OD as per VFSS • Inclusion: ≥65 years; prescribed dysphagia rehabilitation for >3 weeks • Exclusion: no cough provoked on exposure to a citric acid mist for <90 sec; inability to remain still for 15 min stimulation	n = 43 • Treatment group 1 (22), 51.2% NMES at sensory level • Sham group 2 (21), 48.8% Sham NMES	Treatment group: Age 82.7 ± 8.0 45.5% male Primary reason for admission: Dysphagia rehabilitation 63.6%, aspiration pneumonia 27.3%, other 9.1% Sham group 2: Age 86.0 ± 6.7 38.1% male Primary reason for admission: Dysphagia rehabilitation 42.9%, aspiration pneumonia 33.3%, other 23.8% NS differences between groups
Meng, et al. [40] • Country: China	• OD as per water swallow test (WST) by SLT, plus VFSS for those with the test score of grade II or above • Inclusion: 18–85 year olds with stroke <6 months ago; alert, orientated, cooperative; dysphagia confirmed with VFSS • Exclusion: presence of severe cardiac or pulmonary dysfunction, implanted cardiac pacemaker, dementia, aphasia; limited ability to follow instructions; severe aspiration; inability to swallow at all	n = 30 • Treatment group 1 (10), 33.3% NMES (supra and infrahyoid muscles stimulation) + DT [Denoted as 'Meng et al. (2018a)' in Figure 4 and Figure 5] • Treatment group 2 (10), 33.3% NMES (suprahyoid muscles stimulation) + DT [Denoted as 'Meng et al. (2018b)' in Figure 4 and 5] • Treatment group 3 (10), 33.3% DT	Treatment group 1: Age 65.2 ± 10.7 70% male 80% infarction, 20% haemorrhage. Treatment group 2: Age 67.2 ± 15.8 60% male 70% infarction, 30% haemorrhage. Treatment group 3: Age 64.4 ± 9.0 70% male 70% infarction, 30% haemorrhage. NS differences between groups
Nam, et al. [41] • Country: Korea	• OD as per VFSS • Inclusion: subacute stroke or brain injury; VFSS showing aspiration or penetration and decreased laryngeal elevation • Exclusion: chronic dysphagia	n = 50 • Treatment group 1 (25), 50% NMES (suprahyoid muscles stimulation) + DT • Treatment group 2 (25), 50% NMES (supra and infrahyoid muscles stimulation) + DT	Treatment group 1: Age 62.3 ± 11.4 52% male Location of lesion: cortex 13, subcortex 6, brainstem 5, cerebellum 1 Treatment group 2: Age 60.9 ± 12.3 56% male Location of lesion: cortex 10, subcortex 8, brainstem 6, cerebellum 1 NS differences between groups
Oh, et al. [42] • Country: Korea	• OD as per VFSS • Inclusion: post-stroke dysphagia for <6 months; presence of voluntary swallow; Korean MMSE score ≥20 • Exclusion: implanted cardiac pacemaker; severe communication disorder; tracheostomy; Hx of seizure or epilepsy; unstable medical conditions; skin problems associated with electrode placement	n = 26 • Treatment group 1 (14), 54% [Denoted as 'Oh et al. (2019a)' in Figure 4] NMES (suprahyoid muscles stimulation) + DT • Treatment group 2 (12), 46% NMES (infrahyoid muscles stimulation) + DT [Denoted as 'Oh et al. (2019b) in Figure 4]	Treatment group 1: Age 56.3 ± 13.3 50% male Site of stroke lesion: middle cerebral artery (8), midbrain (1), frontal lobe (2), internal capsule (2), corona radiate (1) Treatment group 2: Age 58.7 ± 14.8 41.7% male Site of stroke lesion: middle cerebral artery (7), midbrain (1), frontal lobe (1), internal capsule (2), corona radiate (1) NS differences between groups

Table 2. Cont.

Study, Country	Inclusion/Exclusion Criteria	Sample (N), Group	Group Descriptives (Mean ± SD) Age, Gender, Medical Diagnoses
Ortega, et al. [43], Country: Spain	• OD as per VFSS • Inclusion: ≥70 years with oropharyngeal dysphagia; PAS > 2 • Exclusion: active neoplasm or infectious process; epilepsy or convulsive disorders; gastroesophageal reflux disease; implanted electrodes or pacemakers; severe dementia; current participation in another trial	n = 38 • Treatment group 1 (19), 50% Chemical sensory stimulation with TRPV1 agonist (capsaicin) • Treatment group 2 (19), 50% NMES	Treatment group 1: Age 81.2 ± 5.6 42.1% male Dysphagia cause: elderly (8), stroke (8), neurodegenerative disease (3) Treatment group 2: Age 79.8 ± 4.8 47.4% male Dysphagia cause: elderly (7), stroke (8), neurodegenerative disease (3) NS difference between groups.
Park, et al. [44], Country: Korea	• OD as per VFSS • Inclusion: >1 month post stroke, adequate cognition. Exclusion: SAH, carotid stenosis, unable to perform NMES (as per observation and palpation)	n = 18 • Treatment group 1 (9), 50% NMES + DT (Effortful swallow) • Treatment group 2 (9), 50% NMES at sensory level + DT (Effortful swallow)	Treatment group 1: Age 68.7 ± 12.8 56% intracranial haemorrhage (ICH), 44% infarct. Treatment group 2: Age 62.0 ± 17.2 78% ICH, 22% infarct. Gender reported at cohort level: 88% male. NS differences between groups
Park, et al. [45], Country: Korea	• OD as per VFSS • Inclusion: stroke; onset >6months; able to swallow against resistance applied by electrical stimulation; able to actively participate; MMSE ≥ 24 • Exclusion: psychiatric disorders or dementia; cardiac pacemaker; severe communication disorder; epilepsy; unstable medical condition; skin problems affecting electrode placement	n = 50 • Treatment group 1 (25), 50% NMES + DT (Effortful swallow) [Denoted as 'Park et al. (2016a)' in Figure 4] • Treatment group 2 (25), 50% NMES at sensory level + DT (Effortful swallow) [Denoted as 'Park et al. (2016b)' in Figure 4]	Treatment group 1: Age 54 ± 11.93 48% male Infarct = 14, haemorrhage = 11 Treatment group 2: Age 55.8 ± 12.23 56% male Infarct = 12, haemorrhage = 13 NS differences between groups
Park, et al. [46], Country: Korea	• OD as per VFSS • Inclusion: Parkinson's disease, adequate cognition (MMSE score > 20); age < 75 years; ability to swallow voluntarily; and Hoehn and Yahr scale < 3 points • Exclusion: other neurological disease: deep brain stimulation treatment; neck pain or neck surgery; implanted electronic devices; severe communication problem; severe dyskinesia of the head and neck; history of seizure/epilepsy	n = 18 • Treatment group 1 (9), 50% NMES + effortful swallow • Treatment group 2 (9), 50% NMES at sensory level + DT (effortful swallow)	Treatment group: Age 63.44 ± 13.55 55% male Treatment group 2: 54.67 ± 13.82 33% male NB. Patients' medical diagnosis: stroke (Table 1) [Error?] NS differences between groups
Permsirivanich, et al. [47], Country: Thailand	• OD as per VFSS • Inclusion: stroke; dysphagia with safe swallow as per VFSS • Exclusion: not listed	n = 23 • Treatment group 1 (11), 48% DT (full program) • Treatment group 2 (12), 52% NMES + DT (restricted program)	Treatment group 1: Age 64.7 ± 9.4 36.4% male Type of stroke: infarction 81.8%, haemorrhage 18.2% Treatment group 2: Age 64.5 ± 8.8 41.7% male Type of stroke: infarction 75%, haemorrhage 25% NS differences between groups

Table 2. *Cont.*

Study • Country	Inclusion/Exclusion Criteria	Sample (N) • Group	Group Descriptives (Mean ± SD) Age, Gender, Medical Diagnoses
Ryu, et al. [48] • Country: Korea	• OD confirmed via VFSS and patients on a restricted diet • Inclusion: surgical with or without (chemo)radiation for head and neck cancer, stable vital signs, able to participate in treatment • Exclusion: <20 years, cognitive impairment, history of cerebrovascular disease, serious psychologic disorder, cardiac pacemaker, unable to tolerate electrical stimulation	$n = 26$ • Treatment group 1 (14), 53.8% NMES + DT • Sham/Treatment group 2 (12), 46.2% Sham NMES + DT	Treatment group 1: Age 63.4 ± 7.3 100% male Larynx ca = 6 Hypopharynx ca = 3 Oropharynx = 4 Oral = 1 T1-T2 = 6 T3-T4 = 8 Sham/Treatment group 2: Age 60.8 ± 12.0 92% male Larynx ca = 5 Hypopharynx ca = 1 Oropharynx = 4 Oral = 2 T1-T2 = 7 T3-T4 = 4 Unknown = 1 Statistical difference between groups = NR
Simonelli, et al. [49] • Country: Italy	• OD definition as per clinical swallow exam (confirmed by instrumental exam) • Inclusion: Age: 18–85 years; first-time stroke (confirmed by MRI); presence of dysphagia for 3 weeks > 3 months, with preservation of cough reflex; feeding tube-dependence, FOIS ≤ 2; stable underlying disease process • Exclusion: Cognitive impairment or mental depression; concomitant neurodegenerative disease; unstable cardiopulmonary status; head & neck tumour, surgery, or radiotherapy; cardiac pacemaker or history of seizures or epilepsy; previous swallowing therapy	$n = 33$ • Treatment group 1 (17), 51.5% NMES + DT • Treatment group 2 (16), 48.5% DT	Treatment group 1: Age 67.2 ± 16.2 62.5% male (10?) Left CVA (4), right CVA (6), Other (6) Treatment group 2: Age 72.4 ± 12.3 37.5% male Left CVA (6), right CVA (6), Other (3) NS differences between groups.
Song, et al. [50] • Country: Korea	• OD as per VFSS or rehabilitation doctor • Inclusion: Cerebral palsy (CP) diagnosis by rehabilitation doctor • Exclusion: Vision or hearing disorders, seizure disorders, pacemaker	$n = 20$ • Treatment group 1 (10), 50% NMES + DT (Oral sensorimotor treatment) • Sham/Treatment group 2 (10), 50% Sham NMES + DT (Oral sensorimotor treatment)	Treatment group 1: Age = 6.20 ± 2.78 70% male CP type: Hemiplegia = 2 Diplegia = 5 Quadriplegia = 3 Flaccid = 0 Sham/Treatment group 2: Age = 6.00 ± 2.40 60% male CP type: Hemiplegia = 4 Diplegia = 3 Quadriplegia = 2 Flaccid = 1 NS differences between groups.

Table 2. Cont.

Study • Country	Inclusion/Exclusion Criteria	Sample (N) • Group	Group Descriptives (Mean ± SD) Age, Gender, Medical Diagnoses
Sproson, et al. [51] • Country: UK	OD as per VFSS Inclusion: medically stable; >1 month post-stroke; no other neurological disease; dysphagia incorporating reduced laryngeal elevation (confirmed by VFSS) Exclusion: <18 years; pacemaker; serious cardiac disease; severe cognitive/communication difficulties; lesions/infections in the treatment site	n = 24 • Treatment group 1 (12), 50% NMES + DT • Usual care group 2 (12), 50% Usual care (Different from DT)	Treatment group 1: Age 76 ± 11.4 67% male 33% >1 stroke event Time post-stroke 17.3 months ± 25.0 Usual care group 2: Age 79 ± 11.4 66.7% male 33% >1 stroke event Time post-stroke 9.1 months ± 20.5 Significant difference between groups = NR.
Terré and Mearin [52] • Country: Spain	OD as per VFSS demonstrating aspiration Inclusion: >18 years, acquired brain injury (stroke, TBI); <6 months since insult; able to understand and follow instructions for treatment; medically stable Exclusion: previous stroke or TBI; previous dysphagia secondary to other aetiology; no other metabolic or neurological diseases	n = 20 • Treatment group 1 (10), 50% NMES + DT • Sham/Treatment group 2 (10), 50% Sham NMES + DT	Treatment group 1: Age 46.0 ± 16 60% male 70% stroke, (haemorrhagic = 5, ischaemic = 2) 30% TBI Sham/Treatment group 2: Age 51 ± 23 60% male 70% stroke (haemorrhagic = 6, ischaemic = 1) 30% TBI Significant difference between groups = NR.
Umay, et al. [53] • Country: Turkey	OD as per clinical swallow evaluation and FEES Inclusion: aged 45–75 years, <1 month post stroke (MRI confirmed), admitted to rehabilitation hospital Exclusion: haemorrhagic infarction or bilateral involvement, malignancy, head and/or neck surgery, previous stroke, pulmonary or swallowing disorder, gastroesophageal reflux, dementia or psychiatric disorder, and smoking	n = 98 • Treatment group 1 (58), 59% NMES at sensory level + DT • Sham/Treatment group 2 (40), 41% Sham NMES + DT	Treatment group 1: Age 61.03 ± 10.05 70.7% male 87.9% middle cerebral artery (MCA) stroke, 12.1% posterior inferior cerebellar (PICA) stroke Sham/Treatment group 2: Age 62.40 ± 9.93 87.5% male 87.5% middle cerebral artery (MCA) stroke, 12.5% posterior inferior cerebellar (PICA) stroke NS difference between groups.
Umay, et al. [54] • Country: Turkey	OD as per Paediatric Eating Assessment Tool-10 and FEES. Inclusion: Children aged 2–6 years with cerebral palsy Exclusion: maxillary, head or neck surgery or botulinum toxin treatment, structural oropharyngeal abnormality, oesophageal dysphagia and/or gastroesophageal reflux disease, medical and/or physical therapy for dysphagia, severe cognitive, visual, auditory, and sensory impairments, drug use due to seizure or spasticity, serious pulmonary or cardiac disease, bleeding risk	n = 102 • Treatment group 1 (52), 51% NMES at sensory level + DT • Sham/Treatment group 2 (50), 49% Sham NMES + DT	Treatment group 1: Age 51.97 ± 24.46 months 56% male Motor function status as per GMFCS (I = walks with no limitations, V = wheelchair). I = 0 II = 7 III = 10 IV = 22 V = 13 Sham/Treatment group 2: Age 47.95 ± 23.18 months 46% male I = 0 II = 11 III = 11 IV = 16 V = 12 NS difference between groups.

Table 2. Cont.

Study • Country	Inclusion/Exclusion Criteria	Sample (N) • Group	Group Descriptives (Mean ± SD) Age, Gender, Medical Diagnoses
Xia, et al. [55] • Country: China	• OD as per Standardised Swallow Assessment (SSA) and VFSS • Inclusion: cerebral infarction or haemorrhage (diagnosed by CT or MRI); no pulmonary diseases; 40–80 years old; cognitively intact and able to cooperate • Exclusion: None	$n = 120$ • Treatment group 1 (40), 33.3% DT • Treatment group 2 (40), 33.3% NMES [Denoted as 'Xia et al. (2011a)' in Figure 4 and 5] • Treatment group 3 (40), 33.3% NMES + DT [Denoted as 'Xia et al. (2011b)' in Figure 4 and Figure 5]	Treatment group 1: Age 65.32 ± 14.29 62.5% male 42.5% haemorrhage, 45% infarct, 12.5% other stroke. Treatment group 2: Age 66.40 ± 15.63 57.5% male 35% haemorrhage, 55% infarct, 10% other stroke. Treatment group 3: Age 65.85 ± 14.63 70% male 32.5% haemorrhage, 62.5% infarct, 0.5% other stroke. NS difference between groups.
Zeng, et al. [56] • Country: China	• OD as per Kubota water-drinking test • Inclusion: first-onset stroke (confirmed via MRI); able to actively cooperate; no significant cognitive disorder, aphasia, or other diseases affecting understanding • Exclusion: critical condition or vital organ failure; cardiac pacemaker; metal implants or internal orthotics; comorbidities of malignant tumours, skin damage, heart disease, acute seizure/epilepsy, peripheral nerve damage	$n = 112$ • Treatment group 1 (59), 52.7% DT • Treatment group 2 (53), 47.3% NMES + DT	Treatment group 1: Age 66.13 ± 13.03 73.5% male NIHSS score = 4.25 ± 2.45 Treatment group 2: Age 67.92 ± 12.31 69.4% male NIHSS score = 5.02 ± 2.32 NS differences between groups at baseline.
Zhang, et al. [57] • Country: China	• OD as per VFSS • Inclusion: primary diagnosis of medullary infarction confirmed via CT/MRI; onset <1 month; age 40–80 years; no severe cognitive impairment • Exclusion: unstable vital signs, inflammatory markers; cardiac pacemaker or other electrical implants; dysphagia caused by structural lesions; skin lesions or metal implants in area of treatment; a history of epilepsy, malignancies, or other neurologic disease; pregnancy; spastic paralysis	$n = 82$ • Treatment group 1 (27), 32.9% DT • Treatment group 2 (28), 34.2% NMES at sensory level + DT • Treatment group 3 (27), 32.9% NMES at motor level + DT	Treatment group 1: Age 62.6 ± 8.7 62.9% male Time since infarct: 21.3 ± 4.1 days Treatment group 2: Age 61.3 ± 7.1 57.1% male Time since infarct: 22.1 ± 4.0 days Treatment group 3: Age 62.2 ± 9.2 70.3% male Time since infarct: 20.6 ± 4.3 days NS differences between groups.

Pharyngeal Electrical Stimulation (PES)—$n = 8$

Study • Country	Inclusion/Exclusion Criteria	Sample (N) • Group	Group Descriptives (Mean ± SD) Age, Gender, Medical Diagnoses
Bath, et al. [58] • Country: UK, Spain, Germany, Denmark, France	• OD as per Toronto bedside swallowing screening test (TorBSST) fail + VFSS with PAS ≥ 3 • Inclusion: stroke (ischaemic or haemorrhagic); >18 years; alert/rousable • Exclusion: previous dysphagia, dysphagia due to another condition, implanted pacemaker/compromised cardio-pulmonary status, receiving oxygen, advanced dementia, distorted oropharyngeal anatomy, pregnant/breastfeeding mother	$n = 162$ • Treatment group: (87) 54% PES • Sham group: (75) 56% Sham PES	Treatment group: Age = 74.4 ± 11.2 Male = 55.2% Ischaemic stroke = 89.5% Haemorrhagic = 10.5% PAS >2 in 90.8% Sham group: Age = 74.9 ± 12.6 Male = 61.3% Ischaemic stroke = 88% Haemorrhagic = 10.7% (Non-stroke = 1.3%) PAS > 2 in 92% NS difference between groups

Table 2. Cont.

Study Country	Inclusion/Exclusion Criteria	Sample (N) Group	Group Descriptives (Mean ± SD) Age, Gender, Medical Diagnoses
Dziewas, et al. [59] Country: Germany, The Netherlands, Italy, Austria, UK	• OD not defined • Inclusion: ≥18 years, tracheostomy due to severe dysphagia after stroke (haemorrhagic or ischaemic); minimum 48 h mechanical ventilation, sedation free (min 3 days), Richmond Agitation Sedation Scale (RASS > −1) • Exclusion: infratentorial stroke, pre-existing dysphagia, or other diseases causing dysphagia; participation in other study affecting PES, presence of a cardiac pacemaker/implantable defibrillator, nasal deformity, previous oesophageal surgery, any difficult/unsafe nasogastric tube placement, need for high levels of oxygen supply (>2 L/min), emergency treatment, or <3 months' life expectancy	n = 69 • Treatment group (35), 50.7% PES • Sham group (34), 49.3% Sham PES 2nd open label treatment: Delayed group (n = 30) - Sham group still with a tracheostomy received late treatment; Retreat group (n = 16) PES group still with a tracheostomy received a 2nd treatment	Treatment group: Age = 61.7 ± 13 Male = 69% Sham group: Age = 66.8 ± 10.3 Male = 59% NS differences between groups
Essa, et al. [60] Country: UK	• OD as per VFSS or FEES • Inclusion: First stroke, anterior cerebral circulation or brainstem; ≤6 weeks post onset; medically stable • Exclusion: advanced dementia; other neurological reasons for dysphagia; previous dysphagia; cardiac pacemaker or defibrillator; compromised cardiac or respiratory status; significant structural abnormalities of the mouth or throat	n = 16 • Treatment group (8), 50% Pharyngeal electrical stimulation (PES) • Sham group (8), 50% Sham PES	Treatment group: Age 58.6 ± 13.4 62.5% male Stroke type: infarct (7), bleed (1) Sham group: Age 70.5 ± 11.8 62.5% male Stroke type: infarct (7), bleed (1) NS differences between groups.
Fraser, et al. [61] Country: UK	• OD as per VFSS • Inclusion: acute hemispheric stroke • Exclusion: no details given	n = 16 • Treatment group (10), 62.5% PES • Sham group (6), 37.5% Sham PES	Descriptive statistics only Treatment group: Age range 65–93 60% male Sham group: Age range 56–78 66.6% male Statistical difference between groups = NR
Jayasekeran, et al. [62] Country: UK	• OD as per VFSS >3. • Inclusion: healthy volunteers for protocol 1; study 2—admitted with anterior circulation cerebral infarct or haemorrhage • Exclusion: dementia, pacemaker or implantable cardiac defibrillator, unstable cardiopulmonary status, severe receptive aphasia, distorted oropharyngeal anatomy, dysphagia from conditions other than stroke	Protocol 1 (active or sham PES on virtual lesion) n = 11 (+2 for reversal of swallowing behaviour) Patients their own controls. Protocol 2 (PES with varying dose) n = 22 • Group 0 (6), 27.2% • Group 3 (4), 18.2% • Group 5 (4), 18.2% • Group 9 (4), 18.2% • Group 15 (4), 18.2% Protocol 3 (active or sham PES in acute stroke) n = 28 • Treatment group (16), 57% • Sham group (12), 43%	Protocol 1: Age range 24–47 yrs 45.5% male (no data on treatment and sham groups separately) Protocols 2 and 3: Age 74 ± 10 68% male (No consistent data on treatment and sham groups separately for both protocols) Difference between groups NS

Table 2. *Cont.*

Study • Country	Inclusion/Exclusion Criteria	Sample (N) • Group	Group Descriptives (Mean ± SD) Age, Gender, Medical Diagnoses
Restivo, et al. [63] • Country: Italy	OD as per VFSS Inclusion: Patients with stable multiple sclerosis (MS) with dysphagia for >2 months; no dysphagia intervention in the preceding 3 months; >18 years; Expanded Disability Status Scale (EDSS) < 7.5 Exclusion: neurologic disease other than MS; age >60 years; concomitant illness or upper gastrointestinal disease; inability to give informed consent because of cognitive impairment	$n = 20$ • Treatment group (10), 50% Pharyngeal stimulation • Sham group (10), 50% Sham pharyngeal stimulation	Cohort demographics supplied, no group descriptives given. Mean age = 39.7 ± 6.5 years 35% male Relapsing-remitting MS = 14, Secondary progressive MS = 6 Mean EDSS = 5.7 ± 0.8; mean disease duration = 9.8 ± 2.4 years; mean dysphagia duration = 22.0 ± 7.4 months Statistical difference between groups = NR
Suntrup, et al. [64] • Country: Germany	OD as per FEES Inclusion: tracheostomised, weaned off mechanical ventilation, unable to be decannulated due to severe persistent dysphagia Exclusion: pre-existing dysphagia; presence of implanted electronic devices of any kind	$n = 30$ • Treatment group (20), 66.6% Pharyngeal stimulation • Sham group (10), 33.3% Sham pharyngeal stimulation	Treatment group: Age 63.0 ± 14.5 years 45% male 90% ischaemic, 10% haemorrhagic stroke. 70% supratentorial, 30% infratentorial Sham group: Age: 66.7 ± 14.5 years 60% male 80% ischaemic, 20% haemorrhagic stroke. 90% supratentorial, 10% infratentorial Difference between groups NS
Vasant, et al. [65] • Country: UK	OD as per TOR-BSST confirmed by MBS or FEES with most (but not all) patients Inclusion: dysphagia following anterior or posterior cerebral circulation infarct (ischemic and haemorrhagic) <6 weeks ago; medically stable at inclusion; no history of intubation/tracheotomy Exclusion: advanced dementia, other neurological conditions causing dysphagia, previous history of dysphagia, presence of cardiac pacemaker or implanted cardiac defibrillator, other severe cardiac or respiratory conditions, significant oral/pharyngeal structural abnormalities, continuous oxygen requirements	$n = 35$ at 2 weeks post treatment, $n = 33$ at 3 months post treatment. • Treatment group (15), 48.4% PES • Sham group (16), 51.6% Sham PES	Treatment group: (median) age = 71 Interquartile range (IQR) =56–79. 50% male NIHSS: median score = 10.0 (IQR= 5.2, 18.5) Sham group: (median) age = 71 (IQR = 61–78) 72% male NIHSS: median score = 12.5 (IQR = 9.2, 16.8) No other stroke, site of lesion details reported. NS differences between groups.
Combined Neurostimulation Interventions—$n = 4$			
Cabib, et al. [66] • Country: Spain	OD as per VFSS Inclusion: >3 months post unilateral stroke, stable medical condition Exclusion: neurodegenerative disorders, epilepsy, drug dependency, brain or head trauma or surgery, structural causes of OD, pacemaker or metallic body implants, and pregnancy or lactation	$n = 36$ • Treatment group 1 (12), 33.3%. rTMS • Treatment group 2 (12), 33.3% Capsaicin • Treatment group 3 (12), 33.3% PES	Treatment group 1: Age 70.0 ± 8.6 75% male 0% haemorrhage, 100% infarct. Treatment group 2: Age 74.3 ± 7.8 58% male 8% haemorrhage, 92% infarction Treatment group 3: Age 70.0 ± 14.2 92% male 25% haemorrhage, 75% infarction Difference between groups NS

Table 2. Cont.

Study • Country	Inclusion/Exclusion Criteria	Sample (N) • Group	Group Descriptives (Mean ± SD) Age, Gender, Medical Diagnoses
Lim, et al. [67] • Country: Korea	• OD as per VFSS • Inclusion: primary diagnosis unilateral cerebral infarction or haemorrhage (CT or MRI); stroke onset <3 months; patients who could maintain balance during evaluation + treatment; and adequate cognitive function to participate • Exclusion: could not complete VFSS/failed the examination; presence of dysphagia pre stroke; history of prior stroke, epilepsy, tumor, radiotherapy in the head and neck, or other neurological diseases; unstable medical condition; and contraindication to magnetic or electrical stimulation	n = 47 • Treatment group 1 (15), 32% DT • Treatment group 2 (14), 30% DT + rTMS • Treatment group 3 (18), 38% DT + NMES	Treatment group 1: Age 62.5 ± 8.2 60% male 34% haemorrhage, 66% infarction Treatment group 2: Age 59.8 ± 11.8 43% male 71% haemorrhage, 29% infarction Treatment group 3: Age 66.3 ± 15.4 67% male 66% haemorrhage, 44% infarction Difference between groups NS
Michou, et al. [68] • Country: UK	• OD as per diagnoses made by SLT (confirmed with VFSS at start of treatment) • Inclusion: post stroke dysphagia for >6 weeks • Exclusion: Hx of dementia, cognitive impairment, epilepsy, head&neck surgery; neurological defects prior to stroke; cardiac pacemaker or defibrillator in-situ; severe concomitant medical conditions; structural oropharyngeal pathology; intracranial metal; pregnancy; medications acting on CNS	n = 18 • Treatment group 1 (6), 33.3% Pharyngeal electrical stimulation (PES) • Treatment group 2 (6), 33.3% Paired associative stimulation (PAS) • Treatment group 3 (6), 33.3% Repetitive transcranial magnetic stimulation (rTMS)	Treatment group: Avg age 60.3 83% male Treatment group 2: Avg age 67.3 100% male Treatment group 3: Avg age 67.8 66.7% male Overall: 63 ± 15 weeks post stroke with 7.6 ± 1 on NIHHS Statistical difference between groups = NR
Zhang, et al. [69] • Country: China	• OD as per DOSS by a well trained doctor • Inclusion: stroke as per MRI <2 months earlier; aged 50–75 yrs; normal consciousness, stable vital signs, presence of dysdipsia and dysphagia • Exclusion: brain trauma or other central nervous system disease; unstable arrhytmia, fever, infection, epilepsy, or use of sedative drugs; poor cooperation due to serious aphasia or cognitive disorders; contraindications to magnetic or electrical stimulation	n = 64 • Treatment group 1 (16), 25%. Sham rTMS + NMES • Treatment group 2 (16), 25% Ipsilateral rTMS + NMES • Treatment group 3 (16), 25% Contralateral rTMS + NMES • Treatment group 4 (16), 25% Bilateral rTMS + NMES	Treatment group 1: Age 55.9 ± 8.9 43% male 61.5% subcortical, 38.5% brainstem Treatment group 2: Age 56.8 ± 9.7 54% male 30.8% subcortical, 69.2% brainstem Treatment group 3: Age 56.5 ± 10.1 50% male 58.3% subcortical, 41.7% brainstem Treatment group 4: Age 53.1 ± 10.6 31% male 61.5% subcortical, 38.5% brainstem * All data given on participants that finished the trial and follow-up period (n = 52)

[a] NMES is at motor stimulation level unless explicitly mentioned. Notes. CNS—central nervous system; CP—cerebral palsy; CT—computed tomography; CVA—cerebrovascular accident; DOSS—dysphagia outcome and severity scale; DT—dysphagia therapy; FEES—fiberoptic endoscopic evaluation of swallowing; FOIS—functional oral intake scale; ICH—intracranial haemorrhage; MMSE—Mini-Mental State Exam; MRI—magnetic resonance imaging; MS—multiple sclerosis; NIHSS—National Institutes of Health Stroke Scale; NMES—neuromuscular electrical stimulation; OD—oropharyngeal dysphagia; OST—oral sensorimotor treatment; PAS—penetration–aspiration score; PES—pharyngeal electrical stimulation; rTMS—repetitive transcranial magnetic stimulation; sEMG—surface electromyography; SLT—Speech and Language Therapist; TBI—traumatic brain injury; tDCS—transcranial direct current stimulation; TOR-BSST—Toronto Bedside Swallowing Screening test; VFSS—videofluoroscopic swallowing study.

Table 3. Outcome of NMES and PES interventions for people with oropharyngeal dysphagia.

Study	Intervention Goal	Procedure, Delivery and Dosage Per Intervention Group	Outcome Measures	Intervention Outcomes/Conclusions
NeuroMuscular Electrical Stimulation (NMES) [a]—$n = 30$				
Beom, et al. [28]	To investigate the effectiveness of NMES to suprahyoid muscle compared with NMES to infrahyoid muscle in brain-injured (stroke) patients with dysphagia	Procedure: • NMES as per VitalStim therapy training manual 10–15 sessions, 30 min each, over 2–3 weeks • DT during NMES sessions, as per videofluoroscopy swallow study (VFSS) Treatment group 1: • NMES to the suprahyoid muscles (4 electrodes) 60 Hz pulse frequency, 500 ms pulse interval, using Stimplus Treatment group 2: • NMES to the suprahyoid muscles (2 electrodes) and infrahyoid muscles (2 electrodes) 80 Hz pulse frequency, 700 ms pulse interval, using Vitalstim	Primary outcomes: FDS [b], SFS; aspiration/penetration based off VFSS pre and post treatment. Secondary outcome: N/R	• No statistically significant differences between groups • Both treatments showed significant improvement in FDS ($p < 0.001$) and SFS ($p < 0.001$), and non-significant improvements in penetration or aspiration
Bülow, et al. [29]	To evaluate and compare the outcome of NMES versus traditional swallowing therapy (TT) in stroke patients	Procedure: • NMES as per VitalStim therapy training manual (Placement 3B) • 15 sessions, 60 min each, 5 days/week for 3 weeks • Diet modifications as per SLT recommendations Treatment group 1: • NMES to supra & infra hyoid 4.5–25 mA (mean = 13 mA) Treatment group 2: • clinician determined manoeuvres/ treatment techniques	Primary outcomes: Patient reported VAS (swallowing complaints); VFSS measure [b] (performed day of last treatment). Secondary outcome: N/R	• No statistically significant differences between groups • VAS = No significant improvement for NMES. Significant improvement ($p < 0.01$) noted for combined group effect • VFSS parameters = No significant improvement for NMES nor combined group effect
El-Tanawy, et al. [30]	Assess the effect of NMES and physical therapy program on severe poststroke dysphagia	Treatment group 1: • Standard medical treatment • NMES: 30 min of 80 Hz frequency 0–150 V amplitude stimulation, intensity 0–25 mA at motor level. Electrodes placed horizontally on the submental region 1 cm lateral to the midline above hyoid bone and the other 1 cm latero-posterior to the midline just below the hyoid bone. • Physical therapy program (45 min, range of oromotor and oral stimulation exercises—unclear if these were individualised) • 3 times a week for 6 weeks (plus 3 times daily independently) Control group 2: Standard medical treatment only	Primary outcomes: Swallowing variables (OTT, hyoid elevation, laryngeal elevation, oesophageal sphincter opening, aspiration/penetration) as per VFSS. Secondary outcome: N/R	• OTT significantly improved in Treatment group 1 post intervention ($p = 0.001$) • Significantly higher number of patients in Treatment group 1 who had lower aspiration/penetration rate ($p = 0.008$), improved hyoid elevation ($p = 0.002$) and laryngeal elevation ($p = 0.001$). • No differences seen in oesophageal sphincter opening

Table 3. Cont.

Study	Intervention Goal	Procedure, Delivery and Dosage Per Intervention Group	Outcome Measures	Intervention Outcomes/Conclusions
Guillén-Solà, et al. [31]	Assess the therapeutic effectiveness of NMES and inspiratory and expiratory muscle training (IEMT) in dysphagic subacute stroke patients, compared to standard swallow therapy (DT)	Procedure: DT, IEMT, NMES Delivery and dosage: DT: 5 days a week. Self-management education, individualised oral exercises, compensatory techniques based on VFSS IEMT: 5 sets of 10 respirations twice a day 5 days per week for 3 weeks. Loads were set to 30% of max insp and exp pressures, increased weekly by 10 cm H_2O Sham IEMT: same frequency, but with set workloads of 10 cm H_2O NMES: 40 min a day 5 days per week for 3 weeks at 80 Hz on suprahyoid muscles	Primary outcomes: Max inspiratory + expiratory muscle function (MicroRPM), dysphagia severity (VFSS, PAS), respiratory complications. Secondary outcomes: Swallowing parameter changes as per voice changes, coughing, desaturation (>3%), piecemeal deglutition, oropharyngeal residue (V-VST), FOIS, DOSS. (Not reported in study) Assessed at baseline, 3 weeks post (by V-VST, and 3 months post intervention (VFSS).	Respiratory muscle strength: • Positive treatment effect in the IEMT group at 3 weeks only Dysphagia severity: • No significant differences for PAS scores between groups • Improved safety at 3 weeks for IEMT and NMES; improved efficacy at 3 months for IEMT Respiratory complications: • No adverse effects reported 15.5% with lung infection (4 in DT, 3 in NMES, 2 in IEMT) throughout the follow-up period
Heijnen, et al., [32]	To compare the effects of traditional speech therapy exercises to those combined with NMES on motor or sensory level on dysphagia and quality of life of patients with Parkinson's Disease	Procedure: • NMES with VitalStim protocol • DT included oromotor exercises, swallow manoeuvres and strategies • 13–15 sessions, 30 min each, on five consecutive days a week over 3–5 weeks Treatment group 1 • DT Treatment group 2 • DT • NMES to the suprahyoid muscle • Stimulation to motor level Treatment group 3 • DT • NMES to the suprahyoid muscle • Stimulation to sensory level	Primary outcomes: Health related quality of life (SWAL-QOL; MDADI). Secondary outcomes: Dysphagia severity (single-item Dysphagia Severity Scale)	• No significant differences between groups • Significant improvement ($p < 0.001$) on Dysphagia Severity Scale for all groups. Restricted positive effects on QOL

Table 3. *Cont.*

Study	Intervention Goal	Procedure, Delivery and Dosage Per Intervention Group	Outcome Measures	Intervention Outcomes/Conclusions
Huang, et al. [33]	To compare functional dysphagia recovery in acute stroke patients using traditional dysphagia therapy, NMES or the two combined	Procedure: • NMES, DT • 10 sessions, 3 x a week, 60 min each • VitalStim protocol with electrode placement in a vertical line with one above and one below the thyroid notch • Intensity level individual—determined once patient felt a tingling sensation and a muscle contraction • DT: oromotor exercises, compensatory techniques, thermal-tactile stimulation, swallow manoeuvres individualised as per VFSS Treatment group 1 • DT Treatment group 2 • NMES Treatment group 3 • DT + NMES • DT performed during NMES	Primary outcomes: FOIS, PAS, FDS as per VFSS before and after treatment. Secondary outcome: N/R	• No significant differences between groups post therapy in FOIS or PAS scales • For FDS, 2 of 4 scales were significantly different (improved) in Treatment group 3 ($p = 0.03$) compared with Treatment groups 1 and 2 • Significant differences in FOIS before and after therapy in all 3 groups ($p = 0.03$; $p = 0.01$; $p = 0.005$) • Significant differences in PAS before and after therapy in treatment groups 1 and 3 ($p = 0.04$ for both)
Huh, et al. [34]	To investigate the effect of different electrode placement in NMES in poststroke dysphagia rehabilitation	Procedure: • NMES (VitalStim protocol with stimulation at motor level) + effortful swallow • five 20 min sessions weekly for four weeks Treatment group 1 • NMES with horizontal electrode placement • One pair of electrodes on the suprahyoid muscles, second pair on the infrahyoid muscles Treatment group 2 • NMES with horizontal + vertical electrode placement • One pair horizontally on the suprahyoid muscles, second pair vertically on the infrahyoid muscles Treatment group 3 • NMES with vertical electrode placement along the midline from hyoid bone down to below the thyroid cartilage	Primary outcomes: VFSS performed at baseline and post treatment. • FDS—both oral phase (FDS-O) and pharyngeal phase (FDS-p) separately, also • DOSS [b] Secondary outcome: N/R	• Treatment Group 1 scores for FDS and FDS-p were significantly higher than those in Groups 2 and 3 • No statistically significant differences between groups in FDS-O or DOSS scores post treatment • All groups showed significant improvement in FDS ($p < 0.01$) and DOSS ($p < 0.01$) scores post treatment • Horizontal electrode placement on the suprahyoid and infrahyoid muscles was found to be more beneficial for dysphagia recovery

Table 3. Cont.

Study	Intervention Goal	Procedure, Delivery and Dosage Per Intervention Group	Outcome Measures	Intervention Outcomes/Conclusions
Jing, et al. [35]	To investigate the effect of NMES on post stroke dysphagia	Procedure: • NMES, DT • Treatment for consecutive 10 days • Both groups received general medical treatment, and DT (exercises for tongue, mouth and facial muscle function; sensory stimulation; vocal cord; chewing training; therapeutic feeding) Treatment group 1: • VitalStim as per protocol, though intensity of 6 to 21 mV. Electrode placement selected based on the patient's dysphagia presentation: (a) vertical distribution on each side of the midline with lowest electrode just above the superior thyroid notch (b) 1st channel horizontally and close to the surface of the hyoid bone with 2nd channel horizontally along the midline just below the superior thyroid notch (c) 1st channel vertically below the chin and 2nd channel vertically along the buccal branch of the facial nerve Treatment group 2: • Intensity of swallow rehabilitation exercises NR	Primary outcomes: Swallow efficacy, swallow function scores, laryngeal elevation, severity of aspiration, amount of food intake, residue scores. All based on Rattans dysphagia classification criteria. Secondary outcome: N/R	• Efficacy, laryngeal elevation and severity of aspiration in the treatment group were significantly better post treatment than in the control group ($p < 0.05$) • Swallow function scores improved in both groups, but more pronounced in the treatment group ($p < 0.05$) • Amount of food intake or residue scores were not significantly different between the two groups
Langmore, et al. [36]	To investigate the efficacy of NMES combined with swallow exercises in improving dysphagia post radiotherapy for head & neck cancer	Procedure: • NMES (BMR NeuroTech 2000 default settings with minor alterations) or sham • Electrodes placed supra-hyoid region. • Home-based protocol, performed 2 x day, 6 days/week, for 12 weeks (3 training sessions to ensure competence). 16–20 min per session • DT during treatment sessions: 10 x super-supraglottic, 10x Mendelsohn, 10 x effortful swallows Sham/Treatment group: • Sham-NMES delivered via a similar device with wires inside the equipment disconnected. Same session structure and intensity of treatment	Primary outcome: Swallowing function as measured by PAS on VFSS. Secondary outcomes: OPSE, hyoid excursion, diet measured by the PSS, and quality of life as measured by HNCI. Assessments were performed prior to, midway through (week 7) and at the end of the treatment (week 13).	• Mean PAS: greater improvement in the sham group ($p = 0.027$). No other outcomes showed a significant difference between the two groups. Treatment group: • No significant change in PAS score • Significant decrease in the anterior hyoid excursion ($p = 0.038$) • No significant differences in OPSE • Significant improvement in diet (total PSS score, $p < 0.001$) and HNCI quality of life scores for eating ($p < 0.001$) and speech ($p = 0.016$) Sham/Treatment group: • Significant improvement in PAS score ($p < 0.001$) • No significant differences in OPSE • Significant improvement in diet (total PSS score, $p = 0.046$) and HNCI quality of life scores for eating ($p = 0.003$) and speech ($p = 0.001$)

Table 3. Cont.

Study	Intervention Goal	Procedure, Delivery and Dosage Per Intervention Group	Outcome Measures	Intervention Outcomes/Conclusions
Lee, et al. [37]	To compare early NMES combined with DT versus DT only on dysphagia outcomes in acute/subacute ischaemic stroke patients with moderate to severe dysphagia	Procedure: • DT in both groups included thermal-tactile stimulation with any combination of lingual strengthening exercises, laryngeal adduction-elevation exercises, and swallow manoeuvres by SLP • 60 min/day for 15 days Treatment group 1: • NMES simultaneously with DT for first 30 min max tolerable intensity (120% of the mean threshold value) on both suprahyoid muscles. Pulse rate of 80 Hz with 700 microsec duration • 30 min a day, 5 days per week for 3 weeks Treatment group 2: DT only, as per above	Primary outcome: FOIS[b] as per VFSS at 3, 6, and 12 weeks post treatment. Secondary outcome: N/R	• FOIS: Both groups showed significant improvement in FOIS 3 & 6 weeks post treatment • Treatment group 1 showed significant improvement at 12 weeks • FOIS: significantly greater improvement in treatment group 1 (at all timepoints) when compared to the treatment group 2 ($p < 0.05$)
Li, et al. [38]	To assess whether adding NMES to the conventional swallow therapy improves post-stroke dysphagia	Procedure: • NMES with VitalStim, electrical current level approx 7 mA. No other stimulation data given • Electrodes placed supra-hyoid (top electrodes) and infra-hyoid (bottom electrodes) • 4 weeks of treatment, 1 h sessions, 5 x week • DT included basic training of organs related to food intake and swallowing (no further details given) and direct food intake training (intake environment, body posture for swallowing and removal of residue) Treatment group 1: • NMES + DT Treatment group 2: • NMES Treatment group 3: • DT	Primary outcomes: VAS to compare the differences of muscle pain pre and post treatment; SSA, sEMG, OTT, PTT, LCD and Standardised swallowing PAS were measured using VFSS. Secondary outcome: N/R	• SSA scores significantly higher in Treatment Group 1 ($p < 0.01$) compared to groups 2 and 3 • Significant decrease in OTT and PTT for liquid and paste bolus ($p < 0.05$ for both) in Treatment Group 1 compared to Groups 2 and 3 • No change in LCD • Significant increase in max amplitude of sEMG signal in Treatment Group 1 compared to Groups 2 and 3 • No significant changes between Groups 2 and 3 • SSA scores and maximum amplitude of sEMG signal increased significantly within each group

Table 3. *Cont.*

Study	Intervention Goal	Procedure, Delivery and Dosage Per Intervention Group	Outcome Measures	Intervention Outcomes/Conclusions
Maeda, et al. [39]	To investigate the effect of transcutaneous electrical sensory stimulation (TESS) without muscle contraction in patients undergoing dysphagia rehabilitation	Procedure: • Sensory stimulation or sham, plus usual treatment (details NR) for both groups using Gentle Stim (J Craft, Osaka, Japan). Beat frequency of 50 Hz, other details NR • 2 pairs of electrodes (frequencies of 2000 and 2050 Hz). Anterior electrodes placed at the edge of the thyroid cartilage and the posterior electrodes 4 cm from the ipsilateral electrode along the mandible • 15 min of twice daily intervention, 5 days per week for 2 weeks Treatment group: • Stimulation intensity set at 3.0 mA Sham group: • Stimulation intensity set at 0.1 mA	Primary outcomes: Cough latency time against 1% citric acid mist. Secondary outcomes: FOIS, oral nutritional intake outcomes measured at study entry, and after the 2nd and 3rd week following treatment initiation	• No statistically significant differences were found between or within groups • Changes in cough latency time and FOIS scores indicated better outcomes in the TESS group, based on substantial effect sizes
Meng, et al. [40]	To assess the effectiveness of surface NMES with various electrode placements on patients with post-stroke dysphagia	Procedure: • All groups received DT 30 min per treatment, 5 × week. 10 sessions • NMES with VitalStim (Treatment Groups 1 and 2) for 30 min prior to daily DT • NMES as per VitalStim with minimum degree of stimulation to induce visible muscle contraction • DT combination of therapeutic exercises, compensatory manoeuvres and diet texture modifications. It remains unclear whether these were standard or individual according to VFSS results Treatment Group 1: Electrode placement: 1 pair of electrodes on the surface of both sides of suprahyoid, and another pair on surface of upper and lower edge of thyroid cartilage Treatment Group 2: Electrode placement 2 pairs of electrodes on the surface of suprahyoid (geniohyoid + mylohyoid) Treatment Group 3: DT	Primary outcomes: VFSS pre and post treatment. Hyoid excursion, DOSS[b], WST and RSST. Secondary outcome: N/R	• WST, RSST and DOSS scores improved significantly more for Treatment Groups 1 and 2 compared to Control Group ($p < 0.05$) • Differences not statistically different between treatment group 1 and 2 • WST, RSST and DOSS improved significantly in all groups comparing pre-and post-treatment ($p < 0.05$) • VFSS: only increased anterior movement of the hyoid improved statistically significantly and only in Treatment Group 2, pre-post treatment ($p = 0.006$)

Table 3. Cont.

Study	Intervention Goal	Procedure, Delivery and Dosage Per Intervention Group	Outcome Measures	Intervention Outcomes/Conclusions
Nam, et al. [41]	To assess the effect of repeated sessions of NMES with two different electrode placements on dysphagia following brain injury	Procedure: • Hyolaryngeal electrical stimulation • 10–15 sessions over 2–3 weeks, one session daily for 30 min • Both groups also received simultaneous DT—individual swallow manoeuvres based on VFSS findings Treatment Group 1: • Electrode placement on the suprahyoid muscles • Stimulation delivered using Stimplus (Cuber-Medic Corp., Iksan, South Korea) • Pulse frequency 60 Hz with 500 ms pulse interval Treatment Group 2: • Electrode placement on the suprahyoid and infrahyoid muscles • Stimulation delivered using VitalStim (Chattanooga Group, Hixson, TN, USA) as per VitalStim protocol	Primary outcomes: Motion analysis of the hyolaryngeal excursion according to VFSS conducted before and after the treatment Secondary outcome: N/R	• No significant differences between groups • Treatment Group 1 showed a significant increase in the maximal anterior excursion of the hyoid ($p = 0.008$) and the anterior excursion velocity ($p = 0.017$) • Treatment Group 2 showed a significant increase in the maximal superior excursion and the maximal absolute excursion distance of laryngeal elevation ($p = 0.013$ for both)
Oh, et al. [42]	To identify the effects of NMES with two different electrode placements on post-stroke dysphagia	Procedure: • NMES with VitalStim, as per protocol • 30 min/day, 5 days/week for 4 weeks • Effortful swallow performed during stimulation • Both groups received DT—unclear if this was individualised Treatment group 1: • Electrode placement on the suprahyoid muscles Treatment group 2: • Electrode placement on the infrahyoid muscles DT included thermal-tactile stimulation, various exercises, manoeuvres, modified food material, viscosity and posture	Primary outcomes: VDS, PAS [b] and FOIS Secondary outcome: N/R	• PAS improved more in Treatment Group 1 compared to Group 2 ($p = 0.036$). No other significant differences between groups. • Treatment Group 1: • Significant improvement in VDS ($p = 0.001$), PAS ($p = 0.002$) and FOIS ($p = 0.014$) • Treatment Group 2: • Significant improvement in VDS ($p = 0.002$), PAS ($p = 0.045$) and FOIS ($p = 0.026$) NB. Data as per Table 2 (inconsistencies between text vs table)

Table 3. *Cont.*

Study	Intervention Goal	Procedure, Delivery and Dosage Per Intervention Group	Outcome Measures	Intervention Outcomes/Conclusions
Ortega, et al. [43]	To evaluate the effectiveness of two different sensory stimulation treatments on oropharyngeal dysphagia in the elderly	Procedure: • Sensory stimulation for 2 weeks Treatment group 1: • Chemical sensory stimulation with a natural TRPV1 (capsaicin) agonist solution. • Treatment was taken by patients three times a day before each meal and 5 days per week (Mon-Fri) for 2 weeks Treatment group 2: • Electrical stimulation using the thyroid position (VitalStim, as per protocol) • Intensity 75% of the motor threshold • Once a day 5 days per week (Mon-Fri) for 2 weeks	Primary outcome: VFSS measurements, PAS (measured before and 5 days after the treatment) Secondary outcomes: EAT-10, V-VST,	• No between group differences reported • Treatment group 1: Significant improvement in EAT-10 scores ($p = 0.016$), and safety based on VFSS ($p = 0.019$) • Treatment group 2: Significant improvement in safety ($p = 0.019$) and penetrations ($p = 0.044$) based on VFSS
Park, et al. [44]	To determine whether effortful swallow training combined with surface electrical stimulation as a form of resistance training has an effect on post-stroke dysphagia	Procedure: NMES with VitalStim, 2 sets of electrodes placed on infrahyoid muscles (working against resistance) • 3 sets of 20 min exercise/week over 4 weeks Treatment group 1: • Effortful swallow + NMES (treatment level) • NMES as per VitalStim protocol, intensity increased until muscle activation Treatment group 2: • Effortful swallow + NMES (non-treatment level)	Primary outcome: Hyolaryngeal excursion (max anterior hyoid displacement, max vertical hyoid displacement), maximum vertical laryngeal displacement, UES opening (width), PAS (as per VFSS), pre and post treatment. Secondary outcome: N/R	• Between groups significant difference post treatment NR • Treatment group 1: Significant increase in laryngeal elevation ($p > 0.05$). NS increase in vertical hyoid motion and UES opening • Treatment group 2: NS difference between any pre-post measures

Table 3. Cont.

Study	Intervention Goal	Procedure, Delivery and Dosage Per Intervention Group	Outcome Measures	Intervention Outcomes/Conclusions
Park, et al. [45]	To investigate the effects of effortful swallowing combined with NMES on hyoid bone movement and swallowing function in stroke patients	Procedure: NMES (VitalStim, as per protocol), electrodes placed on infrahyoid muscles (targeting sternohyoid muscle, working against resistance) Delivery and dosage: 30 min per session, 5 sessions a week for 6 weeks. Treatment group 1: <ul><li>Effortful swallow + NMES (treatment level)</li><li>NMES intensity gradually increased until grabbing sensation</li></ul> Treatment group 2: <ul><li>Effortful swallow + NMES (placebo level)</li><li>Sensory NMES intensity gradually increased until tingling sensation</li></ul>	Primary outcomes: As per VDS pre and post treatment (6 weeks). Kinematics of the hyoid bone (analysed with Image J Program); swallow function (as per VDS and PAS [b]); VDS measures: Oral phase (lip closure, bolus formation, mastication, apraxia, tongue to palate contact, premature bolus loss and OTT); Pharyngeal phase (pharyngeal triggering, vallecular residues, pyriform sinus resides, laryngeal elevation, pharyngeal wall coating, pharyngeal transit time and aspiration). Secondary outcome: N/R	<ul><li>Significantly greater improvements shown by the treatment group versus the placebo group</li></ul> Treatment group 1: <ul><li>Significant improvements post treatment for VDS total score ($p < 0.01$), VDS pharyngeal phase ($p < 0.01$), vertical and horizontal hyoid bone displacement ($p < 0.01$) and PAS ($p < 0.01$). Improvement for VDS oral phase = NS.</li></ul> Treatment group 2: <ul><li>Vertical and anterior hyoid elevation = NS ($p = 0.06$, $p = 0.09$ respectively)</li><li>Significant improvement in total VDS score ($p = 0.02$) and oral phase (0.04). Pharyngeal phase improvement = NS ($p = 0.07$)</li><li>PAS improvement = NS ($p = 0.06$)</li></ul>
Park, et al. [46]	To identify the effect of effortful swallowing combined with neuromuscular electrical stimulation NMES in treating dysphagia in Parkinson's disease	Procedure: NMES (VitalStim) 5 days/week, for 4 weeks, 30 min each session <ul><li>During stimulation, patient produced effortful swallow (saliva)</li><li>Infrahyoid electrode placement</li><li>After NMES, patients received 30 min DT (orofacial exercises, thermal tactile stimulation and manoeuvres)</li></ul> Treatment group 1: <ul><li>NMES + effortful swallow</li></ul> Treatment group 2: <ul><li>Sensory NMES + effortful swallow</li><li>Stimulation applied at 1.0 mA, no increase</li></ul>	Primary outcome: Kinematics of the hyoid bone (analysed with Image J Program); swallow function (as per VDS and PAS [b]) Secondary outcomes: VDS measures: Oral phase (lip closure, bolus formation, mastication, apraxia, tongue to palate contact, premature bolus loss and OTT); Pharyngeal phase (pharyngeal triggering, vallecular residues, pyriform sinus resides, laryngeal elevation, pharyngeal wall coating, pharyngeal transit time and aspiration)	<ul><li>Hyoid bone movement: Significant improvement ($p < 0.05$) with vertical and horizontal movement versus sensory NMES</li><li>PAS: Significant improvement ($p < 0.05$) as compared with sensory NMES</li><li>No significant difference between groups with any VDS parameters</li></ul>

Table 3. Cont.

Study	Intervention Goal	Procedure, Delivery and Dosage Per Intervention Group	Outcome Measures	Intervention Outcomes/Conclusions
Permsirivanich, et al. [47]	To compare the treatment outcomes between dysphagia rehabilitation exercises and NMES in post-stroke dysphagia	Procedure: • Treatment administered 5 days a week (Mon-Fri) for 4 weeks • Both groups received diet modifications and oromotor exercises if weakness present Treatment group 1: • Swallowing rehabilitation exercises • Individual based on VFSS findings, may have included thermal stimulation, head & neck positioning and swallow manoeuvres Treatment group 2: • NMES using VitalStim, as per protocol • Vertical electrode placement—from 1mm above the thyroid notch down past the thyroid notch • Treatment level at grabbing sensation • 60 min per session	Primary outcomes: Changes in FOIS [b], complications related to treatment and number of therapy sessions. VFSS only performed pre-treatment. Secondary outcome: N/R	• Improvement in FOIS was significantly greater for Treatment group 2 ($p < 0.001$) • No complications related to treatment, no significant difference in the number of sessions received
Ryu, et al. [48]	To evaluate the effect of NMES on dysphagia following treatment for head and neck cancer	Procedure: 1. 30 min of NMES (VitalStim) or transcutaneous electrical stimulation (TENS) 2. Followed by 30 min DT (oral motor exercises, pharyngeal swallowing exercises, use of compensatory strategies during meals, thermal/tactile stimulation, Mendelsohn manoeuvre and diet-texture modifications) 3. 5 days per week for 2 weeks Treatment group 1: • Electrodes placed horizontally immediately above the thyroid notch (Chanel 1), and parallel below notch (Chanel 2) • NMES as per VitalStim protocol Sham/Treatment group 2: Sham stimulation using low intensity TENS	Primary outcome measures: FDS, CDS, ASHA-NOMS and MDADI Secondary outcome: N/R	• Significant difference ($p = 0.04$) between the treatment and sham group post intervention for FDS only • No significant difference between groups for CDS, ASHA-NOMS nor MDADI
Simonelli, et al. [49]	To investigate the effect of laryngopharyngeal NMES on poststroke dysphagia	Procedure: NMES and/or DT. Treatment 30 min twice daily, 5 days/week for 8 weeks, by SLTs Treatment group 1: NMES (VitalStim) plus DT. Electrode placement 3B (two electrodes were placed just at or above the level of the thyroid notch over the thyrohyoid muscle) Treatment group 2: DT included oral-facial, lingual, laryngeal adduction-elevation exercises, effortful swallow maneuver, Mendelsohn maneuver, Masako maneuver, Shaker exercises and thermal stimulation plus compensatory strategies	Primary outcome: FOIS, PAS [b], the Pooling score and the presence of oropharyngeal secretion as per FEES. Secondary outcomes: Diet taken by mouth; the need for postural compensations and the duration of the dysphagia training.	• Significant difference between groups for FOIS ($p = 0.15$), PAS ($p = 0.003$) and presence of oropharyngeal secretions ($p = 0.048$), with significantly greater improvements in the NMES group. • No difference in pooling score. • Significant difference between groups for all secondary outcomes, with significant improvements for the NMES group ($p < 0.01$)

Table 3. *Cont.*

Study	Intervention Goal	Procedure, Delivery and Dosage Per Intervention Group	Outcome Measures	Intervention Outcomes/Conclusions
Song, et al. [50]	To investigate the effects of NMES and oral sensorimotor treatment (OST) on dysphagia in children with CP	Procedure: OST followed by NMES (20min) with thickened fluid, delivered by occupational therapist • Electrodes placed approximating suprahyoid muscles (Chanel 1) and infrahyoid muscles (Chanel 2) • 2 x week for 8 weeks Treatment group 1: • OST = sensory stimulation to cheeks, chin, lips, tongue and palate using fingers, vibrator, ice-stick • 20 min NMES (Simplus DP 200) 3–5 mA, 80 Hz of 300 milliseconds with 1-s interval Sham/Treatment group: • OST + sham-NMES (device not switched on)	Primary outcomes: (1) BASOFF: jaw closure, lip closure over a spoon, tongue control, lip closure while swallowing, swallowing food without excess loss, chewing food (tongue/jaw control), sipping liquids, swallowing liquids without excess loss, and swallowing food without coughing; (2) ASHA-NOMS. Secondary outcome: N/R	• Significant difference ($p < 0.05$) between groups for total BASOFF scores post treatment • Significant improvements for the treatment group 1 including lip closure while swallowing, swallowing food without excess loss, sipping liquid, swallowing liquid without excess loss, swallowing without cough, and total score • No significant changes between or within groups for ASHA-NOMS scores
Sproson, et al. [51]	To investigate the efficacy of the Ampcare Effective Swallowing Protocol (ESP), combining NMES with swallow-strengthening exercises, compared with usual care in the treatment of dysphagia post-stroke	Procedure: NMES to suprahyoid muscles via AmpCare ESP Treatment group 1: • 30 min, 5 days/week, 4 weeks • NMES pulse rate 30Hz with three sets of 10 min exercises (a) chin to chest against resistance + effortful swallow, (b) chin to chest + Mendelsohn + effortful swallow, (c) chin to chest against resistance + jaw opening-closing + effortful swallow Usual Care Group 2: • Usual care varied from periodic reviews primarily focusing on posture and diet modification to weekly visits with home-practise regimes. These regimes included exercises and postural adaptations based on VFSS findings	Primary outcomes: (1) FOIS and PAS[b] immediately post treatment as per VFSS; (2) FOIS, PAS and SWAL-QOL 1 month follow-up. Secondary outcome: N/R	• No significant difference between groups for any of the outcome measures • Descriptive statistics reported • FOIS: 62% of NMES patients improved (versus 50% of standard care) • PAS: Variable results reported • SWAL-QOL: 83% of NMES patients improved (versus 38% of standard care)
Terré, et al. [52]	To evaluate the effectiveness of neuromuscular electrical stimulation NMES treatment in patients with oropharyngeal dysphagia secondary to acquired brain injury	Procedure: NMES (VitalStim), or sham, + traditional dysphagia therapy, • 60 min, 5 days/week for 4 weeks Treatment group 1: • Stimulation as per VitalStim protocol • Electrode placement: submental/suprahyoid region and infra hyoid region • Plus DT (individualised from VFSS): diet modification, supraglottic, Mendelsohn manoeuvre, oromotor exercises Sham/Treatment group 2: Sham NMES + DT • Electrode placement = chin region and lateral to thyroid with minimal stimulus (2.5 mA) to top electrode • Sham stimulation with DT	Primary outcome: FOIS Secondary outcomes: VFSS parameters, pharyngo-esophageal manometry Assessed at 1 month (immediately post therapy) and at 3 months.	• Significant difference between groups at 1 month (greater improvement with treatment group). No significant difference between groups at 3 months. Secondary outcomes: • VFSS: Statistically fewer patients from treatment group aspirated (nectar and pudding) at 1 month. No significant difference at 3 months. • Pharyngo-esophageal manometry: difference between groups not reported

Table 3. *Cont.*

Study	Intervention Goal	Procedure, Delivery and Dosage Per Intervention Group	Outcome Measures	Intervention Outcomes/Conclusions
Umay, et al. [53]	To evaluate the effects of sensory electrical stimulation (SES) to bilateral masseter muscles in early stroke patients with dysphagia	Procedure: Sensory level electrical stimulation (Intelect Advanced) with galvanic stimulation to bilateral masseter muscles for 60 min, 5 days/week, for 4 weeks Treatment group 1: • Sensory stimulation established when patient reported tingling sensation. Electrical current level 4–6 mA • Combined with DT: dietary modification, and oromotor exercises, though not during stimulation Sham/Treatment group 2: • Electrode placement without stimulation • DT as per above	Primary outcomes: Bedside dysphagia score (from water swallow test, pulse oximetry), total dysphagia score, MASA, NEDS. Secondary outcome: N/R	• Significant difference between groups post treatment = NR • Pre-post treatment changes (improvements) were significantly greater in the treatment group with bedside dysphagia score ($p = 0.015$), total dysphagia score ($p = 0.001$), MASA ($p = 0.004$) and NEDS ($p = 0.001$)
Umay, et al. [54]	To investigate the effects of sensory-level electrical stimulation NMES treatment applied to bilateral masseter muscles at the lowest current level combined with conventional dysphagia rehabilitation in children with CP who had any oropharyngeal dysphagia symptoms	Procedure: • Sensory-level NMES (with Intelect Advanced) 30 min/day, 5 days/week for 4 weeks DT given separately, 30 min/day, 5 days/week for 4 weeks Treatment group 1: • Sensory-level ES + DT • Sensory-level ES to bilateral masseter muscles, at lowest current level where child showed signs of discomfort (sensory threshold). No oropharyngeal exercises or swallow training performed at the same time. • DT by rehabilitation specialist: daily care for oral hygiene, thermal (cold) and tactile stimulation, head and trunk positioning and dietary modification. Oral motor exercises included for children who could participate. Sham/Treatment group 2: • Sham ES + DT • Sham ES = same electrode placement, no stimulus • DT as per above	Primary outcome: Ped EAT-10, FEES; Secondary outcomes: Clinical Feeding Evaluation.	• Significantly greater improvement for treatment group versus sham with both Ped EAT-10 and FEES. (Though difference between groups post therapy not reported). Secondary outcomes: • Statistically greater changes (effect size) for clinical feeding parameters: drooling, tongue movements, chewing and feeding duration for the treatment group versus sham

Table 3. Cont.

Study	Intervention Goal	Procedure, Delivery and Dosage Per Intervention Group	Outcome Measures	Intervention Outcomes/Conclusions
Xia, et al. [55]	To investigate the effects of VitalStim therapy coupled with conventional swallowing training on recovery of post-stroke dysphagia	Treatment group 1: • Standard swallow therapy (DT). Schedule not reported • Direct and indirect OD training related to food intake and swallowing, body posture and removal of pharyngeal food residue Treatment group 2: • NMES (VitalStim), 30 min, 2 × day. 5 days/week for 4 weeks Treatment group 3: • DT + VitalStim • Schedule not reported	Primary outcome: Dysphagia Rating Scale [b] (as per VFSS); Secondary outcomes: Maximum amplitude of surface electromyography (sEMG) signals of hyoid muscles; SWAL-QOL.	• Primary outcomes: All 3 groups significantly improved post treatment. Significant greater improvement ($p < 0.01$) for group 3 (DT + VitalStim) versus other 2 groups (DT only group and VitalStim only group). • Secondary outcomes. SWAL-QOL and sEMG signals significantly increased in all groups. Significant difference between DT + VitalStim (greater improvement) versus DT group and VitalStim group.
Zeng, et al. [56]	To observe the improvement of swallow function and negative affect disorders in patients with cerebral infarction and dysphagia by NMES	Procedure: 1. NMES and/or swallow training 2. NMES via YS1002T Glossopharyngeal Nerve and Muscle Electrical Stimulator (Changzhou Yasi Medical Instruments Co) 3. Stimulation pulse width of 800 ms, intensity 28 mA 4. Swallow training included: massage to cheeks, tongue, retropharyngeal wall, pharyngopalatine arch and lips with frozen cotton swabs or fingers soaked in ice water. Followed by an empty swallow. Treatment group 1: 5. Swallow training only 6. Dose/schedule not reported Treatment group 2: 7. Swallow training + NMES 8. NMES for 20 min period in intervals of 3 s, daily for 12 days. After a 2 day break, NMES for another 12 days.	Primary outcome: Swallow function as per Kubota water-drinking test; Secondary outcomes: Negative affect disorders as per Hamilton anxiety scale and depression scale test.	• Primary outcomes: Both groups improved swallow function post treatment, significantly greater improvements ($p = 0.035$) for group 2 (swallow training + NMES) • Secondary outcomes: Anxiety and depression subscales and scores improved significantly only in treatment group 2. Significant difference between the groups post treatment for anxiety scales ($p = 0.001$) and depression scales (0.033).

Table 3. Cont.

Study	Intervention Goal	Procedure, Delivery and Dosage Per Intervention Group	Outcome Measures	Intervention Outcomes/Conclusions
Zhang, et al. [57]	To evaluate and compare the effects of NMES acting on the sensory input versus motor muscle in treating patients with dysphagia with medullary infarction	Procedure: • Electrical stimulation via vocaSTIM-master + 2 surface electrodes, placed submentally. • Pulse width = 100 ms; frequency = 120 Hz. • 20 min, 2 × day, 5 days/week for 4 weeks. Treatment group 1: • Standard swallowing therapy (DT): postural adjustment, diet modification, thermal-tactile stimulation, oromotor exercises, swallow manoeuvres • Dosage and schedule not reported Treatment group 2, DT + sensory NMES: • Stimulation intensity 0–15 mA, increasing to 'sensory input'. Treatment group 3, DT + motor NMES: • Stimulation intensity 0–60 mA, increasing to maximal tolerable level.	Primary outcomes: WST, FOIS, SWAL-QOL, SSA. Secondary outcome: N/R	• All treatment groups improved significantly ($p < 0.01$) pre-post across all outcome measures • Significantly greater treatment effect was noted for DT + sensory NMES compared to other two treatment groups, across all measures ($p = 0.01$–0.04) • Significantly greater treatment effect was noted for DT + motor NMES compared to DT only
Pharyngeal Electrical Stimulation (PES)—n = 8				
Bath, et al. [58]	Assess the efficacy of PES in treating subacute poststroke dysphagia	Procedure: PES (Phagenyx) catheter + standard stroke care • 3 days, 10 min/day • Standard stroke care included thrombolysis; rehabilitation; antihypertensive agents; if indicated, oral antithrombotic, lipid-lowering agents and carotid endarterectomy (ischemic stroke patients) Treatment group: • 10 min stimulation, PES (mA) at 75% of difference between max tolerance level and threshold level Sham: • Phagenyx catheter inserted, no stimulation after threshold and max tolerance level obtained	Primary outcome: PAS [b] (via VFSS), assessed at 2 and 12 weeks post treatment. 3–7 bolus per VFSS. Secondary outcome: At 2, 6 and 12 weeks = DSRS, function (Barthel Index), dependency (modified Rankin Scale), impairment (NIHSS), quality of life (EQ-5D), nutritional measures and serious adverse events (chest infections, pneumonia, death).	• No significant difference ($p = 0.60$) in dysphagia improvement between treatment and sham group • Treatment group: PAS mean = 3.7 (2.0) • Sham group: PAS mean = 3.6 (1.9) • Authors conclude: PES is safe but did not improve dysphagia. May be impacted by PES 'under-treatment'/suboptimal dose

Table 3. Cont.

Study	Intervention Goal	Procedure, Delivery and Dosage Per Intervention Group	Outcome Measures	Intervention Outcomes/Conclusions
Dziewas, et al. [59]	Assess the safety and efficacy of PES in accelerating dysphagia rehabilitation and enabling decannulation of tracheostomised stroke patients	Procedure: PES (Phagenyx) • 10 min/day, 3 consecutive days Treatment group: • 10 min stimulation calculated using patient's perceptual threshold and max tolerated threshold Sham group: • Phagenyx catheter inserted, no stimulation after threshold and max tolerance obtained Open label PES group: • Following post-treatment assessment, all patients who had not improved were offered active PES treatment as per above schedule	Primary outcome: Readiness for decannulation 24–72 h after treatment (determined by FEES protocol) Secondary outcomes: delayed improvement in Open label group; recannulations (between 2–30 days post decannulation/discharge); DSRS; FOIS; stroke severity as per modified Rankin Scale and NIHSS; LOS, SLT plan, number and type of adverse events.	Primary outcomes: 17/35 patients (49%) ready for decannulation versus sham 3/34 (9%) patients. Significant difference ($p < 0.001$) between groups Secondary outcomes: Open-label PES (a) Retreated group = 4/15 (27%) ready for decannulation (b) Sham/delayed treatment group = 16/30 (53%) ready for decannulation. No significant differences between groups.
Essa, et al. [60]	Assess if The Brain Derived Neurotrophic Factor (BDNF) genotype can influence swallowing recovery post PES in stroke patients	Procedure: • PES • Once a day for 10 min on 3 consecutive days Treatment group • PES—0.2 ms pulses, 280 V with 5Hz frequency at 75% max tolerated intensity Sham group Sham PES	Primary outcome: DSRS. Assessed at baseline, 2 weeks and 3 months post treatment. Secondary outcome: N/R	• No between group statistics reported • In the treatment group, the genotype Met carriers of the BDNF gene had significant improvement in DSRS by 3 months post intervention ($p = 0.009$), when compared to those homozygous for the Val allele • No significant improvement in the Sham group • Data support the notion that the presence of the Met allele might be a predictor of improved long-term outcomes for dysphagia after PES
Fraser, et al. [61]	To assess the effect of PES on swallow function in hemispheric stroke patients	Procedure: • PES • Single session of 10 min • 5 Hz with max tolerated intensity for treatment group Sham group received no stimulation	Primary outcomes: PTT, swallowing response time, PAS Secondary outcome: N/R	Between group statistics = NR • Treatment group showed a significant pre-post reduction in pharyngeal transit time, swallowing response time and PAS (all $p < 0.01$) • No difference in pre-post (change) outcomes for the sham group

Table 3. Cont.

Study	Intervention Goal	Procedure, Delivery and Dosage Per Intervention Group	Outcome Measures	Intervention Outcomes/Conclusions
Jayasekeran, et al. [62]	To examine the role of PES in expediting human swallowing recovery after experimental (virtual) and actual (stroke) lesions	Agent: PES Protocol 1—active or sham PES with virtual lesion. Patients their own controls. The two studies (active or sham) took place at least 1 week apart. Protocol 2—PES with varying treatment intensity (times/day) and dose (total number of days) • Group 0—no stimulation • Group 3—once/day for 3 days • Group 5—once/day for 5 days • Group 9—3 times/day for 3 days • Group 15—3 times/day for 5 days Protocol 3—active or sham PES with acute stroke. Once daily on three consecutive days.	Primary outcomes: Protocol 1 Cortical excitability, swallow timeliness Protocol 2 PAS[b] Protocol 3 PAS[b], swallow timing, DSRS, LOS at hospital, Barthel Index. For protocols 2 and 3, VFSS conducted before treatment, and again weeks later. Secondary outcome: N/R	Protocol 1 • Active PES abolished the effects of virtual lesion by reversing the direction of excitability. Active PES reversed the direction of cortical excitability in both hemispheres ($p = 0.42$). • Active PES abolished the behavioural effects of the virtual lesion ($p = 0.02$), increasing the number of correctly timed swallows by 65% Protocol 2 • Intensity (times/day): Compared to control, once/day stimulation (groups 3 and 5) produced the greatest reduction in aspiration ($p = 0.04$) • Dose: Compared to control, total of 3 days of stimulation (groups 3 and 9) showed the greatest reduction in aspiration scores ($p = 0.038$) Protocol 3 • Reduction of PAS post intervention for the active PES group compared to sham = NS ($p = 0.49$) • No significant changes in swallow timing for either group • Significantly reduced DSRS in the PES group ($p = 0.04$) • NS shorter stay in hospital for the PES group ($p = 0.38$)
Restivo, et al. [63]	To investigate whether intraluminal electrical pharyngeal stimulation facilitates swallowing recovery in dysphagic multiple sclerosis (MS) patients	Procedure: PES (bipolar platinum pharyngeal ring electrodes built into 3 mm-diameter intraluminal catheter) using constant/current electrical simulator (DS7) • Stimulation 10 min, 5 consecutive days Treatment group: • 5 Hz pharyngeal stimulation (mA calculated using sensory threshold and pain thresholds, mean = 14.2 ± 0.6 mA) Sham: • Same catheter, no stimulation	Primary outcome: PAS via VFSS at pre-treatment (T0), immediately after treatment (T1), after two (T2), and four (T3) weeks of PES. Secondary outcomes: sEMG measure of: (1) duration of laryngeal excursion; (2) duration of the sEMG activity of suprahyoid/submental muscles; (3) duration of the inhibition of the CP muscle; and (4) interval between onset of suprahyoid/submental muscles and onset of laryngeal elevation.	• Significant difference between treatment and sham group immediately and 4 week post treatment, for PAS ($p < 0.0001$) and all secondary measures ($p < 0.0001$) • Treatment group improved significantly across all measures, sham group did not

Table 3. *Cont.*

Study	Intervention Goal	Procedure, Delivery and Dosage Per Intervention Group	Outcome Measures	Intervention Outcomes/Conclusions
Suntrup, et al. [64]	To assess the effectiveness of PES on swallowing function of severely dysphagic tracheostomised patients	Procedure: PES (Phagenyx) catheter system and base station, stimuli of 0.2 ms pulse duration at a frequency of 5 Hz with 280 V • Stimulation 10 min, 5 consecutive days Treatment group: • Stimuli of 0.2 ms pulse duration at a frequency of 5 Hz with 280 V Sham: • Same catheter, no stimulation Another treatment session was offered to participants who were not eligible for tracheostomy decannulation post the first treatment session.	Primary outcome: Eligibility for decannulation Secondary outcomes:FOIS at discharge; mRS; LOS in ICU and hospital; time from stimulation to discharge.	• 75% of the treatment group participants were able to be decannulated post Tx compared to 20% of sham group ($p < 0.01$) • No significant differences in the secondary outcomes between groups A further 71.4% of participants were able to be decannulated post second round of treatment
Vasant, et al. [65]	To assess the effectiveness of PES on swallowing in poststroke dysphagia, with clinical effects in longer-term follow-up	Procedure: PES (Gaeltec catheter) inserted nasally or orally (patient preference) • 10 min stimulation for 3 consecutive days Treatment group: • PES: stimuli delivered (0.2 ms pulses, maximum 280 V) at defined optimal parameters (5 Hz frequency and an intensity [current] 75% of maximum patient toleration Additional DT as determined by SLP assessment (details not supplied) Sham: • PES catheter insitu, no stimulation. • DT by SLP.	Primary outcome: DSRS at 2 weeks post treatment. Secondary outcomes: DSRS at 3 months, feeding method, PAS [b] (as per MBS/FEES), number of adverse events (chest infections, death).	• Primary outcome: significant difference between groups NR Treatment group effects (DSRS measures) were noted at 2 weeks and 3 months post treatment, though not significant ($p = 0.26$ and 0.97 respectively) • No significant difference reported between groups for most secondary outcomes

Table 3. Cont.

Study	Intervention Goal	Procedure, Delivery and Dosage Per Intervention Group	Outcome Measures	Intervention Outcomes/Conclusions
Combined Neurostimulation Interventions—n = 4				
Cabib, et al. [66]	To investigate the effect of repetitive transcranial magnetic stimulation (rTMS) of the primary sensory cortex (A), oral capsaicin (B) and intra-pharyngeal electrical stimulation (IPES; C) on post stroke dysphagia	Procedure: All patients received both treatment and sham, cross over active/sham in visits 1 week apart (randomised). Assessment occurred immediately prior to treatment and within 2 h post treatment. Treatment group 1: rTMS (Magstim rapid stimulator) • Stimulation (90% of threshold) bilaterally to motor hotspots for pharyngeal cortices • 5 Hz train of 50 pulses for 10 sec × 5 (total 250 pulses), 10 sec between trains • Sham = coil tilted 90 degrees. Treatment group 2: Capsaicin stimulus (10−5 M) or placebo (potassium sorbate) were administered once in a 100 mL solution Treatment group 3: PES via two-ring electrode naso-pharyngeal catheter (Gaeltec Ltd) • 10 min stimulation at 75% tolerance threshold (0.2 ms of duration) and 5 Hz • Sham = 30 seconds of above stimulation then no stimulation	Primary outcomes: Effect size pre-post treatment for neurophysiological variables (pharyngeal and thenar RMT and MEP). Secondary outcomes: Effects on the biomechanics of swallow (PAS ^{b}, impaired efficiency + more) VFSS before and after treatment	• Between group differences (post treatment) not reported Primary outcomes: • No significant differences in pre-post pharyngeal RMTs with any of the active or sham conditions • Combined analysis (interventions grouped together) showed significantly shorter latency times, increased amplitude, and area of the thenar MEP in the contralesional hemisphere Secondary outcomes: (VFSS) • No significant change/difference in effect size across any of the treatment or sham groups
Lim, et al. [67]	To investigate the effect of low-frequency repetitive transcranial magnetic stimulation (rTMS) and neuromuscular electrical stimulation (NMES) on post-stroke dysphagia	Procedure: • DT: oropharyngeal muscle-strengthening, exercise for range of motion of the neck/tongue, thermal tactile stimulation, Mendelson manoeuvre, and food intake training for 4 weeks Treatment group 1: • DT 4 weeks • Intensity NR Treatment group 2: • DT + rTMS via Magstim 200 (Magstim, Whiteland, UK) • Stimulation to pharyngeal motor cortex, contralateral hemisphere • 1 Hz stimulation, 100% intensity of resting motor threshold • 20 min/day, (total 1200 pulses a day), 5 × week for 2 weeks Treatment group 3: • DT + NMES (Vitalstim) • 300 ms, 80 Hz (100 ms in interstimulus intervals). Intensity between 7–9 mA, depending on patient compliance • Stimulation to supra and infra hyoid region • 30 min/day, 5 days/week, 2 weeks	Primary outcomes: VFSS baseline, 2 weeks + 4 weeks post treatment (for semi-solids and liquids) FDS, PTT, PAS. Secondary outcome: N/R	Difference between groups post treatment = NR FDS outcome: • For semi-solids all groups improved, no significant difference in pre-post change, between groups • For liquids, the rTMS and NMES improved significantly compared to DT, 2 weeks post treatment ($p = 0.016$ and $p < 0.001$, respectively) • No significant difference in the change from baseline to the 4th week evaluation among groups ($p = 0.233$) PAS outcome: • For semi-solids all groups improved, no significant difference in pre-post PAS change, between groups • For liquids, the rTMS and NMES improved significantly compared to DT, 2 weeks post treatment ($p = 0.011$ and $p = 0.014$, respectively) • No significant difference in the change from baseline to the 4th week evaluation among groups ($p = 0.540$)

Table 3. *Cont.*

Study	Intervention Goal	Procedure, Delivery and Dosage Per Intervention Group	Outcome Measures	Intervention Outcomes/Conclusions
Michou, et al. [68]	To compare the effects of a single application of one of three neurostimulation techniques (PES, paired stimulation, rTMS) on swallow safety and neurophysiological mechanisms in chronic post-stroke dysphagia	Procedure: • Single application of neurostimulation • All patients received real and sham treatment in randomised order on two different days Treatment group 1: • PES • Frequency of 5 Hz for 10 min. Intensity set at 75% of the difference between perception and tolerance thresholds Treatment group 2: • Paired associative stimulation: • Pairing a pharyngeal electrical stimulus (0.2 ms pulse) with a single TMS pulse over the pharyngeal M1 at MT intensity plus 20% of the stimulator output. The 2 pulses were delivered repeatedly every 20 s with an inter-stimulus interval of 100 ms for 10 min. Treatment group 3: • rTMS • Stimuli to pharyngeal motor cortex with the TMS coil. Frequency of 5 Hz, intensity 90% of resting thenar motor threshold in train of 250 pulses, in 5 blocks of 50 with 10 s between-blocks pause.	Primary Outcome: VFSS before and after treatment (PAS [b]) Secondary outcomes: Percentage change in cortical excitability; OTT, pharyngeal response time, PTT, airway closure time and upper oesophageal opening time as per VFSS	• Treatment group 1 (PES): significant excitability increase immediately post-Tx in the unaffected hemisphere (real vs sham $p = 0.043$) and in the affected hemisphere 30 min post-Tx (real vs sham $p = 0.04$) With Paired Stimulation, cortical excitability increased 30 min post-Tx in the unaffected side ($p = 0.043$) compared to sham, and immediately post-Tx in the affected hemisphere following contralateral Paired stimulation ($p = 0.027$) • Treatment group 2 (paired neurostimulation): an overall increase in corticobulbar excitability in the unaffected hemisphere ($p = 0.005$) with an associated 15% reduction in aspiration ($p = 0.005$) when compared to sham Pharyngeal response time was significantly shorter post treatment with real stimulation compared to sham ($p = 0.007$) • Treatment group 3 (rTMS): an increase in excitability in the unaffected hemisphere, but no significant difference compared to sham. No change in the affected hemisphere. Corticobulbar excitability of pharyngeal motor cortex was beneficially modulated by PES, Paired Stimulation and to a lesser extent by rTMS

Table 3. Cont.

Study	Intervention Goal	Procedure, Delivery and Dosage Per Intervention Group	Outcome Measures	Intervention Outcomes/Conclusions
		Procedure: 9. 10 rTMS (sham or real) and 10 NMES sessions Mon-Fri during 2 weeks 10. NMES: 30 min once daily using a battery powered handheld device (HL-08178B; Changsha Huali Biotechnology Co., Ltd., Changsha, China), vertical placement of electrodes. Pulse width of 700 ms, frequency 30–80 Hz, current intensity 7–10 mA. 11. rTMS delivered by figure-of-eight coil (CCY-IV; YIRUIDE Inc., Wuhan, China) during NMES with a sequence of HF-rTMS over the affected hemisphere followed by LF-rTMS over the unaffected hemisphere. 12. HF-rTMS parameters: 10 Hz, 3 s stimulation, 27 s interval, 15 min, 900 pulses, and 110% intensity of resting motor threshold (rMT) at the hot spot. 13. LF-rTMS parameters: 1 Hz, total of 15 min, 900 pulses, and 80% intensity of rMT at the hot spot.		Compared with group 2 or 3 in the affected hemisphere, group 4 displayed a significantly greater % change (p 0.017 and p 0.024, respectively). All groups displayed significant improvements in SSA and DD scores after treatment and at 1-month follow-up. The % change in cortical excitability increased over time in the affected or unaffected hemisphere in treatment groups 1, 2 and 4 ($p < 0.05$). In Group 3, the % change in cortical excitability in the unaffected hemisphere significantly decreased after the stimulation course ($p < 0.05$). Change in SSA and DD scores in group 4 was markedly higher than that in the other three groups at the end of stimulation (p 0.02, p 0.03, and p 0.005) and still higher than that in group 1 at the 1-month follow-up (p 0.01).
Zhang, et al. [69]	To determine whether repetitive transcranial magnetic stimulation (rTMS) combined with neuromuscular electrical stimulation (NMES) effectively ameliorates dysphagia and how rTMS protocols (bilateral vs. unilateral) combined with NMES can be optimized	Treatment group 1: Sham rTMS + NMES • 10 Hz sham rTMS delivered to the hot spot for the mylohyoid muscle at the ipsilesional hemisphere followed by 1 Hz sham rTMS over the corresponding position of the contralesional hemisphere. • Delivered using a vertical coil tilt, generating the same noise as real rTMS without cortical stimulation. Treatment group 2: Ipsilateral rTMS + NMES 10 Hz real rTMS was delivered to the hot spot for the mylohyoid muscle at the ipsilesional hemisphere followed by 1 Hz sham rTMS over the corresponding position of the contralesional hemisphere. Treatment group 3: Contralateral rTMS + NMES 10 Hz sham rTMS was delivered to the hot spot for the mylohyoid muscle at the ipsilesional hemisphere followed by 1-Hz real rTMS over the corresponding position of the contralesional hemisphere Treatment group 4: Bilateral rTMS + NMES 10 Hz real rTMS was delivered to the hot spot for the mylohyoid muscle at the ipsilesional hemisphere followed by 1-Hz real rTMS over the corresponding position of the contralesional hemisphere	Primary outcome: cortical excitability (amplitude of the motor evoked potential) Secondary outcomes: SSA and DD.	

[a] NMES is at motor stimulation level unless explicitly mentioned. [b] Data included in meta-analyses. Notes. ASHA-NOMS—American speech-language-hearing association national outcome measurement system; BASOFF—behavioural assessment scale of oral functions in feeding; BI—Barthel index; CDS—clinical dysphagia scale; CNS—central nervous system; CP—cerebral palsy; CT—computed tomography; CVA—cerebrovascular accident; DD—degree of dysphagia; A-DHI-Arabic dysphagia handicap index; DOSS—dysphagia outcome and severity scale; DSRS-dysphagia severity rating scale; DT—dysphagia therapy; EAT-10—eating assessment tool-10; EES—electrokinesiographic/electromyographic study of swallowing; EQ-5D—European Quality of Life Five Dimension; FDS—functional dysphagia scale; FOIS—functional oral intake scale; FEDSS—fiberoptic endoscopic dysphagia severity scale; FEES-fiberoptic endoscopic evaluation of swallowing; HNCI—head neck cancer inventory; IADL—instrumental activities of daily living; ICH—intracranial haemorrhage; ICU—intensive

care unit; LPM—laryngeal-pharyngeal mechanogram; MASA—Mann assessment of swallowing ability; MDADI—M.D. Anderson dysphagia inventory; LCD—laryngeal closure duration; LOS—length of stay; MBS—modified barium swallow; MBSImp—modified barium swallow impairment profile; MEG—magnetoencephalography; MMSE—mini-mental state exam; MEP—motor evoked potentials; MRI—magnetic resonance imaging; mRS—modified rankin scale; MS—multiple sclerosis; NEDS—neurological examination dysphagia score; NIHSS—national institutes of health stroke scale; NIHSS—National Institutes of Health Stroke Scale; NMES—neuromuscular electrical stimulation; NS—not significant; OD—oropharyngeal dysphagia; OPSE—oropharyngeal swallow efficiency; OST—oral sensorimotor treatment; OTT—oral transit time; PAS—penetration–aspiration score; PED EAT-10 pediatric eating assessment tool-10;PES–pharyngeal electrical stimulation; PESO— pharyngoesophageal segment opening; PPS—performance status scale; PTT—pharyngeal transit time; RMT—resting motor threshold; RSST—repetitive saliva swallowing test; rTMS—repetitive transcranial magnetic stimulation; SAH—subarachnoid haemorrhage; SAPP—swallowing activity and participation profile; SDQ—swallowing disturbance questionnaire; sEMG—surface electromyography; SFS—swallow function score; SHEMG— electromyographic activity of the submental/suprahyoid muscles complex; SI—similarity index; SLT–speech and language therapist; SSA—standardised swallowing assessment; SWAL-QOL—swallowing quality of life; TBI—traumatic brain injury; tDCS—transcranial direct current stimulation; TOR-BSST—Toronto bedside swallowing screening test; UES—upper esophageal sphincter; UPDRS—unified Parkinson's disease rating scale; VAS—visual analogue scale; VFSS—videofluoroscopic swallowing study; VVS-T—volume viscosity swallow test; WST—water swallow test.

Peripheral Neurostimulation Interventions. Across the 42 included studies, 30 studies reported on NMES and eight studies reported on PES. Four studies used another type of neurostimulation (i.e., rTMS) in addition to NMES or PES, either within the same group or different treatment groups.

Participants (Table 2). The 42 studies included a total of 2281 participants (mean 54.3; SD 39.1). The sample sizes ranged from the smallest sample of 16 participants [60,61] to the largest sample of 162 participants [36]. By intervention type, samples were characterized as follows: NMES total 1706, mean 56.9, SD 38.9, range 18–135; PES total 410, mean 51.3, SD 49.0, range 16–162; and combined neurostimulation total 165, mean 41.3, SD 19.3, range 18–64. The mean age of participants across all studies was 61.8 years (SD 15.3), with one study reporting age range only (65–93 years) [61]. Participant mean age across all studies ranged from 4.2 years [54] to 84.4 years [39]. The mean age of participants by intervention group was: NMES 60.9 years (SD 16.9), PES 64.7 years (SD 11.9), and combined neurostimulation 63.8 years (SD 6.4).

Across all studies, 61.0% (SD 13.5) of participants were male and one study did not report gender distribution [30]. Percentage of males by intervention group was NMES 62.6% (SD 14.0), PES 56.7% (SD 9.6), and other/combined 65.4% (SD 12.3). Most studies included stroke patients ($n = 31$), while three studies included mixed populations [28,41,43] and one study reported OD without further underlying medical diagnosis [39]. Other diagnoses by intervention group were: Parkinson's disorder ($n = 2$) [32,46], cerebral palsy ($n = 2$) [50,54], and head and neck cancer ($n = 2$) [36,48] in NMES; and multiple sclerosis ($n = 1$) [63] in PES.

Across the 42 studies, VFSS was most frequently used to confirm participant's diagnosis of OD ($n = 31$), whereas six studies used FEES [49,53,54,60,64,65]. Several of these studies combined instrumental assessment with either a screen ($n = 2$) [58,65] or clinical assessment ($n = 6$) [49,50,53–55,68]. One study used either clinical assessment or VFSS [50]. One study used a single screen [56], three studies used clinical assessment only [35,38,59], and one study used both [33]. The studies were conducted across 14 countries, with studies most frequently conducted in Korea ($n = 11$), China ($n = 7$), the UK ($n = 7$), Spain ($n = 4$), Italy ($n = 2$), Turkey ($n = 2$), and Germany ($n = 2$).

Outcome Measures (Table 2). Outcomes measures varied greatly across all studies included in the review, covering several domains within the area of OD. The Penetration Aspiration Score was the most reported outcome measure (PAS; 18 studies), followed by Functional Oral Intake Scale (FOIS; 12 studies), Functional Dysphagia Scale (FDS; 5 studies), Dysphagia Severity Rating Scale (DSRS; 5 studies), Swallowing Quality of Life questionnaire (SWAL-QOL; 4 studies), and Dysphagia Outcome and Severity Scale (DOSS; 3 studies).

NMES Intervention ($n = 30$: Tables 2 and 3). In total, 22 studies included two study arms or groups, whereas eight studies included three groups [31–34,38,40,55,57]. All but five NMES studies [29,39,43,53,54] combined neurostimulation with simultaneous DT consisting of a wide range of behavioural interventions (e.g., head and body positioning, bolus modification, oromotor exercises, or swallow manoeuvres). Six studies included a NMES only group without DT [29,33,38,39,43,55], with five of these studies using NMES at motor stimulation level [29,33,38,43,55] and one study using NMES at sensory stimulation level [39]. An additional seven studies included a treatment arm with NMES at sensory stimulation level combined with DT [32,44–46,53,54,57]. All other participants in NMES groups received stimulation at motor level. Five studies compared different NMES electrode positions [28,34,40–42] and seven studies included a sham stimulation group [36,39,48,50,52–54].

Control groups included mostly sham NMES stimulation and/or DT. Only one study included a control group receiving neither DT nor NMES [30], and one study included usual care across different healthcare settings as the comparison group [51].

PES Intervention (*n* = 8: Tables 2 and 3). All eight studies compared PES to a sham version of the treatment [58–65]. None of the studies included other treatment groups (e.g., DT) or control groups (e.g., usual care or no treatment).

Combined Neurostimulation Interventions (*n* = 4: Tables 2 and 3). Three studies in the combined intervention group compared three different treatments. Of these, one study compared PES, paired associative stimulation (PAS) and rTMS [68], a second study compared DT, rTMS combined with DT, and NMES combined with DT [67], and a third study compared rTMS, PES and capsaicin stimulation [66]. A fourth study combined NMES stimulation with sham rTMS or rTMS stimulating different hemispheres (ipsilesional, contralesional or bilateral) [69].

5.3. Risk of Bias Assessment and Methodological Quality

The tau values from the Begg and Mazumdar rank correlation were 0.101 (two-tailed $p = 0.589$) and < 0.000 (two-tailed $p > 0.999$) for NMES and PES, respectively. The NMES meta-analysis incorporates data from 16 studies, which yielded a z-value of 4.107 (two-tailed $p < 0.001$). The fail-safe N is 55 indicating 55 'null' studies need to be located and included for the combined two-tailed *p*-value to exceed 0.050. Therefore, there would need to be 3.4 missing studies for every observed study for the effect to be nullified. The PES meta-analysis incorporates data from five studies yielding a z-value of 1.156 (two-tailed $p < 0.248$). Since the combined result is not statistically significant, the fail-safe N (which addresses the concern that the observed significance may be spurious) is not relevant. Both of these procedures (i.e., Begg and Mazumdar rank correlation and fail-safe N) indicate the absence of publication bias.

Figures 2 and 3 present, respectively, the risk of bias summary per domain for all included studies combined and for individual studies. The majority of studies had low risk of bias with very few exceptions.

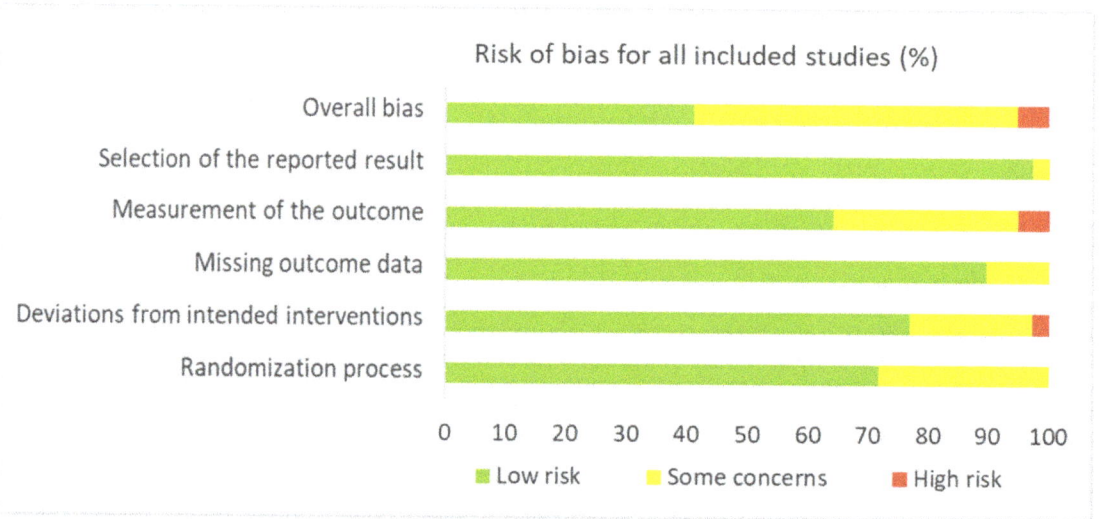

Figure 2. Risk of bias summary for all included studies (*n* = 42) in accordance with RoB-2.

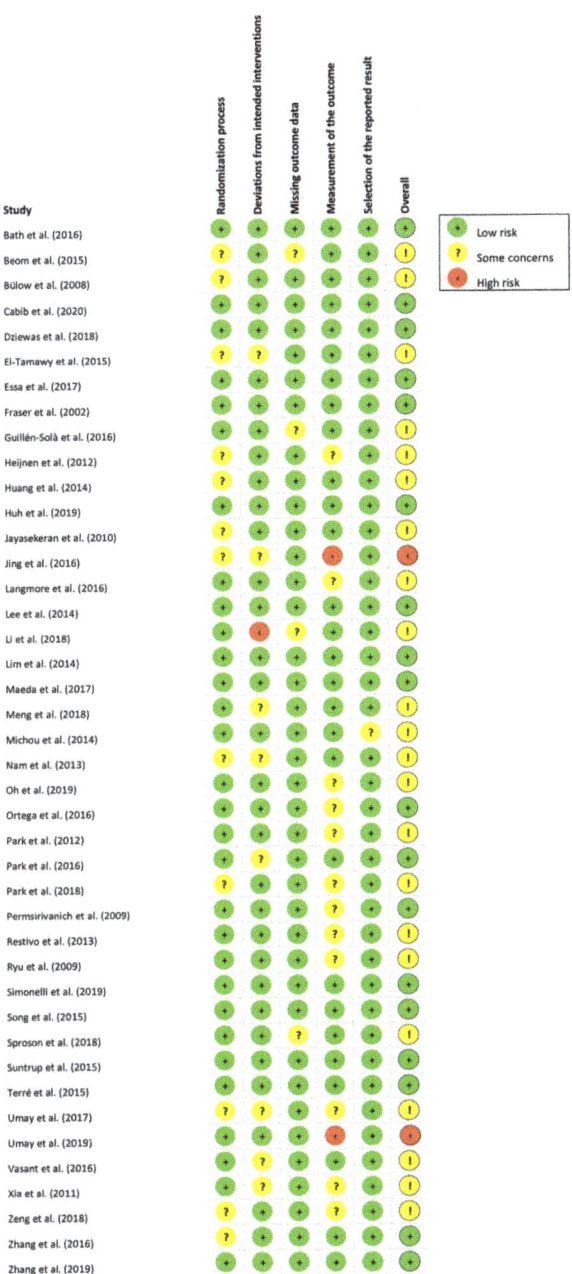

Figure 3. Risk of bias summary for individual studies (*n* = 42) in accordance with RoB-2.

6. Meta-Analysis: Effects of Interventions

6.1. Neuromuscular Electrical Stimulation (NMES) Meta-Analysis

Eleven studies were included in the NMES meta-analysis [28,29,34,37,40,42,45,47,49,51,55], of which six studies included two or three different intervention groups [28,34,40,42,45,55]. A total of 20 studies were excluded from meta-analysis for the following reasons: in three studies, OD diagnosis was not confirmed by instrumental assessment (VFSS or FEES); five studies provided insufficient data for meta-analyses; and, twelve studies were excluded to reduce heterogeneity: six studies including subject populations with medical diagnoses other than stroke (i.e., children with cerebral palsy, head and neck cancer patients, patients with Parkinson's disease, and elderly), five studies because of outcome measures (e.g., kinematic or biomechanical variables in VFS recordings), and one study using sensory NMES stimulation.

Overall within-group analysis (Figure 4). A significant, large pre-post intervention effect size was calculated using a random-effects model ($z(17) = 6.477$, $p < 0.001$, Hedges' $g = 1.272$, and 95% CI = 0.887–1.657). Pre-post intervention effect sizes ranged from 0.000 to 3.826. In 13 of the 18 NMES intervention groups, effect sizes were large (Hedges' $g > 0.8$), indicating that NMES accounted for a significant proportion of standardized mean difference for these studies. Between-study heterogeneity was significant ($Q(17) = 106.7$, and $p < 0.001$), with I^2 showing that heterogeneity accounted for 84.1% of variation in effect sizes across studies.

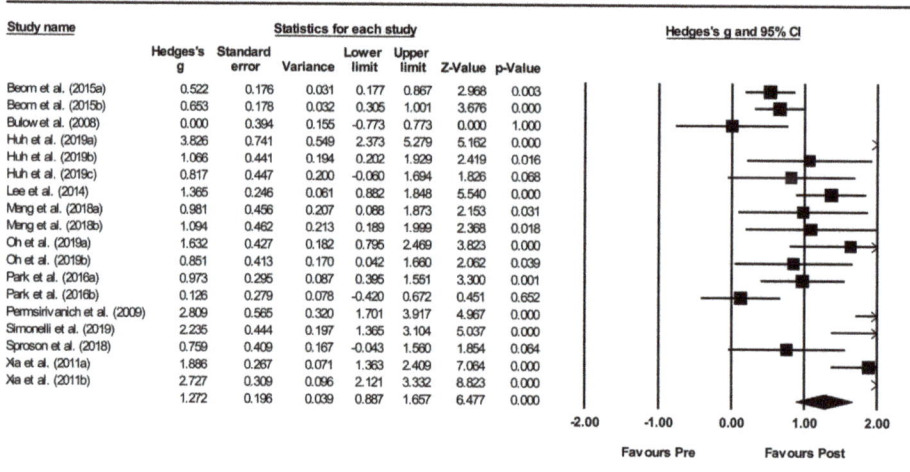

Figure 4. Neuromuscular electrical stimulation (NMES) within intervention group pre-post meta-analysis [28,29,34,37,40,42,45,47,49,51,55]. Note. Refer to Table 2 for explanation of the subgroups.

Overall between-group analysis (Figure 5). A significant, small post-intervention between-group total effect size in favour of NMES was calculated using a random-effects model ($z(8) = 2.589$, $p = 0.010$, Hedges' $g = 0.433$, and 95% CI = 0.105–0.760). Between-study heterogeneity was significant ($Q(8) = 18.0$, and $p = 0.021$), with I^2 showing that heterogeneity accounted for 55.6% of variation in effect sizes across studies.

Between-subgroup analyses. Subgroup analyses (Table 4) were conducted to compare diagnostic groups. Treatment effects were highest (moderate) for stroke patients, while other groups showed no significant effect sizes. For all other subgroup analyses, only stroke patients were included to improve homogeneity between studies. Subgroup analyses between studies compared intervention types (NMES, NMES + DT), time between pre- and post-intervention measurement, outcome measures, total stimulation times, electrodes configurations, pulse durations, and pulse rates (Table 4). NMES as an adjunctive treatment to DT showed significant, moderate positive treatment effects, whereas NMES alone showed non-significant effects. Effect sizes comparing time between pre- and post-treatment measurements showed no clear results. Although no effects could be identified at 2 weeks, a significant, positive effect size was found at 7 weeks. When comparing effect sizes based on outcome measures, the only significant effect found was a significant, large effect size for oral intake. The non-significant effects sizes for visuoperceptual evaluation of instrumental assessment ranged between negligible negative to moderate positive effects. Total stimulation time subgroup analyses showed significant, moderate positive treatment effects for longer stimulation times (>100 min). Shorter stimulation times did not result in significant effects. Comparisons for electrode configurations showed significant, moderate positive effects sizes for infrahyoid configuration. Electrode configuration based on patients' characteristics, including OD outcome scores, indicated non-significant moderate effects, whereas both suprahyoid combined with infrahyoid and suprahyoid configurations resulted in negligible effects. Final comparisons between studies using different pulse durations did not suggest a linear relationship, whereas pulse rate comparisons indicated that studies using higher frequencies showed increased significant, positive moderate effect sizes.

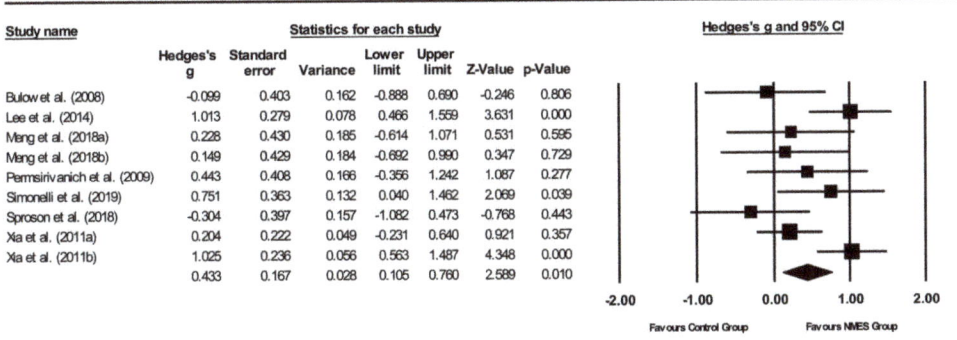

Figure 5. NMES between group post meta-analysis [29,37,40,47,49,51,55]. Note. Refer to Table 2 for explanation of the subgroups.

6.2. Pharyngeal Electrical Stimulation (PES) Meta-Analysis

Five studies using PAS in adult stroke patients were included in the meta-analyses [58,62,65,66,68]. Three studies were excluded from meta-analyses for the following reasons: overlap in participant population between studies, insufficient data for meta-analyses, and no confirmation of OD diagnosis prior to treatment.

Overall within-group analysis. The pre-post intervention effect sizes for the included studies ranged from 0.265 (small effect) [66] to 0.802 (large effect) [62], with an overall moderate effect size of 0.527 (Figure 6). As one study, however, did not provide PAS data for all included participants [65], a sensitivity analysis was conducted for both PAS and DSRS, indicating minimal differences in effect sizes.

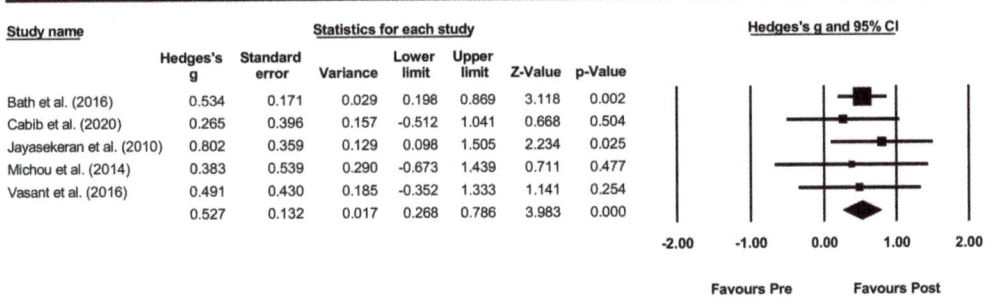

Figure 6. PES within intervention group pre-post meta-analysis [58,62,65,66,68].

Table 4. Between subgroup meta-analyses for NMES and pharyngeal electrical stimulation (PES) comparing intervention groups of included studies.

Neurostimulation	Subgroup	Hedges' g	Lower Limit CI	Upper Limit CI	Z-Value	p-Value
NMES	Diagnostic groups					
	Aged dysphagia [>65 yrs] (n = 1)	0.291	−0.299	0.881	0.966	0.334
	Cerebral palsy (children) (N = 2)	0.264	−0.088	0.616	1.470	0.142
	Head and neck cancer (n = 2)	0.281	−0.610	1.172	0.618	0.536
	Parkinson's disease (n = 2)	0.000	−0.359	0.359	0.000	1.000
	Stroke (n = 9)	0.433	0.105	0.760	2.589	0.010 *
	Intervention types					
	NMES (n = 2)	0.134	−0.247	0.515	0.688	0.492
	NMES + DT (n = 7)	0.648	0.398	0.897	5.086	<0.001 *
	Time between pre-post (days)					
	14 (n = 1)	−0.099	−0.888	0.690	−0.246	0.806
	21 (n = 1)	1.013	0.466	1.559	3.631	<0.001 *
	28 (n = 6)	0.342	−0.062	0.746	1.657	0.098
	56 (n = 1)	0.751	0.040	1.462	2.069	0.039 *
	Outcome measures					
	DOSS (n = 2)	0.188	−0.407	0.784	0.621	0.535
	FOIS (n = 2)	0.805	0.268	1.343	2.937	0.003 *
	PAS (n = 2)	0.235	−0.799	1.269	0.446	0.656
	VFSS-scale 1 (n = 1)	−0.099	−0.888	0.690	−0.246	0.806
	VFSS-scale 2 (n = 2)	0.611	−0.193	1.415	1.489	0.137
	Total stimulation time (min)					
	Low [< 500 min] (N = 4)	0.317	−0.304	0.938	0.999	0.318
	Medium [500–100 min] (N = 1)	−0.099	−0.888	0.690	−0.246	0.806
	High [>100 min] (N = 4)	0.607	0.176	1.038	2.761	0.006 *
	Electrodes configuration					
	Infrahyoid (N = 3)	0.771	0.041	1.501	2.069	0.039 *
	Mixed (patient-dependent) (N = 2)	0.617	−0.195	1.429	1.489	0.137
	Suprahyoid and infrahyoid (N = 2)	0.056	−0.0544	0.655	0.182	0.856
	Suprahyoid (N = 2)	−0.100	−0.694	0.493	−0.331	0.740
	Pulse duration (μs)					
	300 (N = 1)	0.751	0.040	1.462	2.069	0.039 *
	350 (N = 3)	0.084	−0.391	0.559	0.348	0.728
	700 (N = 4)	0.680	0.227	1.133	2.944	0.003 *
	Pulse rates (Hz)					
	30 (N = 1)	−0.304	−1.082	0.473	−0.768	0.433
	80 (N = 8)	0.519	0.202	0.836	3.206	0.001 *
PES	Total stimulation time (min)					
	10 (N = 2)	0.300	−0.325	0.925	0.940	0.347
	30 (N = 3)	0.053	0.245	0.351	0.348	0.728

Note. * Significant.

Overall between-group analysis. A non-significant post-intervention between-group total effect size in favour of PES was found using a random-effects model ($z(4) = 0.718$, $p = 0.473$, Hedges' $g = 0.099$, and 95% CI = -0.170–0.368), suggesting no improvement in PAS outcomes following PES neurostimulation (Figure 7). Between-study heterogeneity was non-significant ($Q(4) = 1.8$, and $p = 0.766$).

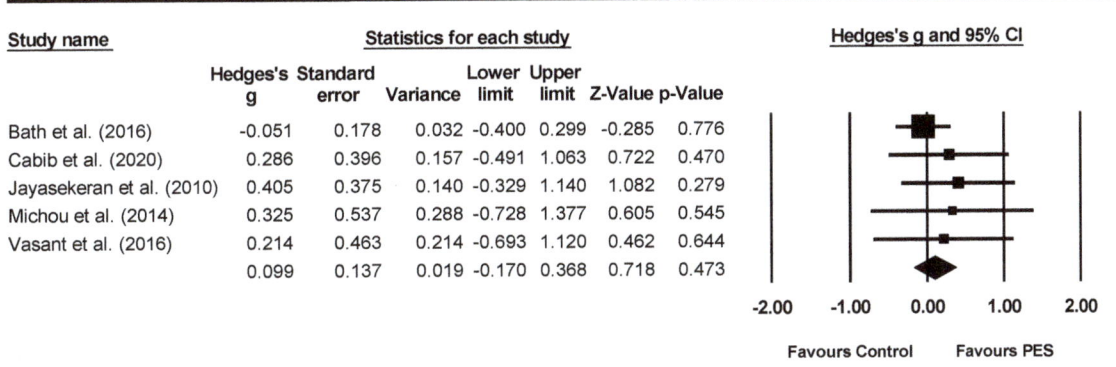

Figure 7. PES between group post meta-analysis [58,62,65,66,68].

Between-subgroup analyses. Subgroup analyses were conducted (Table 4) comparing total stimulation time between studies, favouring shorter stimulation times ($z(1) = 0.940$, $p = 0.347$, Hedges' $g = 0.300$, and 95% CI = -0.325–0.925).

7. Discussion

This study (Part I) aimed to determine the effects of PES and NMES in people with OD without excluding populations based on medical diagnoses. To base findings on the highest level of evidence, only RCTs were included. This systematic review and meta-analysis were conducted using PRISMA procedures as a guide.

7.1. Systematic Review Findings

When comparing RCTs in pharyngeal and neuromuscular electrical stimulation (i.e., PES and NMES), various methodological problems became apparent. Some studies did not define OD or used divergent definitions, whereas other studies applied different inclusion criteria. Most studies included patients with confirmed OD by instrumental assessment, but several studies used screening, patient self-report or clinical assessments instead. Consequently, participant characteristics may differ widely between studies. Despite most studies included stroke patients, meta-analysis comparing diagnostic groups other than stroke was possible for NMES, however this could not be conducted for PES.

Furthermore, the great variety in outcome measures also restricted comparisons by meta-analysis. As heterogeneity between studies indicates that no estimated overall effect by meta-analysis should be determined, combining studies targeting different domains within the area of OD will have similar implications. For instance, meta-analyses based on both patients' self-reported health-related quality of life and visuoperceptual evaluation of instrumental assessments would very likely lead to inappropriate estimated overall effects. Thus, to reduce heterogeneity between outcome measures, some studies were excluded from the meta-analysis. This strong focus on reducing heterogeneity between studies when performing meta-analysis also implies that data other than the authors' primary outcomes may have been preferably included in this analysis. For example, the primary outcome for Dziewas, Stellato, Van Der Tweel, Walther, Werner, Braun, Citerio, Jandl, Friedrichs, Nötzel, Vosko, Mistry, Hamdy, McGowan, Warnecke, Zwittag and Bath [59] and Suntrup, Marian, Schröder, Suttrup, Muhle, Oelenberg, Hamacher, Minnerup, Warnecke and Dziewas [64] was readiness for decannulation, which was considered too different from outcomes in the other included studies.

All eight PES studies compared neurostimulation with sham stimulation. However, among the 30 NMES studies, the comparison group variably consisted of usual care, DT, another dysphagia treatment or a combination of treatments. In contrast to PES studies that did not include any DT groups, most NMES studies combined neurostimulation with simultaneous DT. However, DT consisted of a wide range of behavioural interventions, using different treatment dosages, timings, and durations. Moreover, DT was referred to by many different names and acronyms (e.g., dysphagia training, behavioural intervention, classic treatment, or standard care). This suggest that care should be taken with the use of DT as an overarching term to group many different behavioural interventions to estimate overall effect sizes in meta-analyses.

Furthermore, RCTs are characterised by random allocation of participants to intervention groups and blinding or masking the nature of treatment for participants. However, in neurostimulation studies, blinding is frequently not feasible and participants may identify what treatment arm they have been assigned to (e.g., the presence of neurostimulation equipment, the experience of active stimulation). Also, since neurostimulation thresholding in PES is frequently applied in all groups to mask treatment assignment, patients receiving sham stimulation would still have been exposed to a certain level of neurostimulation during thresholding. Those studies not using thresholding in sham groups (e.g., [59,64]) might show larger treatment effect differences when comparing neurostimulation versus sham stimulation.

7.2. NMES

When considering meta-analyses for NMES, the highest effect sizes were found for stroke populations. As existing reviews in NMES [10,12,18,19] excluded other patient populations, no comparisons could be made between clinical populations. In addition, only two reviews conducted meta-analyses [18,19] selecting studies using different inclusion criteria (e.g., excluding comparison groups with active treatment components [18] or excluding chronic stroke patients [19]). Reviews may also prefer different outcome data for meta-analyses, especially in the case of RCTs using a large battery of assessments. As such, total numbers of included studies vary per review, but comparisons between reviews may be falsely estimated due to differences in methodology.

In this systematic review, a wide range in effect sizes was found in NMES RCTs depending on outcome measures used. However, oral intake scales showed highest effects sizes when compared to visuoperceptual evaluation of instrumental assessment or clinical assessment. This might be explained by NMES treatment usually taking place over consecutive weeks, in contrast to other neurostimulation techniques (e.g., PES or rTMS) that may be restricted to limited sessions over a few days only.

The great heterogeneity between DT groups also impeded comparisons between NMES only, NMES plus DT, and DT-only groups. No RCTs provided adequate DT group data to be included in the meta-analysis. For NMES groups, only two studies were included. As a result, information about the effects of DT is lacking. The negligible effect sizes found for NMES without DT were based on only two studies and the moderate effect sizes for combined NMES and DT were based on a total of seven studies.

Most studies performed NMES at motor stimulation level, whereas only a few studies included a group receiving NMES at sensory stimulation level. As none of these latter studies could be included in meta-analyses, no further details are available on comparisons between effect sizes for sensory versus motor stimulation. Also, terminology was confusing as sensory stimulation was sometimes referred to as sham stimulation [39].

NMES studies showed marked variation in the technical parameters and protocols applied. When comparing electrode configurations, both hyoid and combined hyoid and suprahyoid configurations showed negligible effects, whereas infrahyoid configurations resulted in moderate effects. A study using patient-dependent configurations showed promising results as well [55]. However, it remained unclear which criteria were used to decide on individual configurations. Furthermore, reporting on many technical parameters proved to be either incomplete or unclear for several studies (e.g., data on pulse duration, pulse rate, or stimulation time). As technical parameters may depend on medical device manufacturers, comparisons between brands may be warranted. For example, when considering pulse duration, a clear distinction in effect sizes is found between one study using a lower pulse rate—indicating a negative effect size—versus eight studies using higher pulse rates with moderate effect sizes.

7.3. PES

Compared to NMES, fewer PES studies were identified and thus a more limited meta-analysis was conducted. RCTs included stroke populations, except for one study that included patients with multiple sclerosis [63]. All studies compared active PES with sham treatment in stroke patients and used mostly visuoperceptual evaluation of radiographic recordings of the swallowing act as an outcome measure. Meta-analysis identified a non-significant post-intervention between-group total effect size in favour of PES. This finding seemed in line with findings by Chiang, Lin, Hsiao, Yeh, Liang and Wang [19], but this comparison is limited as it is based on only two studies. Additionally, Bath, Lee and Everton [18] reported that PES studies did not show an effect for many outcome measures (e.g., post-treatment proportions of participants with dysphagia, swallowing ability, penetration and aspiration scores or nutrition). However, in contrast to previous reviews, Cheng, Sasegbon and Hamdy [7] found a significant, moderate effect size in favour of PES when conducting meta-analysis. Again, inclusion criteria between reviews differed. For example, two studies [59,64] were excluded from meta-analysis in this review as well as the reviews by Chiang, Lin, Hsiao, Yeh, Liang and Wang [19] and Bath, Lee and Everton [18], but were included in the review by Cheng, Sasegbon and Hamdy [7]. This may have impacted the overall effect size as both PES studies showed significant treatment effects.

7.4. Moderators

Differences between NMES and PES studies made comparisons between RCTs difficult and hindered meta-analyses. Studies used different participant inclusion criteria in relation to underlying medical diagnoses or chronicity of stroke and used a large variety of outcome measures covering different domains within the area of OD. Outcome measures may also lack responsiveness, thus lack sensitivity to change during treatment. Moreover, studies varied significantly in technical parameters of neurostimulation. The number of studies and participants restricted the ability of statistical analyses to consider how each variable may have impacted the effects of neurostimulation.

Studies frequently neglected to report on potential moderators of stimulation effects in sufficient detail. For example, stroke severity and OD severity are inextricably linked and may moderate stimulation effects, yet only very few studies provided data on stroke severity. Similar problems occur when the chronicity of a stroke is not reported or the possibility of spontaneous recovery is ignored. This is especially true during NMES treatment, which may span a period of several weeks. In addition, no consensus was reached regarding the optimal moment for outcome measurement. Consequently, in this review, between-subgroup meta-analyses were conducted using post-intervention data only, so that the possibility of spontaneous recovery during the intervention period was taken into consideration.

7.5. Limitations

Despite a rigorous reviewing process following PRISMA guidelines and the use of RoB 2 to reduce bias, this review is subject to some limitations. Only RCTs published in English were included in this current study. Thus, some RCTs may have been excluded based on language criteria when their findings could have contributed to the current meta-analysis. Furthermore, meta-analyses included mostly stroke studies, thereby not providing effect sizes for other diagnostic patient populations. However, the main limitation of this review originates from the high degree of heterogeneity between studies, making comparisons across studies challenging. As such, generalisations and meta-analyses should be interpreted with care.

8. Conclusions

Meta-analyses for RCTS in NMES found a significant, large pre-post intervention effect size and significant, small post-intervention between-group effect size in favour of NMES. For PES studies, the meta-analyses showed a significant, moderate effect size for pre-post intervention, whereas overall between-group analysis did not result in significant treatment effects. Based on these results, NMES seems to have a more promising outcome compared to PES. However, only careful generalisations and interpretations of these meta-analyses can be made due to the NMES studies showing high heterogeneity in protocols and experimental variables, including potential moderators, and featuring inconsistent methodological reporting.

There is a need for more RCTs with larger sample sizes in addition to the standardisation of protocols and guidelines for reporting. These changes would better facilitate comparisons of studies and help to determine intervention effects more definitively. Delphi studies involving international experts might allow for a consensus to be reached, thus supporting future research, comparability and generalisability.

Supplementary Materials: The following supporting information can be downloaded at: https://www.mdpi.com/article/10.3390/jcm11030776/s1, Table S1: PRISMA 2020 for Abstracts Checklist; Table S2: PRISMA 2020 Checklist.

Author Contributions: Conceptualization: R.S., R.C., A.-L.S., L.B., S.H. Formal analysis: R.S., R.C. Methodology: R.S., R.C. Project administration: R.S., R.C. Validation: R.S., R.C. Writing—review & editing: R.S., R.C., A.-L.S., L.B., S.H., B.J.H., L.R., S.W.-G. All authors have read and agreed to the published version of the manuscript.

Funding: This research received no external funding.

Conflicts of Interest: The authors declare no conflict of interest.

References

1. Speyer, R. (Ed.) *Behavioural Treatment of Oropharyngeal Dysphagia*; Springer: Berlin, Germany, 2018.
2. Speyer, R.; Cordier, R.; Kim, J.H.; Cocks, N.; Michou, E.; Wilkes-Gillan, S. Prevalence of drooling, feeding and swallowing problems in cerebral palsy across the lifespan: Systematic review and meta-analysis. *Dev. Med. Child Neurol.* **2019**, *61*, 1249–1258. [CrossRef] [PubMed]
3. Takizawa, C.; Gemmell, E.; Kenworthy, J.; Speyer, R. A Systematic Review of the Prevalence of Oropharyngeal Dysphagia in Stroke, Parkinson's Disease, Alzheimer's Disease, Head Injury, and Pneumonia. *Dysphagia* **2016**, *31*, 434–441. [CrossRef] [PubMed]
4. Jones, E.; Speyer, R.; Kertscher, B.; Denman, D.; Swan, K.; Cordier, R. Health-related quality of life in oropharyngeal dysphagia. *Dysphagia* **2018**, *33*, 141–172. [CrossRef] [PubMed]
5. Wang, Z.; Wu, L.; Fang, Q.; Shen, M.; Zhang, L.; Liu, X. Effects of capsaicin on swallowing function in stroke patients with dysphagia: A randomized controlled trial. *J. Stroke Cerebrovasc. Dis.* **2019**, *28*, 1744–1751. [CrossRef] [PubMed]
6. Quiroz-González, S.; Torres-Castillo, S.; López-Gómez, R.E.; Estrada, I.J. Acupuncture points and their relationship with multireceptive fields of neurons. *J. Acupunct. Meridian Stud.* **2017**, *10*, 81–89. [CrossRef]
7. Cheng, I.; Sasegbon, A.; Hamdy, S. Effects of neurostimulation on poststroke dysphagia: A synthesis of current evidence from randomised controlled trials. *Neuromodulation Technol. Neural Interface* **2021**, *24*, 1388–1401. [CrossRef]
8. Michou, E.; Sasegbon, A.; Hamdy, S. Neurostimulation for the treatment of dysphagia after stroke: Behavioural treatment of oropharyngeal dysphagia. In *Dysphagia: Diagnosis and Treatment*, 2nd ed.; Ekberg, O., Ed.; Medical Radiology: Diagnostic Imaging; Springer: Berlin/Heidelberg, Germany, 2019.
9. Carnaby, G.D.; LaGorio, L.; Silliman, S.; Crary, M. Exercise-based swallowing intervention (McNeill Dysphagia Therapy) with adjunctive NMES to treat dysphagia post-stroke: A double-blind placebo-controlled trial. *J. Oral Rehabil.* **2020**, *47*, 501–510. [CrossRef]
10. Alamer, A.; Melese, H.; Nigussie, F. Effectiveness of Neuromuscular Electrical Stimulation on Post-Stroke Dysphagia: A Systematic Review of Randomized Controlled Trials. *Clin. Interv. Aging* **2020**, *15*, 1521–1531. [CrossRef]
11. Baijens, L.W.J.; Speyer, R.; Passos, V.L.; Pilz, W.; Van Der Kruis, J.; Haarmans, S.; Desjardins-Rombouts, C. Surface electrical stimulation in dysphagic parkinson patients: A randomized clinical trial. *Laryngoscope* **2013**, *123*, E38–E44. [CrossRef]
12. Clark, H.; Lazarus, C.; Arvedson, J.; Schooling, T.; Frymark, T. Evidence-Based Systematic Review: Effects of Neuromuscular Electrical Stimulation on Swallowing and Neural Activation. *Am. J. Speech Lang. Pathol.* **2009**, *18*, 361–375. [CrossRef]

13. Dionisio, A.; Duarte, I.C.; Patricio, M.; Castelo-Branco, M. Transcranial magnetic stimulation as an intervention tool to recover from language, swallowing and attentional deficits after stroke: A systematic review. *Cerebrovasc. Dis.* **2018**, *18*, 176–183. [CrossRef] [PubMed]
14. Liao, X.; Xing, G.; Guoqiang, X.; Jin, Y.; Tang, Q.; He, B.; McClure, M.A.; Liu, H.; Chen, H.; Mu, Q. Repetitive transcranial magnetic stimulation as an alternative therapy for dysphagia after stroke: A systematic review and meta-analysis. *Clin. Rehabil.* **2017**, *31*, 289–298. [CrossRef]
15. Marchina, S.; Pisegna, J.M.; Massaro, J.M.; Langmore, S.E.; McVey, C.; Wang, J.; Kumar, S. Transcranial direct current stimulation for post-stroke dysphagia: A systematic review and meta-analysis of randomized controlled trials. *J. Neurol.* **2021**, *268*, 293–304. [CrossRef] [PubMed]
16. Momosaki, R.; Kinoshita, S.; Kakuda, W.; Yamada, N.; Abo, M. Noninvasive brain stimulation for dysphagia after acquired brain injury: A systematic review. *J. Med. Investig.* **2016**, *63*, 153–158. [CrossRef] [PubMed]
17. Pisegna, J.M.; Kaneoka, A.; Pearson, W.G.; Kumar, S.; Langmore, S.E. Effects of non-invasive brain stimulation on post-stroke dysphagia: A systematic review and meta-analysis of randomized controlled trials. *Clin. Neurophysiol.* **2016**, *127*, 956–968. [CrossRef]
18. Bath, P.M.; Lee, H.S.; Everton, L.F. Swallowing therapy for dysphagia in acute and subacute stroke (Review). *Cochrane Database Syst. Rev.* **2018**, *10*, CD000323.
19. Chiang, C.-F.; Lin, M.-T.; Hsiao, M.-Y.; Yeh, Y.-C.; Liang, Y.-C.; Wang, T.-G. Comparative Efficacy of Noninvasive Neurostimulation Therapies for Acute and Subacute Poststroke Dysphagia: A Systematic Review and Network Meta-analysis. *Arch. Phys. Med. Rehabil.* **2019**, *100*, 739–750.e4. [CrossRef]
20. Page, M.J.; McKenzie, J.E.; Bossuyt, P.M.; Boutron, I.; Hoffmann, T.C.; Mulrow, C.D.; Moher, D. The PRISMA 2020 statement: An updated guideline for reporting systematic reviews. *BMJ* **2021**, *372*, n71. [CrossRef] [PubMed]
21. Page, M.J.; Moher, D.; Bossuyt, P.M.; Boutron, I.; Hoffmann, T.C.; Mulrow, C.D.; McKenzie, J.E. PRISMA 2020 explanation and elaboration: Updated guidance and exemplars for reporting systematic reviews. *BMJ* **2021**, *372*, n160. [CrossRef] [PubMed]
22. Sterne, J.A.; Savović, J.; Page, M.J.; Elbers, R.G.; Blencowe, N.S.; Boutron, I.; Cates, C.J.; Cheng, H.Y.; Corbett, M.S.; Eldridge, S.M.; et al. RoB 2: A revised tool for assessing risk of bias in randomised trials. *BMJ* **2019**, *366*, l4898. [CrossRef]
23. Borenstein, M.; Hedges, L.; Higgins, J.; Rothstein, H. *Comprehensive Meta-Analysis*; Biostat: Englewood, NJ, USA, 2014; Volume 3.
24. Higgins, J.P.T.; Thompson, S.G.; Deeks, J.J.; Altman, D.G. Measuring inconsistency in meta-analyses. *BMJ* **2003**, *327*, 557–560. [CrossRef] [PubMed]
25. Cohen, J. *Statistical Power Analysis for the Behavioural Sciences*, 2nd ed.; Routledge: New York, NY, USA, 1988.
26. Begg, C.B.; Mazumdar, M. Operating Characteristics of a Rank Correlation Test for Publication Bias. *Biometrics* **1994**, *50*, 1088–1101. [CrossRef] [PubMed]
27. Rosenthal, R. The file drawer problem and tolerance for null results. *Psychol. Bull.* **1979**, *86*, 638–664. [CrossRef]
28. Beom, J.; Oh, B.-M.; Choi, K.H.; Kim, W.; Song, Y.J.; You, D.S.; Kim, S.J.; Han, T.R. Effect of Electrical Stimulation of the Suprahyoid Muscles in Brain-Injured Patients with Dysphagia. *Dysphagia* **2015**, *30*, 423–429. [CrossRef] [PubMed]
29. Bülow, M.; Speyer, R.; Baijens, L.; Woisard, V.; Ekberg, O. Neuromuscular Electrical Stimulation (NMES) in Stroke Patients with Oral and Pharyngeal Dysfunction. *Dysphagia* **2008**, *23*, 302–309. [CrossRef] [PubMed]
30. El-Tamawy, M.S.; Darwish, M.H.; El-Azizi, H.S.; Abdelalim, A.M.; Taha, S.I. The influence of physical therapy on oropharyngeal dysphagia in acute stroke patients. *Egypt. J. Neurol. Psychiatry Neurosurg.* **2015**, *52*, 201–205.
31. Guillén-Solà, A.; Sartor, M.M.; Soler, N.B.; Duarte, E.; Barrera, M.C.; Marco, E. Respiratory muscle strength training and neuromuscular electrical stimulation in subacute dysphagic stroke patients: A randomized controlled trial. *Clin. Rehabilitation* **2017**, *31*, 761–771. [CrossRef]
32. Heijnen, B.J.; Speyer, R.; Baijens, L.W.J.; Bogaardt, H.C.A. Neuromuscular electrical stimulation versus traditionaltherapy in patients with Parkinson's Disease and propharyngeal dysphagia: Effects on quality of life. *Dysphagia* **2012**, *27*, 336–345. [CrossRef] [PubMed]
33. Huang, K.-L.; Liu, T.-Y.; Huang, Y.-C.; Leong, C.-P.; Lin, W.-C.; Pong, Y.-P. Functional Outcome in Acute Stroke Patients with Oropharyngeal Dysphagia after Swallowing Therapy. *J. Stroke Cerebrovasc. Dis.* **2014**, *23*, 2547–2553. [CrossRef]
34. Huh, J.; Park, E.; Min, Y.; Kim, A.; Yang, W.; Oh, H.; Nam, T.; Jung, T. Optimal placement of electrodes for treatment of post-stroke dysphagia by neuromuscular electrical stimulation combined with effortful swallowing. *Singap. Med. J.* **2020**, *61*, 487–491. [CrossRef]
35. Jing, Q.; Yang, X.; Reng, Q. Effect of Neuromuscular Electrical Stimulation in Patients with Post-Stroke Dysphagia. *Med. Sci. Technol.* **2016**, *57*, 1–5. [CrossRef]
36. Langmore, S.E.; McCulloch, T.M.; Krisciunas, G.P.; Lazarus, C.L.; Van Daele, D.J.; Pauloski, B.R.; Rybin, D.; Doros, G. Efficacy of electrical stimulation and exercise for dysphagia in patients with head and neck cancer: A randomized clinical trial. *Head Neck* **2015**, *38*, E1221–E1231. [CrossRef] [PubMed]
37. Lee, K.W.; Kim, S.B.; Lee, J.H.; Lee, S.J.; Ri, J.W.; Park, J.G. The Effect of Early Neuromuscular Electrical Stimulation Therapy in Acute/Subacute Ischemic Stroke Patients with Dysphagia. *Ann. Rehabil. Med.* **2014**, *38*, 153–159. [CrossRef] [PubMed]
38. Li, L.; Li, Y.; Huang, R.; Yin, J.; Shen, Y.; Shi, J. The value of adding transcutaneous neuromuscular electrical stimulation (VitalStim) to traditional therapy for post-stroke dysphagia: A randomized controlled trial. *Eur. J. Phys. Rehabil. Med.* **2014**, *51*, 200–206.

39. Maeda, K.; Koga, T.; Akagi, J. Interferential current sensory stimulation, through the neck skin, improves airway defense and oral nutrition intake in patients with dysphagia: A double-blind randomized controlled trial. *Clin. Interv. Aging* **2017**, *12*, 1879–1886. [CrossRef]
40. Meng, P.; Zhang, S.; Wang, Q.; Wang, P.; Han, C.; Gao, J.; Yue, S. The effect of surface neuromuscular electrical stimulation on patients with post-stroke dysphagia. *J. Back Musculoskelet. Rehabil.* **2018**, *31*, 363–370. [CrossRef]
41. Nam, H.S.; Beom, J.; Oh, B.-M.; Han, T.R. Kinematic Effects of Hyolaryngeal Electrical Stimulation Therapy on Hyoid Excursion and Laryngeal Elevation. *Dysphagia* **2013**, *28*, 548–556. [CrossRef]
42. Oh, D.-H.; Park, J.-S.; Kim, H.-J.; Chang, M.-Y.; Hwang, N.-K. The effect of neuromuscular electrical stimulation with different electrode positions on swallowing in stroke patients with oropharyngeal dysphagia: A randomized trial. *J. Back Musculoskelet. Rehabil.* **2020**, *33*, 637–644. [CrossRef]
43. Ortega, O.; Rofes, L.; Martin, A.; Arreola, V.; López, I.; Clavé, P. A Comparative Study Between Two Sensory Stimulation Strategies After Two Weeks Treatment on Older Patients with Oropharyngeal Dysphagia. *Dysphagia* **2016**, *31*, 706–716. [CrossRef]
44. Park, J.-W.; Kim, Y.; Oh, J.C.; Lee, H.-J. Effortful Swallowing Training Combined with Electrical Stimulation in Post-Stroke Dysphagia: A Randomized Controlled Study. *Dysphagia* **2012**, *27*, 521–527. [CrossRef]
45. Park, J.-S.; Oh, D.-H.; Hwang, N.-K.; Lee, J.H. Effects of neuromuscular electrical stimulation combined with effortful swallowing on post-stroke oropharyngeal dysphagia: A randomised controlled trial. *J. Oral Rehabil.* **2016**, *43*, 426–434. [CrossRef] [PubMed]
46. Park, J.S.; Oh, D.H.; Hwang, N.K.; Lee, J.H. Effects of neuromuscular electrical stimulation in patients with Parkinson's disease and dysphagia: A ran-domized, single-blind, placebo-controlled trial. *Neurorehabilitation* **2018**, *42*, 457–463. [CrossRef] [PubMed]
47. Permsirivanich, W.; Tipchatyotin, S.; Wongchai, M.; Leelamanit, V.; Setthawatcharawanich, S.; Sathirapanya, P.; Boonmeeprakob, A. Comparing the effects of rehabilitation swallowing therapy vs. neuromuscular electrical stimu-lation therapy among stroke Pptients with persistent pharyngeal dysphagia: A randomized controlled study. *Med. J. Med. Assoc. Thail.* **2009**, *92*, 259.
48. Ryu, J.S.; Kang, J.Y.; Park, J.Y.; Nam, S.Y.; Choi, S.H.; Roh, J.L.; Kim, S.Y.; Choi, K.H. The effect of electrical stimulation therapy on dysphagia following treatment for head and neck cancer. *Oral Oncol.* **2009**, *45*, 665–668. [CrossRef] [PubMed]
49. Simonelli, M.; Ruoppolo, G.; Iosa, M.; Morone, G.; Fusco, A.; Grasso, M.G.; Gallo, A.; Paolucci, S. A stimulus for eating. The use of neuromuscular transcutaneous electrical stimulation in patients affected by severe dysphagia after subacute stroke: A pilot randomized controlled trial. *Neurorehabilitation* **2019**, *44*, 103–110. [CrossRef] [PubMed]
50. Song, W.J.; Park, J.H.; Lee, J.H.; Kim, M.Y. Effects of Neuromuscular Electrical Stimulation on Swallowing Functions in Children with Cerebral Palsy: A Pilot Randomised Controlled Trial. *Hong Kong J. Occup. Ther.* **2015**, *25*, 1–6. [CrossRef]
51. Sproson, L.; Pownall, S.; Enderby, P.; Freeman, J. Combined electrical stimulation and exercise for swallow rehabilitation post-stroke: A pilot randomized control trial. *Int. J. Lang. Commun. Disord.* **2018**, *53*, 405–417. [CrossRef] [PubMed]
52. Terré, R.; Mearin, F. A randomized controlled study of neuromuscular electrical stimulation in oropharyngeal dysphagia secondary to acquired brain injury. *Eur. J. Neurol.* **2015**, *22*, 687-e44. [CrossRef]
53. Umay, E.K.; Yaylaci, A.; Saylam, G.; Gundogdu, I.; Gurcay, E.; Akcapinar, D.; Kirac, Z. The effect of sensory level electrical stimulation of the masseter muscle in early stroke patients with dysphagia: A randomized controlled study. *Neurol. India* **2017**, *65*, 734. [CrossRef]
54. Umay, E.; Gurcay, E.; Ozturk, E.A.; Akyuz, E.U. Is sensory-level electrical stimulation effective in cerebral palsy children with dysphagia? A randomized controlled clinical trial. *Acta Neurol. Belg.* **2020**, *120*, 1097–1105. [CrossRef]
55. Xia, W.; Zheng, C.; Lei, Q.; Tang, Z.; Hua, Q.; Zhang, Y.; Zhu, S. Treatment of post-stroke dysphagia by vitalstim therapy coupled with conventional swallowing training. *J. Huazhong Univ. Sci. Technol.* **2011**, *31*, 73–76. [CrossRef] [PubMed]
56. Zeng, Y.; Yip, J.; Cui, H.; Guan, L.; Zhu, H.; Zhang, W.; Du, H.; Geng, X. Efficacy of neuromuscular electrical stimulation in improving the negative psychological state in patients with cerebral infarction and dysphagia. *Neurol. Res.* **2018**, *40*, 473–479. [CrossRef]
57. Zhang, M.; Tao, T.; Zhang, Z.-B.; Zhu, X.; Fan, W.-G.; Pu, L.-J.; Chu, L.; Yue, S.-W. Effectiveness of Neuromuscular Electrical Stimulation on Patients with Dysphagia with Medullary Infarction. *Arch. Phys. Med. Rehabil.* **2016**, *97*, 355–362. [CrossRef] [PubMed]
58. Bath, P.M.; Scutt, P.; Love, J.; Clavé, P.; Cohen, D.; Dziewas, R.; Hamdy, S. Pharyngeal electrical stimulation for treatment of dysphagia in subacute stroke: A randomised controlled trial. *Stroke* **2016**, *47*, 1–19. [CrossRef] [PubMed]
59. Dziewas, R.; Stellato, R.; van der Tweel, I.; Walther, E.; Werner, C.J.; Braun, T.; Citerio, G.; Jandl, M.; Friedrichs, M.; Nötzel, K.; et al. Pharyngeal electrical stimulation for early decannulation in tracheotomised patients with neurogenic dysphagia after stroke (PHAST-TRAC): A prospective, single-blinded, randomised trial. *Lancet Neurol.* **2018**, *17*, 849–859. [CrossRef]
60. Essa, H.; Vasant, D.H.; Raginis-Zborowska, A.; Payton, A.; Michou, E.; Hamdy, S. The BDNF polymorphism Val66Met may be predictive of swallowing improvement post pharyngeal electrical stimulation in dysphagic stroke patients. *Neurogastroenterol. Motil.* **2017**, *29*, e13062. [CrossRef] [PubMed]
61. Fraser, C.; Power, M.; Hamdy, S.; Rothwell, J.; Hobday, D.; Hollander, I.; Tyrell, P.; Hobson, A.; Williams, S.; Thompson, D. Driving Plasticity in Human Adult Motor Cortex Is Associated with Improved Motor Function after Brain Injury. *Neuron* **2002**, *34*, 831–840. [CrossRef]
62. Jayasekeran, V.; Singh, S.; Tyrrell, P.; Michou, E.; Jefferson, S.; Mistry, S.; Gamble, E.; Rothwell, J.; Thompson, D.; Hamdy, S. Adjunctive functional pharyngeal elctrical stimulation reverses swallowing disability after brain lesions. *Gastroentrology* **2010**, *138*, 1737–1746. [CrossRef]

63. Restivo, D.A.; Casabona, A.; Centonze, D.; Ragona, R.M.; Maimone, D.; Pavone, A. Pharyngeal Electrical Stimulation for Dysphagia Associated with Multiple Sclerosis: A Pilot Study. *Brain Stimul.* **2013**, *6*, 418–423. [CrossRef] [PubMed]
64. Suntrup, S.; Marian, T.; Schröder, J.B.; Suttrup, I.; Muhle, P.; Oelenberg, S.; Hamacher, C.; Minnerup, J.; Warnecke, T.; Dziewas, R. Electrical pharyngeal stimulation for dysphagia treatment in tracheotomized stroke patients: A randomized controlled trial. *Intensiv. Care Med.* **2015**, *41*, 1629–1637. [CrossRef] [PubMed]
65. Vasant, D.H.; Michou, E.; O'Leary, N.; Vail, A.; Mistry, S.; Hamdy, S.; Greater Manchester Stroke Research Network. Pharyngeal electrical stimulation in dysphagia poststroke: A prospective, randomized single-blinded interventional study. *Neurorehabilit. Neural Repair* **2016**, *30*, 866–875. [CrossRef] [PubMed]
66. Cabib, C.; Nascimento, W.; Rofes, L.; Arreola, V.; Tomsen, N.; Mundet, L.; Palomeras, E.; Michou, E.; Clavé, P.; Ortega, O. Short-term neurophysiological effects of sensory pathway neurorehabilitation strategies on chronic post-stroke oropharyngeal dysphagia. *Neurogastroenterol. Motil.* **2020**, *32*, 1–14. [CrossRef] [PubMed]
67. Lim, K.-B.; Lee, H.-J.; Yoo, J.; Kwon, Y.-G. Effect of Low-Frequency rTMS and NMES on Subacute Unilateral Hemispheric Stroke with Dysphagia. *Ann. Rehabil. Med.* **2014**, *38*, 592–602. [CrossRef]
68. Michou, E.; Mistry, S.; Jefferson, S.; Tyrrell, P.; Hamdy, S. Characterizing the Mechanisms of Central and Peripheral Forms of Neurostimulation in Chronic Dysphagic Stroke Patients. *Brain Stimul.* **2014**, *7*, 66–73. [CrossRef]
69. Zhang, C.; Zheng, X.; Lu, R.; Yun, W.; Yun, H.; Zhou, X. Repetitive transcranial magnetic stimulation in combination with neuromuscular electrical stimulation for treatment of post-stroke dysphagia. *J. Int. Med. Res.* **2019**, *47*, 662–672. [CrossRef] [PubMed]

Journal of
Clinical Medicine

Review

Neurostimulation in People with Oropharyngeal Dysphagia: A Systematic Review and Meta-Analysis of Randomised Controlled Trials—Part II: Brain Neurostimulation

Renée Speyer [1,2,3,*], Anna-Liisa Sutt [4,5], Liza Bergström [6,7], Shaheen Hamdy [8], Timothy Pommée [9], Mathieu Balaguer [9], Anett Kaale [1,10] and Reinie Cordier [2,11]

1. Department Special Needs Education, University of Oslo, 0318 Oslo, Norway; anett.kaale@isp.uio.no
2. Curtin School of Allied Health, Faculty of Health Sciences, Curtin University, Perth, WA 6102, Australia; reinie.cordier@northumbria.ac.uk
3. Department of Otorhinolaryngology and Head and Neck Surgery, Leiden University Medical Centre, 1233 ZA Leiden, The Netherlands
4. Critical Care Research Group, The Prince Charles Hospital, Brisbane, QLD 4032, Australia; annaliisasp@gmail.com
5. School of Medicine, University of Queensland, Brisbane, QLD 4072, Australia
6. Remeo Stockholm, 128 64 Stockholm, Sweden; liza.bergstrom@regionstockholm.se
7. Speech Therapy Clinic, Danderyd University Hospital, 182 88 Stockholm, Sweden
8. Faculty of Biology, GI Sciences, School of Medical Sciences, Medicine and Health, University of Manchester, Manchester M13 9PL, UK; shaheen.hamdy@manchester.ac.uk
9. IRIT, CNRS, Université Paul Sabatier, 31400 Toulouse, France; timothy.pommee@irit.fr (T.P.); mathieu.balaguer@irit.fr (M.B.)
10. Norwegian Centre of Expertise for Neurodevelopmental Disorders and Hypersomnias, Oslo University Hospital, 0424 Oslo, Norway
11. Department of Social Work, Education and Community Wellbeing, Faculty of Health & Life Sciences, Northumbria University, Newcastle upon the Tyne NE7 7XA, UK
* Correspondence: renee.speyer@isp.uio.no

Abstract: *Objective.* To assess the effects of brain neurostimulation (i.e., repetitive transcranial magnetic stimulation [rTMS] and transcranial direct current stimulation [tDCS]) in people with oropharyngeal dysphagia (OD). *Methods.* Systematic literature searches were conducted in four electronic databases (CINAHL, Embase, PsycINFO, and PubMed) to retrieve randomised controlled trials (RCTs) only. Using the Revised Cochrane risk-of-bias tool for randomised trials (RoB 2), the methodological quality of included studies was evaluated, after which meta-analysis was conducted using a random-effects model. *Results.* In total, 24 studies reporting on brain neurostimulation were included: 11 studies on rTMS, 9 studies on tDCS, and 4 studies on combined neurostimulation interventions. Overall, within-group meta-analysis and between-group analysis for rTMS identified significant large and small effects in favour of stimulation, respectively. For tDCS, overall within-group analysis and between-group analysis identified significant large and moderate effects in favour of stimulation, respectively. *Conclusion.* Both rTMS and tDCS show promising effects in people with oropharyngeal dysphagia. However, comparisons between studies were challenging due to high heterogeneity in stimulation protocols and experimental parameters, potential moderators, and inconsistent methodological reporting. Generalisations of meta-analyses need to be interpreted with care. Future research should include large RCTs using standard protocols and reporting guidelines as achieved by international consensus.

Keywords: deglutition; swallowing disorders; RCT; intervention; repetitive transcranial magnetic stimulation; transcranial direct current stimulation; rTMS; tDCS

1. Introduction

Oropharyngeal dysphagia (OD) or swallowing problems is highly prevalent among stroke patients, people with progressive neurological diseases, patients with head and neck cancer, and in frail older persons [1,2]. Prevalence estimates of OD may vary depending on underlying medical diagnoses, but have been reported as high as 80% in stroke and Parkinson's disease [3], and 70% in oncological populations [4]. OD is associated with dehydration, malnutrition, aspiration pneumonia, and increased mortality [5–7], but also leads to decreased health-related quality of life [8].

Treatment and management of OD may vary widely. However, apart from traditional compensatory and rehabilitative strategies including diet modifications, postural adjustments, oromotor training and swallow manoeuvres [9], recent studies report on the possible beneficial effects of non-invasive brain stimulation. Brain neurostimulation aims to modulate cortical excitability and include techniques such as repetitive transcranial magnetic stimulation (rTMS) and transcranial direct current stimulation (tDCS). rTMS uses electromagnetic induction resulting in depolarisation of postsynaptic connections, whereas tDCS uses direct electrical current shifting the polarity of nerve cells [10]. Neurostimulation protocols may vary greatly per study, including different neurostimulation sites, frequencies, stimulation duration and number of different outcome measures are used to objectify treatment effects, and individual responses to stimulation are highly variable [10–12].

Aspiring to improved treatment efficacy in OD management, non-invasive brain stimulation has achieved growing interest over the past decade. Several reviews have been published on rTMS and tDCS [10,12–18], each publication having different inclusion and exclusion criteria and methodology. All previous reviews targeted brain neurostimulation interventions in post-stroke populations except for one review that included patients with acquired brain injury [16]; to date, all reviews on brain stimulation set criteria based on medical diagnoses. Moreover, not all reviews performed meta-analysis [14] and as several neurostimulation trials have only been published recently, earlier reviews will have identified fewer studies.

This is the second paper (Part II) of two companion papers on treatment effects of neurostimulation in people with OD. The first systematic review (Part I) reported on the effects of pharyngeal electrical stimulation (PES) and neuromuscular electrical stimulation (NMES).

The aim of this systematic review (Part II) is to determine the effects of brain neurostimulation (i.e., rTMS and tDCS) in people with OD without excluding populations based on medical diagnoses. Only randomised controlled trials (RCTs) will be included being the highest level of evidence. Meta-analyses will be conducted to summarise results and report on possible moderators of treatment effects.

2. Methods

The methodology and reporting of this systematic review followed the Preferred Reporting Items for Systematic Reviews and Meta-Analyses (PRISMA) 2020 statement and checklist (Supplementary Tables S1 and S2) [19,20]. Adhering to the PRISMA statement and checklist ensures essential and transparent reporting of systematic reviews. The protocol for this review was registered with PROSPERO, the international prospective register of systematic reviews (registration number: CRD42020179842).

2.1. Information Sources and Search Strategies

An electronic database search for extant literature was conducted on 6 March 2021, using the following four databases: CINAHL, Embase, PsycINFO, and PubMed. Publications dates included in the search were 1937–2021, 1902–2021, 1887–2021, and 1809–2021, respectively. Generally, search strategies consisted of combinations of terms related to 'dysphagia' and 'randomised controlled trial'. Both subject headings (e.g., MeSH and Thesaurus terms) and free text terms were used to search databases. The full list of electronic search strategies for each database can be found in Table 1. To identify literature not found utilising these strategies, the reference lists of eligible articles were checked.

Table 1. Search strategies.

Database and Search Terms	Number of Records
Cinahl: ((MH "Deglutition") OR (MH "Deglutition Disorders")) AND (MH "Randomized Controlled Trials")	239
Embase: (swallowing/OR dysphagia/) AND (randomization/or randomized controlled trial/OR "randomized controlled trial (topic)"/OR controlled clinical trial/)	4550
PsycINFO: (swallowing/OR dysphagia/) AND (RCT OR (Randomised AND Controlled AND Trial) OR (Randomized AND Clinical AND Trial) OR (Randomised AND Clinical AND Trial) OR (Controlled AND Clinical AND Trial)).af.	231
PubMed: ("Deglutition" [Mesh] OR "Deglutition Disorders" [Mesh]) AND ("Randomized Controlled Trial" [Publication Type] OR "Randomized Controlled Trials as Topic" [Mesh] OR "Controlled Clinical Trial" [Publication Type] OR "Pragmatic Clinical Trials as Topic" [Mesh])	3039

2.2. Inclusion and Exclusion Criteria

To be eligible for inclusion in this systematic review, studies had to meet the following criteria: (1) participants had a diagnosis of oropharyngeal dysphagia; (2) the study included non-invasive neurostimulation interventions aimed at reducing swallowing or feeding problems; (3) the study included a control group or comparison intervention group; (4) participants were randomly assigned to one of the study arms or groups; and (5) the study was published in English language.

Interventions such as non-electrical peripheral stimulation (e.g., air-puff or gustatory stimulation), pharmacological interventions and acupuncture, were considered out of scope of this review, thus were excluded. Invasive techniques and/or those that did not specifically target OD (e.g., deep-brain stimulation studies after neurosurgical implementation of a neurostimulator) were also excluded. Conference abstracts, doctoral theses, editorials, and reviews were excluded.

2.3. Systematic Review

Methodological Quality and Risk of Bias. The Revised Cochrane risk-of-bias tool for randomised trials (RoB 2) [21] was used to assess the methodological quality of the included studies. The RoB 2 tool identifies domains to consider when assessing where bias may have been introduced into a randomised trial: (1) bias arising from the randomisation process; (2) bias due to deviations from intended interventions; (3) bias due to missing outcome data; (4) bias in measurement of the outcome; and (5) bias in selection of the reported result. For each domain, a series of signalling questions are answered to give a judgement (i.e., "low risk of bias", "some concerns", or "high risk of bias"), which can then be assessed in aggregate to determine a study's overall risk of bias [21].

Data Collection Process. Data were extracted from the included studies using a data extraction form created for this purpose. This form allowed for extraction of data under several categories, relevant to meta-analyses, including participant diagnosis, inclusion and exclusion criteria, sample size, age, gender, intervention goal, intervention agent/delivery/dosage, outcome measures, and treatment outcomes.

Data, Items and Synthesis of Results. Titles and abstracts of included studies were reviewed for eligibility by two independent reviewers. Next, the same two reviewers assessed the selected original articles at a full-text level to determine their eligibility. To ensure rating accuracy, a random selection of one hundred records were scored and discussed over two consecutive group sessions prior to rating the remaining records. Any disagreement between the first two reviewers was resolved by consulting a third reviewer. Assessment of methodology study quality followed an equivalent process. None of the reviewers had formal or informal affiliations with any of the authors of the included studies.

Extracted data were extrapolated and synthesised within the following categories to allow for comparison: participant characteristics, inclusion criteria, intervention conditions, outcome measures and intervention outcomes. Effect sizes and significance of findings were used to assess treatment outcomes.

2.4. Meta-Analysis

Using the extracted data, effect sizes were compared for the following: (1) pre-post outcome measures of OD and (2) mean difference in outcome measures from pre- to post-intervention scores between neurostimulation and comparison controls. Control groups either received no treatment, sham stimulation and/or traditional dysphagia therapy (DT; e.g., compensatory and rehabilitative strategies including diet modifications, postural adjustments, oromotor training and swallow manoeuvres). Only studies using instrumental assessment (e.g., videofluoroscopic swallow study [VFSS] or fiberoptic endoscopic evaluation of swallowing [FEES]) to confirm OD were included.

When selecting what data points to extract, data collected using outcome measures based on visuoperceptual evaluation of instrumental assessment were preferred over clinical non-instrumental assessments. Oral intake measures were only included if no other clinical data were available, whereas screening tools and patient self-report measures were excluded entirely. When selecting outcome measures for meta-analyses, reducing heterogeneity between studies was given priority. Consequently, measures other than the authors' primary outcomes may have been preferred if these measures contributed to greater homogeneity.

Comprehensive Meta-Analysis Version 3.3.070 [22] software was used to complete the meta-analysis, allowing comparison of sample size, effect size, group means and standard deviations of pre- and post-measurements. In the case that no parametric data were available, the reported non-parametric data (i.e., medians, interquartile ranges) were converted into parametric data for meta-analysis purposes. Studies with multiple intervention groups were analysed separately for each experimental-control comparison. If studies included the same participants, only one study was included in the meta-analysis. Where reported data were insufficient, attempts were made to contact authors of individual studies and request additional data.

Using Comprehensive Meta-Analysis, a random-effects model was used to calculate effect sizes. This was due to variations in participant characteristics, sampling, interventions, and measurement, which suggested a low likelihood that studies would have similar true effects. Heterogeneity was estimated using the Q statistic to determine the spread of effect sizes about the mean and I^2 was used to estimate the ratio of true variance to total variance. I^2-values of less than 50%, 50% to 74%, and higher than 75% denote low, moderate, and high heterogeneity, respectively [23]. Effects sizes were generated using the Hedges' g formula for standardised mean difference with a confidence interval of 95%. Effects sizes were interpreted using Cohen's d convention as follows: $d \leq 0.2$ as no or negligible effect; $0.2 < d \leq 5$ as small effect; $0.5 < d \leq 0.8$ as moderate effect; and $d > 0.8$ as large effect [24].

Forest plots of effect sizes for OD outcome scores were generated for both types of neurostimulation (i.e., rTMS and tDCS): (1) pre-post neurostimulation and (2) neurostimulation interventions versus comparison groups. Subgroup analyses were conducted to compare effect sizes as a function of different moderators and neurostimulation types including: outcome measures, total treatment duration, total neurostimulation time, and stimulation characteristics (e.g., pulse range, stimulation current, and stimulation site). To take into consideration the possibility of spontaneous recovery during the intervention period, only between-subgroup meta-analyses were conducted using post-intervention data.

Utilising Comprehensive Data Analysis software, publication bias was evaluated as per the Begg and Muzumdar's rank correlation test and the Fail-safe N test. Begg and Muzumdar's rank correlation test provides information on the rank correlations between standardised effect size and the ranks of their variances [25]. In addition to a tau value, a two-tailed p value is also generated. Where the analysis results in a value of zero, it can be concluded that there is unlikely to be an association between the effect size and ranks of variance. Conversely, the closer to one the tau or p values, the more likely there is to be an association between the effect size and ranks of variance. Therefore, high standard error would be connected to higher effect sizes if publication bias was the result of asymmetry. If larger effects are represented by low values, tau would be over zero; conversely tau would be negative if larger effects are represented by high values.

The Fail-safe N test is a calculation of the quantity of studies with zero effect size that could be incorporated into the meta-analysis prior to the result losing statistical significance, that is, the quantity of excluded studies that would result in the effect being nullified [26]. Results should be treated with care where the fail-safe N is relatively small, however, when it is large, conclusions can be confidently drawn that the treatment effect, while potentially raised by the removal of some studies, is not nil.

3. Results

3.1. Study Selection

A total of 8059 studies were retrieved through the subject heading and free text searches (CINAHL: $n = 239$, Embase: $n = 4550$, PsycINFO: $n = 231$, and PubMed: $n = 3039$). Following removal of duplicates at a title and abstract level ($n = 1113$), a total of 6946 records remained. A total of 261 original articles were assessed at a full-text level, with articles grouped according to type of intervention. At this stage, no studies were excluded based on type of intervention (e.g., behavioural intervention, neurostimulation). Of these, 58 articles on neurostimulation were identified that satisfied the inclusion criteria. Four additional studies were found through reference checking of the included articles. This process resulted in a final number of 24 included studies. Figure 1 presents the flow diagram of the overall reviewing process according to PRISMA.

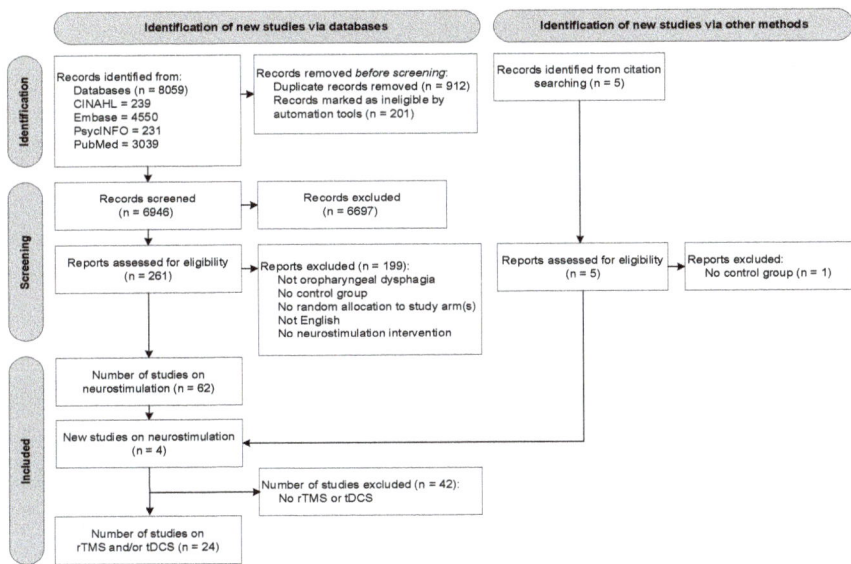

Figure 1. Flow diagram of the reviewing process according to PRISMA.

3.2. Description of Studies

Tables 2 and 3 report detailed descriptions of all included studies. Table 2 includes data on study characteristics including methodological study quality, inclusion and exclusion criteria, and details on participant groups. Information is provided for all study groups (control and intervention groups), medical diagnosis, sample size, age and gender. Table 3 reports on intervention characteristics, including goals, intervention components, outcome measures, intervention outcomes, as well as main conclusions.

Brain stimulation Interventions (Table 2). Across the 24 included studies, eleven studies reported on rTMS and nine studies reported on tDCS. Four studies used another type of neurostimulation (i.e., NMES) in addition to rTMS, either within the same group or over different treatment groups.

Participants (Table 2). The 24 studies included a total of 728 participants (mean 30.3; SD 13.4). The sample sizes ranged from the smallest sample of 14 participants [27] to the largest sample of 64 participants [28]. By intervention type, samples were characterised as follows: *rTMS* total 280, mean 25.5, SD 7.6, range 15–40; *tDCS* total 283, mean 31.4, SD 14.6, range 14–59; and combined neurostimulation total 165, mean 41.3, SD 19.3, range 18–64. The mean age of participants across all studies was 64.6 years (SD 5.8), ranging from 51.8 years [29] to 74.9 years [27]. By intervention group, the mean age of participants was: *rTMS* 63.6 (4.8), *tDCS* 66.2 (SD 6.9), and combined neurostimulation 66.5 years (SD 4.4).

Across all studies 59.6% (SD 12.7) participants were male and two studies did not report gender distribution [29,30]. Percentage of males by intervention group was *rTMS* 61.9% (SD 12.8), *tDCS* 57.5% (SD 10.9), and other/combined 65.4% (SD 12.3). Most studies included stroke patients ($n = 21$), with other diagnoses by intervention group reported as: presbyphagia due to central nervous system disorder ($n = 1$) [31] in *tDCS*; Parkinson's disorder ($n = 1$) [30] and brain injury ($n = 1$) [32] in *rTMS*. All 24 studies used VFSS to confirm participants' diagnosis of OD. The studies were conducted across 12 countries, with the highest number of studies conducted in Korea ($n = 6$), Egypt ($n = 4$), China ($n = 3$), Italy ($n = 2$) and Japan ($n = 2$).

Outcome Measures (Table 3). Outcomes measures varied greatly across all studies included in the review, covering several domains within the area of OD. The Penetration Aspiration Score (PAS) was the most reported outcome measure (8 studies), followed by the Dysphagia Outcome and Severity Scale (DOSS; 7 studies), Functional Oral Intake Scale (FOIS; 3 studies) and Degree of Dysphagia (DD; 3 studies).

rTMS Intervention ($n = 11$: Tables 2 and 3). All but one of the rTMs studies [33] compared rTMS stimulation with sham rTMS. One single study compared rTMS with rTMS combined with DT, and DT only [33]. Three more studies included three arms; two studies compared rTMS using different frequencies versus sham rTMS [32,34], and one study compared bilateral and unilateral rTMS versus sham rTMS [35].

tDCS Intervention ($n = 9$: Tables 2 and 3). Eight studies compared tDCS with sham tDCS [27,29,31,36–41], and one study compared tDCS with theta-burst stimulation (TBS) [31]. All but one study (31) combined both study arms with DT. In one study both groups received simultaneous catheter balloon dilatation in addition to DT [40].

Combined Neurostimulation Interventions ($n = 4$: see Tables 2 and 3). Three studies in the combined intervention group compared three different treatments. Of these, one compared rTMS, PES and paired associative stimulation (PAS) [42], a second compared DT, rTMS combined with DT, and NMES combined with DT [43], and a third compared rTMS, PES and capsaicin stimulation [44]. A fourth study combined NMES stimulation with sham rTMS or rTMS stimulating different hemispheres (ipsilesional, contralesional or bilateral) [45].

Table 2. Study characteristics of studies on rTMS and tDCS interventions for people with oropharyngeal dysphagia.

Study • Author (Year) • Country	Inclusion/Exclusion Criteria	Sample (n) • Groups	Group Descriptives (Mean ± SD) Age, Gender, Medical Diagnoses	Procedure, Delivery and Dosage per Intervention Group [a]
repetitive Transcranial Magnetic Stimulation (rTMS)—n = 11				
Cheng et al. (2017) [46] Hong Kong, China	• OD not defined. Screened face-to-face or via telephone using inclusion criteria • Inclusion: chronic post-stroke (>12 months); ≤80 years; able to follow simple instructions and sit upright for 30 min • Exclusion: previous history of epilepsy; dysphagia, head injury or other neurological disease; neurosurgery; oral/maxillofacial surgery; presence of magnetic implants; medically unstable and on medications that lower neural threshold	n = 15 • Treatment group (11), 73.3% rTMS • Sham group (4), 26.7% Sham rTMS	Treatment group: Age = 65.1 ± 8.3 Male = 64% Sham group: Age = 63.3 ± 7.8 Male = 100% NS difference between groups in age or post-stroke duration.	Procedure: rTMS (Magstim Rapid) daily for 10 days over 2 weeks • rTMS (5 Hz) to the tongue area of the motor cortex of affected hemisphere, identified by MRI, via Magstim coil Treatment group: • Thirty 100-pulse trains of 5 Hz rTMS, with inter-train interval of 15 s • Stimulation at 90% of patient's resting motor threshold Sham: • rTMS via a sham Magstim coil (identical appearance and noise, but no active stimulation) Identical stimulation schedules
Du et al. (2016) [34] China	• OD as per clinical assessment. • Inclusion: first monohemispheric ischaemic stroke <2 months ago; single infarction • Exclusion: other concomitant neurological disease; fever; infection; use of sedatives; severe aphasia or cognitive impairment; inability to complete follow-up; contraindications for stimulation used in study	n = 40 High frequency rTMS • Treatment group 1 (15), 37.5% Low frequency rTMS • Treatment group 2 (13), 32.5% Sham rTMS • Sham group (12), 30.0%	Treatment group 1: Age 58.2 ± 2.8 87% male Treatment group 2: Age 57.9 ± 2.5 54% male Location of lesion: cortical (0), subcortical (9), massive (4) Sham group: Age 58.8 ± 3.4 50% male Location of lesion: cortical (2), subcortical (5), massive (5) Location of lesion: cortical (1), subcortical (10), massive (4) NS differences between groups.	Procedure: • rTMS (MagPro ×100 stimulator) targeting the mylohyoid cortical area of hemisphere ('hot spot'), identified by EMG. Coil angle approximately = 45 degrees. • Daily for 5 consecutive days Treatment group 1, high frequency stimulation: • 3 Hz rTMS for 10 s • Inter-train interval of 10 s, and 40 trains with a total of 1200 pulses at 90% rTMS on the *affected hemisphere* Treatment group 2, low frequency stimulation: • 1 Hz rTMS for 30 s • Inter-train interval of 2 s, and 40 trains with a total of 1200 pulses at 100% rMT on the *unaffected hemisphere* Sham: • Similar conditions to Treatment group 2 to imitate noise of the stimulation with coil rotated 90 degrees away from the scalp

Table 2. *Cont.*

Study • Author (Year) • Country	Inclusion/Exclusion Criteria	Sample (n) • Groups	Group Descriptives (Mean ± SD) Age, Gender, Medical Diagnoses	Procedure, Delivery and Dosage per Intervention Group [a]

Khedr et al. (2009) [47]
• Egypt
	• OD as per swallowing questionnaire confirmed by bedside examination.
	• Inclusion: single thromboembolic non-haemorrhagic infarction of the middle cerebral artery with acute hemiplegia and dysphagia
	• Exclusion: unstable cardiac arrhythmia, fever, infection, hyperglacaemia, prior administration of sedatives, inability to give informed consent due to severe aphasia, anosognosia or cognitive deficits
		n = 26
		• Treatment group (14), 53.8%
		  rTMS
		• Sham group (12), 46.2%
		  Sham rTMS
			Treatment group: Age 58.9 ± 11.7
			Sham group: Age 56.2 ± 13.4
			No group specific descriptors given. Overall, 38.5% male. 14 with right-sided hemiplegia and 12 patients with left-sided hemiplegia. NS difference between groups.
				Procedure:
				• rTMS or sham
				• 5 consecutive days, 10 min at a time
				• A total of 300 3 Hz rTMS pulses at an intensity of 120% resting motor threshold, delivered by Dantec Magilite (TM Copenhagen, Denmark).
				• Figure-of-eight coil placed over oesophageal cortical area of the affected hemisphere, identified by EMG.
				Sham group:
				• Similar parameters producing the same noise, but with the coil rotated away from scalp

Khedr and Abo-Elfetoh (2010) [48]
• Egypt
	• OD as per swallowing questionnaire and bedside swallow screening
	• Inclusion: conscious patient within 1–3 months of first ever ischaemic stroke (LMI or other brainstem infarction with pontomedullary dysfunction); degree of dysphagia from grade III to IV
	• Exclusion: head injury or other neurological disease than stroke; unstable cardiac arrhythmia; fever; infection; hyperglycaemia; epilepsy or prior administration of tranquilisers; presence of intracranial metallic devices or pacemakers; inability to give informed consent
		n = 22
		• Treatment group (11), 50%
		  rTMS
		• Sham group (11), 50%
		  Sham rTMS
			Group statistics given based on infarction type divided into treatment versus sham.
			Lateral medullary infarction group:
			Treatment group (6):
			Age 56.7 ± 16
			100% male
			Sham (5):
			Age: 58 ± 17.5
			100% male
			Other brainstem infarction group:
			Treatment group (5):
			Age: 55.4 ± 9.7
			40% male
			Sham (6):
			Age: 60.5 ± 11
			50% male
			NS difference between groups.
				Procedure:
				• rTMS or sham
				• 5 consecutive days for 10 min
				Treatment group:
				• 10 trains of 10 s 3 Hz stimulation, repeated every minute, delivered by Mag-Lite r25 stimulator (Dantec Medical, Denmark). Intensity set at 130% of resting motor threshold
				• Figure-of-eight coil placed over oesophageal cortical area of both hemispheres, judged to be about 3 cm anterior and 6 cm lateral to the vertex (neurophysiology explorations not performed on participants due to severity of vertigo and dysphagia).
				Sham group:
				• Similar parameters producing the same noise, but with coil rotated away from scalp

Table 2. Cont.

Study • Author (Year) • Country	Inclusion/Exclusion Criteria	Sample (n) • Groups	Group Descriptives (Mean ± SD) Age, Gender, Medical Diagnoses	Procedure, Delivery and Dosage per Intervention Group [a]
Khedr et al. (2019) [30] • Egypt	OD as per Swallowing Disturbance Questionnaire (SDQ) Inclusion: 50–75 years old patients with Parkinson's Disease Exclusion: history of repeated head injury, cerebrovascular accident, encephalitis, oculogyric crisis, supranuclear gaze palsy, exposure to antipsychotics or MPTP (1-methyl-4-phenyl-1,2,3,6-tetrahydropyridine), severe dementia or depression, severe dysautonomia, cerebellar signs, Babiniski sign, strictly unilateral features after 3 years, hydrocephalus, intracranial lesion, contraindications to repetitive transcranial magnetic stimulation (rTMS), inability to give informed consent	n = 30 • Treatment group (19), 63.3% rTMS • Sham group (11), 36.7% Sham rTMS	Treatment group: Age 60.7 ± 8.8 duration of illness 5.7 +/− 3.9 Hoehn and Yahr 3.1 +/− 1.1 Sham group: Age 57.4 ± 10.0 duration of illness 6.5 +/− 3.7 Hoehn and Yahr 3.5 +/− 1.0 Gender distribution not given. NS difference between groups.	Procedure: • rTMS or sham (Magstim 200) • 10 days (5 days per week) followed by 5 booster sessions every month for 3 months • 10 trains of 20 Hz stimulation, each lasting for 10 s with intertrain interval of 25 s. Intensity set at 90% of the RMT. • Stimulation to cortical area: first dorsal interosseous (hand area) for each hemisphere. Location identified from where rTMS elicited MEP's of the highest amplitude. • Both hemispheres stimulated, one at a time during each session. Sham group: • Similar parameters producing the same noise, but with the coil rotated away from scalp

Table 2. Cont.

Study · Author (Year) · Country	Inclusion/Exclusion Criteria	Sample (n) · Groups	Group Descriptives (Mean ± SD) Age, Gender, Medical Diagnoses	Procedure, Delivery and Dosage per Intervention Group [a]
Kim et al. (2011) [32] · Korea	· OD as per VFSS · Inclusions: dysphagia post-brain injury <3 months ago; unilateral hemisphere involvement · Exclusion: prior neurological disease; unstable medical condition; severe cognitive impairment; severe aphasia; history of seizures	· n = 30 · Treatment group 1 (10), 33.3% High frequency rTMS · Treatment group 2 (10), 33.3% Low frequency rTMS · Sham group (10), 33.3% Sham rTMS	Treatment group 1: Age: 69.8 ± 8.0 50% male Stroke (9), TBI (1) Treatment group 2: Age: 66.4 ± 12.3 66.6% male Stroke (10), TBI (0) Sham group: Age: 68.2 ± 12.6 66.6% male Stroke (9), TBI (1) NS difference between groups.	Procedure: · rTMS or sham (Magstim 200) using a figure-eight coil cooled with air · Once a day for 20 min on 10 days (5 times a week for 2 weeks) · All groups received DT, which included oral and facial sensory training, oral and pharyngeal muscle training, compensatory techniques, and NMES[b] on pharyngeal muscles during rTMS. · Stimulation sites identified by evaluation of MEP's of the bilateral mylohyoid muscles. Treatment group 1: · High intensity rTMS · Ipsilateral hemisphere hotspot at 100% of each MEP threshold · At 5 Hz, for 10 s, and repeated every minute for 20 min (total 1000 pulses) Treatment group 2: · Low intensity rTMS · Contralesional hemisphere hotspot at 100% MT · At 1 Hz for 20 min (total 1200 pulses) Sham group: · Similar parameters to high frequency stimulation producing the same noise, but with the coil rotated away from scalp

Table 2. *Cont.*

Study • Author (Year) • Country	Inclusion/Exclusion Criteria	Sample (*n*) • Groups	Group Descriptives (Mean ± SD) Age, Gender, Medical Diagnoses	Procedure, Delivery and Dosage per Intervention Group [a]
Momosaki et al. (2014) [49] • Japan	• OD as per patient reports of swallowing difficulties. • Inclusion: cerebral infarction >6 months ago; mild dysphagia; ≥20 years of age • Exclusion: contraindications to magnetic stimulation; cognitive impairment; major general health problems; malignant tumours; skin disease of the neck; carotid vein thrombosis	*n* = 20 • Treatment group (10), 50% Functional magnetic stimulation • Sham group (10), 50% Sham Functional magnetic stimulation	Treatment group: Age 61 ± 22 80% male Duration post-stroke 19 +/− 8 months Lesion: cerebrum 2, cerebellum 2, brainstem 5, mixed 1 Sham group: Age 66 ± 9 60% male Duration post-stroke 21 +/− 8 months Lesion: cerebrum 1, cerebellum 3, brainstem 2, mixed 4. NS difference between groups.	Procedure: • Single session of Functional Magnetic Stimulation or sham using MagVenture MagProR30 (MagVenture Company) • Stimulation strength was set at 90% of the minimal intensity at which the patient could subjectively feel local pain • High-frequency stimulation of 30 Hz directly to the suprahyoid muscle group, 1200 pulses in total with 10 min in duration. • Location of stimulation site unreported. • Suprahyoid muscle group defined as being at the midpoint of the hyoid bone and the chin. Sham group: Same parameters with the coil held on its lateral side
Park et al. (2013) [50] • Korea	• OD as per VFSS • Inclusion: >1 month post-stroke, • Exclusion: metal implants, pacemaker, history of seizures	*n* = 18 • Treatment group (9), 50% rTMS • Sham group (9), 50% Sham rTMS	Treatment group: Age 73.7 ± 3.8 56% male Infarct = 7, haemorrhage = 2 Right lesion = 6 Sham group: Age 68.9 ± 9.354% male Infarct = 8, haemorrhage = 1 Right lesion = 5 NS difference between groups.	Procedure: rTMS (Magstim Rapid2) • **Stimulation via Magstim coil positioned over pharyngeal hotspot of intact hemisphere. Stimulation site identified by EMG.** • **10 min/day, daily for 2 weeks** Treatment group: • Pharyngeal motor thresholds calculated • 10 trains of 5-Hz stim, each 10 s, repeated every minute Sham group: Same rTMS dosage, however Magstim coil positioned at 90 degree tilt (same noise, no motor cortical stimulation)

Table 2. *Cont.*

Study • Author (Year) • Country	Inclusion/Exclusion Criteria	Sample (n) • Groups	Group Descriptives (Mean ± SD) Age, Gender, Medical Diagnoses	Procedure, Delivery and Dosage per Intervention Group [a]
Park et al. (2017) [35] • Korea	• OD as per VFSS. • Inclusion: subacute stroke (unilateral ischemic or haemorrhagic) <3 months post-stroke; swallowing problems lasting >2 weeks; aspiration and/or penetration on VFSS • Exclusion: dysphagia from other underlying neurological diseases; history of intractable seizure; metallic implants in the brain	n = 33 • Treatment group 1 (11), 33.3% Bilateral rTMS • Treatment group 2 (11), 33.3% Unilateral rTMS • Sham group (11), 33.3% Sham rTMS	Treatment group 1: Age 60.2 ± 13.8 73% male Infarct = 7, haemorrhage = 4 Treatment group 2: Age 67.5 ± 13.4 73% male Infarct = 9, haemorrhage = 2 Sham group: 69.6 ± 8.6 64% male Infarct = 7, haemorrhage = 4 NS difference between groups.	Procedure: rTMS (Magstim Rapid 2) to cortical representation of the mylohyoid muscle, identified by EMG. Applied 10 Hz and 90% of RMT for 5 s with a 55 s inter-train interval. • 10 consecutive rTMS sessions. DT for 30 min each day after rTMS Treatment group 1 (Bilateral rTMS): • rTMS applied at the ipsilesional motor cortex over the mylohyoid hotspot • rTMS applied (same area) to contralesional hemisphere. • DT Treatment group 2 (Unilateral rTMS): • rTMS applied at the ipsilesional motor cortex over the mylohyoid hotspot • Sham rTMS over the contralesional hemisphere • DT Treatment group 3 (Sham): • Sham rTMS was performed with the coil held at 90° to the scalp, with same stimulation (duration, time, intensity, and frequency) to both hemispheres • DT DT included oral sensory training, oral and pharyngeal muscle exercise training, and compensatory techniques.

Table 2. Cont.

Study • Author (Year) • Country	Inclusion/Exclusion Criteria	Sample (n) • Groups	Group Descriptives (Mean ± SD) Age, Gender, Medical Diagnoses	Procedure, Delivery and Dosage per Intervention Group [a]
Tarameshlu et al. (2019) [33] • Iran	• OD as per Mann Assessment of Swallowing Ability (MASA) • Inclusion: >18 years; first-ever stroke; dysphagia >1 month post-stroke • Exclusion: presence of dementia; other neurological diseases; history of recurrent stroke; severe aphasia; severe agitation/unconscious	n = 18 • Treatment group 1 (6), 33.3% rTMS • Treatment group 2 (6), 33.3% DT only • Treatment group 3 (6), 33.3% DT + rTMS	Treatment group 1: Age 55.33 ± 19.55 67% male 67% cortical stroke, 33% subcortical Treatment group 2: Age 74.67 ± 5.92 17% male 83% cortical stroke, 17% subcortical Treatment group 3: Age 66 ± 5.55 67% male 67% cortical stroke, 33% subcortical NS difference between groups.	Treatment group 1: rTMS (Magstim super-rapid stimulator). • Stimulation to intact hemisphere (cortical area for mylohyoid muscles), identified by EMG. Train of 1200 pulses at 1 Hz, stimulus strength at 20% above resting motor threshold. • 20 min daily × 5 consecutive days Treatment group 2: Standard swallow therapy (DT). • Postural changes (chin up, chin down, head tilt, and head rotation), oral motor exercises, swallowing manoeuvers, and strategies to sensory stimulation alerting volume and speed of food presentation, alerting food consistency and viscosity, and downward pressure of the spoon against the tongue • 18 sessions (3 × week) Treatment group 3: Combined rTMS + DT • 5 consecutive days rTMS + 18 sessions DT

Table 2. Cont.

Study • Author (Year) • Country	Inclusion/Exclusion Criteria	Sample (n) • Groups	Group Descriptives (Mean ± SD) Age, Gender, Medical Diagnoses	Procedure, Delivery and Dosage per Intervention Group [a]
Ünlüer et al. (2019) [51] • Turkey	• OD as per VFSS • Inclusion: unilateral hemispheric stroke, chronic (2–6 months) oropharyngeal dysphagia, no prior dysphagia rehabilitation and/or cortical stimulation therapy • Exclusion: previous dysphagia, other neurogenic disease, epilepsy, tumour, head/neck radiotherapy, unstable medical condition, severe cognitive impairment, severe aphasia, contraindication to magnetic or electrical stimulation	n = 28 • Treatment group (15), 53.6% rTMS • Sham group (13), 46.4% Sham rTMS	Treatment group: Age 67.80 ± 11.88 60% male 7% haemorrhage, 93% ischaemic stroke Sham group: Age 69.31 ± 12.89 46% male 8% haemorrhage, 92% ischaemic stroke NS difference between groups.	Procedure: DT for 30–45 min, 3 days/week (+2 days home exercises) for 4 weeks • DT included oropharyngeal muscle strengthening exercises, thermal tactile stimulation, Masako and Mendelson manoeuvres, vocal fold exercises, Shaker exercises, and tongue retraction exercises Treatment group: • DT • Combined rTMS (via MMC-140, 33 kT/s, figure 8 coil) delivered in the final 4th week 20 min daily, 5 consecutive days • rTMS, 1 Hz (at 90% of threshold intensity) applied to the mylohyoid cortical area of the unaffected hemisphere, identified by EMG. Control group: • DT as per above No rTMS delivered in the 4th final week

transcranial Direct Current Stimulation (tDCS)—n = 9

Study	Inclusion/Exclusion Criteria	Sample (n)	Group Descriptives	Procedure, Delivery and Dosage
Ahn et al. (2017) [36] • Korea	• OD as per clinical assessment, confirmed by VFSS pre-treatment • Inclusion: 18–80 years; first stroke, unilateral (subcortical lesion, >6 months ago; able to receive dysphagia therapy 5× a week; no history of abnormal response to brain or electrical stimulation • Exclusion: pre-existing major neurological or psychiatric disease; dementia; other brain lesions; risk factors for transcranial direct current stimulation (tDCS)	n = 26 • Treatment group (13), 50% tDCS + DT • Sham group (13), 50% sham-tDCS + DT	Treatment group: Age 61.6 ± 10.3 69.2% male 38.5% infarction, 61.5% haemorrhage Sham group: Age 66.4 ± 10.7 46.2% male 84.6% infarction, 15.4% haemorrhage Statistical difference between groups = NR	Procedure: • Bihemispheric anodal tDCS 1 mA stimulation (via Neuroconn GmbH), and standard swallow therapy (DT). • 2 anodal electrodes bilaterally to the pharyngeal motor cortices (site location method not described), 2 cathodal references electrodes attached to both supraorbital regions of the contralateral hemisphere. • DT included compensatory methods, behavioural manoeuvres, oromotor exercises and thermal tactile stimulation Treatment group + DT: • Ten 20 min sessions (5 times a week for 2 weeks) Sham + DT: 30 s through 2 anodal electrodes–tingling sensation, but no changes in cortical excitability

Table 2. *Cont.*

Study • Author (Year) • Country	Inclusion/Exclusion Criteria	Sample (n) • Groups	Group Descriptives (Mean ± SD) Age, Gender, Medical Diagnoses	Procedure, Delivery and Dosage per Intervention Group [a]
Cosentino et al. (2020) [31] • Italy	• OD as per clinical assessment and FEES. • Inclusion: presbydysphagia for ≥6 months due to Central ervous System disorder; ≥65 years • Exclusion: unstable medical condition; cognitive impairment; severe dysphagia with inability to swallow liquid or semiliquid boluses; contraindications to stimulation used in study	n = 40 • Treatment group 1 (17), 42.5% tDCS • Treatment group 2 (23), 57.5% Theta-burst stimulation (TBS) Both groups crossed over to sham treatment, also. Order randomised.	Treatment group 1: Age 71.5 ± 5.2 53% male 70.5% primary presbydysphagia, 72.4% secondary presbydysphagia Treatment group 2: Age 75.2 ± 4.8 ($p = 0.025$) 57% male 76.4% primary presbydysphagia, 74.0% secondary presbydysphagia Statistical difference between groups = NR	Procedure: • tDCS or TBS (Transcranial Magnetic Stimulation Unit STM9000, Ates Medica Device) • 5 sessions over 5 consecutive days • Anode electrode placed over the right swallowing motor cortex; cathode positioned over the contralateral orbitofrontal cortex. Optimal location identified as the site where 3/5 consecutive, low intensity magnetic stimuli elicited MEP's of minimum 50 microV from resting contralateral submental muscles complex. Treatment group 1: • tDCS at 1.5 mA (ramped up or down for the first and last 30 s) over 20 min • Sham treatment similar for patient, DC stimulator turned off after 30 s of stimulation Treatment group 2: • TBS: three 50 Hz magnetic pulses repeated every 200 ms for 2 s. Each cycle repeated every 10 s for 20 times (600 pulses in total) Sham treatment parameters set as for real TBS with coil positioned at 90 degrees against the skull

Table 2. Cont.

Study • Author (Year) • Country	Inclusion/Exclusion Criteria	Sample (n) • Groups	Group Descriptives (Mean ± SD) Age, Gender, Medical Diagnoses	Procedure, Delivery and Dosage per Intervention Group [a]
Kumar et al. (2011) [27] • USA	OD as per Dysphagia Outcome and Severity Scale (DOSS) score by SLT. In cases of ambiguity about appropriate DOSS score, VFSS was performed (required with 7 patients) Inclusion: first ischaemic stroke 24–168 h ago, new onset dysphagia with DOSS score ≤5 Exclusion: difficulty following instructions, pre-existing swallowing problems, contraindications to anodal transcranial direct current stimulation (tDCS)	n = 14 (pilot study) • Treatment group (7), 50% tDCS + DT • Sham group (7), 50% Sham tDCS + DT	Treatment group: Average age 79.7 43% male Average NIHHS score 13.6Sham group: Average age 70 57% male Average NIHHS score 13.1Statistical difference between groups = NR	Procedure: • tDCS or sham (via Phoresor; Iomed stimulator) • 5 consecutive days (2 mA for 30 min to the nonlesional hemisphere). Site location identified by MRI or CT. • Electrode placed over the undamaged hemisphere, mid-distance between C3-T3 on left, or C4-T4 on right; reference electrode over the contralateral supraorbital region Concurrent DT–patients sucked on a lemon-flavoured lollipop doing effortful swallows (~60x each session) Sham group + DT: Treatment parameters not described in detail
Pingue et al. (2018) [37] • Italy	OD as per clinical swallow examination and DOSS <5 Inclusion: unilateral stroke < 4 weeks prior to enrolment; age > 18 years; no other muscular or neurological disease or severe disorder of consciousness; mild to severe dysphagia (DOSS <5); National Institutes of Health Stroke Scale (NIHSS) <22 Exclusion: history of dysphagia, other severe clinical conditions (eg, severe infections), potential contraindications to tDCS	n = 40 • Treatment group (20), 50% tDCS + DT • Sham group (20), 50% Sham tDCS + DT	Treatment group: Age 63.5 (range = 54.5–75.25) 40% male Infarct = 11, haemorrhage = 11 (NB. Note numeral errors reported here, n= 20, not 22) Sham group: Age 68.5 (range = 62–73) 40% male Infarct = 4, haemorrhage = 16 NS difference between groups.	Procedure: tDCS by a battery-driven constant current stimulator (HDCkit Newronika, Italy). Stimulation targeted the pharyngeal motor cortex (site location method not described). • 30 min stimulation was applied during swallowing rehabilitation • 10 sessions over 10 days • DT: Direct = compensatory methods, behavioural manoeuvers, supraglottic and effortful swallowing). Indirect approaches = physical manoeuvers, thermal tactile stimulation. Treatment group + DT: 2 mA of anodal tDCS over the lesioned hemisphere and cathodal stimulation to the contralesional hemisphere. Sham + DT: Same protocol except current was delivered for only 30 s through 2 electrodes, producing initial tingling sensation but no cortical excitability.

Table 2. Cont.

Study • Author (Year) • Country	Inclusion/Exclusion Criteria	Sample (n) • Groups	Group Descriptives (Mean ± SD) Age, Gender, Medical Diagnoses	Procedure, Delivery and Dosage per Intervention Group [a]
Sawan et al. (2020) [29] • Egypt	• OD as per bedside swallow assessment as pre-treatment VFSS • Inclusion: acute or subacute carotid system ischaemic stroke; stable, oriented and able to follow commands; presence of dysphagia • Exclusion: pre-existing severe dysphagia; difficulty communicating; impaired cognition; neuro-degenerative disorder; major psychiatric illness; unstable health issues such as severe cardiac disease or renal failure; intracranial devices and/or metal; pacemaker or other implanted electrically sensitive device; chronic drug use that could affect brain activity; epilepsy; pregnancy	n = 40 • Treatment group (20), 50% tDCS + DT (physical therapy program) • Sham group (20), 50% Sham tDCS + DT (physical therapy program)	Treatment group: Age 53.3 ± 5.0 50% unilateral stroke, 50% bilateral stroke Sham group: Age 50.3 ± 5.2 50% unilateral stroke, 50% bilateral stroke NS difference between groups.	Procedure: • tDCS or Sham Stimulation targeted the pharyngeal motor cortex (site location method not described), using neuromodulation technology (Soterix medical Inc, New York, NY, USA). • 30 min stimulation with a constant current of 2 mA intensity • 5 consecutive sessions for 2 weeks • Physical therapy program to improve swallowing; details NR Treatment group + DT: Group 1 (unilateral hemispheric stroke) anode placed on healthy hemisphere with reference electrode over contralateral supraorbital region. Group 2 (bilateral hemispheric stroke) stimulation first applied to the dominant hemisphere, then non-dominant hemisphere. Sham + DT: Same protocol producing tingling sensation but no cortical excitability.
Shigematsu et al. (2013) [28] • Japan	• Severe OD as per clinical swallow examination, confirmed by VFSS and FEES; tube-feeding. • Inclusion: ≥4 weeks post-stroke; admitted to rehabilitation hospital • Exclusion: subarachnoid haemorrhage; history of seizures; severe consciousness disturbance; organic neck disease; history of surgery; no other muscular or neurological disorders.	n = 20 • Treatment group (10), 50% tDCS + DT • Sham group (10), 50% Sham tDCS + DT	Treatment group: Age: 66.9 ± 6.3 70% male; Time post-stroke: 12.9 ± 7.8 Site of lesion: 20% putamen; 20% medulla oblongata; 10% corona radiata; 10% frontotemporal; 10% frontoparietal; 10% pons; 10% thalamus; 10% internal capsule Sham group: Age 64.7 ± 8.9 70% male Time post-stroke: 12.1 ± 9.0 Site of lesion: 40% pons; 20% frontoparietal; 10% putamen; 10% thalamus; 10% internal capsule; 10% caudate nucleus NS difference between groups.	Procedure: stimulation by DC stimulator (NeuroConn) • 1-mA anodal tDCS to ipsilateral pharyngeal motor cortex area, cathode placed contralesional supraorbital region (site location method not described). • 1 × day, 10 days (2 × blocks of 5 days) Simultaneous intensive DT (based on VFSS and FEES) including thermal-tactile stimulation, supraglottic swallow, effortful swallow, Shaker exercise, K-point stimulation, blowing Treatment group + DT: • 20 min tDCS with simultaneous intensive DT Sham + DT: • Same stimulation set-up, for 40 s only • Same intensive DT.

Table 2. Cont.

Study • Author (Year) • Country	Inclusion/Exclusion Criteria	Sample (n) • Groups	Group Descriptives (Mean ± SD) Age, Gender, Medical Diagnoses	Procedure, Delivery and Dosage per Intervention Group [a]

Suntrup-Krueger et al. (2018) [39]
• Germany
	• OD as per FEES
	• Inclusion: dysphagia due to acute ischemic stroke, confirmed by brain imaging; >18 years; >24 h post-stroke onset
	• Exclusion: pre-existing swallowing difficulties, contraindications to tDCS, tracheal cannula, unstable medical condition, inability to stay alert
		$n = 59$
		• Treatment group (29), 49.2%
		  tDCS + DT
		• Sham group (30), 50.8%
		  Sham tDCS + DT
			Treatment group: Age 68.9 ± 11.5
			58.6 % male
			72.4% supratentorial stroke 27.6% infratentorial stroke Sham group: Age 67.2 ± 14.5
			56.7 % male
			80.0% supratentorial stroke 20.0% infratentorial stroke NS difference between groups.
				Procedure: tDCS stimulation delivered by battery-driven constant current stimulator (NeuroConn)
				• 1 mA anodal tDCS, 1 × day, 4 consecutive days. Stimulation to area of the motor cortical swallowing network of intact hemisphere in cortical stroke patients; stimulation applied to right hemisphere in brainstem stroke patients (site location method not described, but rationale provided).
				• Swallow exercises performed during stimulation, if appropriate
				Treatment group + DT:
				• Anodal tDCS for 20 min with simultaneous swallow exercises, if appropriate
				Sham + DT:
				• Stimulation for 30 s only, with electrodes left in place for 20 min

Wang et al. (2020) [40]
• China
	• OD caused by cricopharyngeal muscle dysfunction as per VFSS
	• Inclusion: brainstroke with cricopharyngeal muscle dysfunction, onset duration >1 month prior to enrolment; aspiration as per VFSS; nasogastric tube in-situ; MMSE ≥ 23
	• Exclusion: severely decreased consciousness; history of epilepsy; unstable medical condition; history of previous dysphagia; history of radiotherapy for head and neck diseases; intracranial metallic device
		$n = 28$
		• Treatment group (14), 50%
		  tDCS + DT
		• Sham group (14), 50%
		  Sham tDCS + DT
			Treatment group: Age 61.43 ± 11.24
			79% male
			Time post-stroke: 66.79 ± 38.62 days
			Sham group: Age 62.00 ± 10.46
			71% male
			Time post-stroke: 67.50 ± 47.62 days NS difference between groups.
				Procedure: anodal tDCS + catheter balloon dilatation + standard swallow therapy (based on VFSS, details not described)
				• 20 sessions, 5 × week for 4 weeks
				Treatment group + DT + Balloon dilatation:
				• tDCS via IS300 (Zhineng Electronics Industrial Co.)
				• 1 mA anodal stimulation to oesophageal cortical areas, bilaterally (site location method not described). Each hemisphere stimulated for 20 min (interval of 30 min between).
				• Combined with catheter balloon dilation and standard swallow therapy
				Sham + DT + Baloon dilatation:
				• tDCS anodal stimulation as per treatment except for 30 s only
				Combined with catheter balloon dilation and standard swallow therapy

Table 2. Cont.

Study • Author (Year) • Country	Inclusion/Exclusion Criteria	Sample (n) • Groups	Group Descriptives (Mean ± SD) Age, Gender, Medical Diagnoses	Procedure, Delivery and Dosage per Intervention Group [a]
Yang et al. (2012) [41] • South Korea	OD as per clinical swallow examination (VFSS at baseline) Inclusion: first ever ischemic stroke ≤2 months ago; use of a nasogastric tube Exclusion: bilateral brain lesion; tDCS contraindicators; unstable medical condition; severe language disturbance; neglect, depression, or cognitive deficits (MMSE, ≤10/30 points); history of severe alcohol or drug abuse; taking Na+ or Ca2+ channel blockers or N-methyl-D-aspartate (NMDA) receptor antagonists; previous stroke that resulted in residual disability	n = 16 • Treatment group (9), 56.3% tDCS + DT • Sham group (7), 43.7% Sham tDCS + DT	Treatment group: Age 70.44 ± 12.59 66.7% male 44.4% right lesion, NIHSS = 9.7 ± 5.4 Sham group: Age 70.57 ± 8.46 42.9% male 57.1% right lesion, NIHSS = 13.9 ± 6.3 NS differences between groups.	Procedure: anodal tDCS (Phoresor II) • Stimulation, at 1 mA, to the pharyngeal area of the affected hemisphere (site location method not described). • 5 times/week for 2 weeks • DT = diet modifications, positioning, Mendelsohns manoeuver, supraglottic, effortful swallowing, thermal tactile stimulation and oral motor exercises Treatment group + DT: • 20 min tDCS + simultaneous DT • DT alone, continued for another 10 min Sham + DT: • 30 s tDCS + simultaneous DT • DT alone, continued for another 10 min

Combined Neurostimulation Interventions—n = 4

Study	Inclusion/Exclusion Criteria	Sample (n)	Group Descriptives	Procedure, Delivery and Dosage per Intervention Group [a]
Cabib et al. (2020) [44] • Spain	OD as per VFSS Inclusion: > 3 months post-unilateral stroke, stable medical condition Exclusion: neurodegenerative disorders, epilepsy, drug dependency, brain or head trauma or surgery, structural causes of OD, pacemaker or metallic body implants, and pregnancy or lactation	n = 36 rTMS • Treatment group 1 (12), 33.3% Capsaicin • Treatment group 2 (12), 33.3% PES • Treatment group 3 (12), 33.3%	Treatment group 1: Age 70.0 ± 8.6 75% male 0% haemorrhage, 100% infarction Treatment group 2: Age 74.3 ± 7.8 58% male 8% haemorrhage, 92% infarction Treatment group 3: Age 70.0 ± 14.2 92% male 25% haemorrhage, 75% infarction NS differences between groups, except shorter time since stroke for capsaicin group.	Procedure: All patients received both treatment and sham, cross-over active/sham in visits 1 week apart (randomised). Assessment occurred immediately prior to treatment and within 2 h post-treatment. Treatment group 1: rTMS (Magstim rapid stimulator) • Stimulation (90% of threshold) bilaterally to motor hotspots for pharyngeal cortices, identified by EMG. • 5 Hz train of 50 pulses for 10 s × 5 (total 250 pulses), 10 s between trains • Sham = coil tilted 90 degrees Treatment group 2: Capsaicin stimulus (10^{-5} M) or placebo (potassium sorbate) were administered once in a 100 mL solution Treatment group 3: PES via two-ring electrode naso-pharyngeal catheter (Gaeltec Ltd.) • 10 min stimulation at 75% tolerance threshold (0.2 ms of duration) and 5 Hz Sham = 30 s of above stimulation then no stimulation

Table 2. *Cont.*

Study • Author (Year) • Country	Inclusion/Exclusion Criteria	Sample (n) • Groups	Group Descriptives (Mean ± SD) Age, Gender, Medical Diagnoses	Procedure, Delivery and Dosage per Intervention Group [a]
Lim et al. (2014) [43] • Korea	• OD as per VFSS • Inclusion: primary diagnosis unilateral cerebral infarction or haemorrhage (CT or MRI); stroke onset <3 months; patients who could maintain balance during evaluation + treatment; and adequate cognitive function to participate • Exclusion: could not complete VFSS/failed the examination; presence of dysphagia pre-stroke; history of prior stroke, epilepsy, tumor, radiotherapy in the head and neck, or other neurological diseases; unstable medical condition; and contraindication to magnetic or electrical stimulation	n = 47 • Treatment group 1 (15), 31.9% DT • Treatment group 2 (14), 29.8% DT + rTMS • Treatment group 3 (18), 38.3% DT + NMES	Treatment group 1: Age 62.5 ± 8.2 60% male 34% haemorrhage, 66% infarction Treatment group 2: Age 59.8 ± 11.8 43% male 71% haemorrhage, 29% infarction Treatment group 3: Age 66.3 ± 15.4 67% male 66% haemorrhage, 44% infarction NS difference between groups.	Procedure: • DT: oropharyngeal muscle-strengthening, exercise for range of motion of the neck/tongue, thermal tactile stimulation, Mendelson maneuver, and food intake training for 4 weeks Treatment group 1: • DT 4 weeks • Intensity NR Treatment group 2: • DT + rTMS via Magstim 200 (Magstim, Whiteland, UK) • Stimulation to pharyngeal motor cortex, contralateral hemisphere; optimal stimulation site located by EMG. • 1 Hz stimulation, 100% intensity of resting motor threshold • 20 min/day, (total 1200 pulses a day), 5 × week for 2 weeks Treatment group 3: • DT + NMES (Vitalstim) • 300 ms, 80 Hz (100 ms in interstimulus intervals). Intensity between 7–9 mA, depending on patient compliance. • Stimulation to supra and infra hyoid region • 30 min/day, 5 days/week, 2 weeks

Table 2. *Cont.*

Study · Author (Year) · Country	Inclusion/Exclusion Criteria	Sample (n) · Groups	Group Descriptives (Mean ± SD) Age, Gender, Medical Diagnoses	Procedure, Delivery and Dosage per Intervention Group [a]
Michou et al. (2014) [42] · UK	OD as per diagnoses made by SLT (confirmed with VFSS at start of treatment) Inclusion: post-stroke dysphagia for >6 weeks Exclusion: Hx of dementia, cognitive impairment, epilepsy, head and neck surgery; neurological defects prior to stroke; cardiac pacemaker or defibrillator in-situ; severe concomitant medical conditions; structural oropharyngeal pathology; intracranial metal; pregnancy; medications acting on Central Nervous System.	n = 18 · Treatment group 1 (6), 33.3% Pharyngeal electrical stimulation (PES) · Treatment group 2 (6), 33.3% Paired associative stimulation (PAS) · Treatment group 3 (6), 33.3% rTMS	Treatment group: Avg age 60.3 83% male Treatment group 2: Avg age 67.3 100% male Treatment group 3: Avg age 67.8 66.7% male Overall 63 +/− 15 weeks post-stroke with 7.6 +/− 1 on NIHHS Statistical difference between groups = NR	Procedure: · Single application of neurostimulation using a figure of 8 shaped magnetic coil connected to a Magstim BiStim2 magnetic stimulator (Magstim Co, UK) · All patients received real and sham treatment in randomised order on two different days Treatment group 1: · PES · Frequency of 5 Hz for 10 min. Intensity set at 75% of the difference between perception and tolerance thresholds. Treatment group 2: · Paired associative stimulation: · Pairing a pharyngeal electrical stimulus (0.2 ms pulse) with a single TMS pulse over the pharyngeal MI at MT intensity plus 20% of the stimulator output. The 2 pulses were delivered repeatedly every 20 s with an inter-stimulus interval of 100 ms for 10 min. Treatment group 3: · rTMS · Stimuli to pharyngeal motor cortex, identified by EMG, with the TMS coil. Frequency of 5 Hz, intensity 90% of resting thenar motor threshold in train of 250 pulses, in 5 blocks of 50 with 10 s between-blocks pause.

Table 2. *Cont.*

Study • Author (Year) • Country	Inclusion/Exclusion Criteria	Sample (n) • Groups	Group Descriptives (Mean ± SD) Age, Gender, Medical Diagnoses	Procedure, Delivery and Dosage per Intervention Group [a]
Zhang et al. (2019) [45] • China	• OD as per DOSS by a well-trained doctor • Inclusion: stroke as per MRI <2 months earlier; aged 50–75 years; normal consciousness, stable vital signs, presence of dysdipsia and dysphagia • Exclusion: brain trauma or other central nervous system disease; unstable arrhythmia, fever, infection, epilepsy, or use of sedative drugs; poor cooperation due to serious aphasia or cognitive disorders; contraindications to magnetic or electrical stimulation	n = 64 • Treatment group 1 (16), 25.0%: Sham rTMS + NMES • Treatment group 2 (16), 25.0%: Ipsilateral rTMS + NMES • Treatment group 3 (16), 25.0%: Contralateral rTMS + NMES • Treatment group 4 (16), 25.0%: Bilateral rTMS + NMES	Treatment group 1: Age 55.9 ± 8.9 43% male 61.5% subcortical, 38.5% brainstem Treatment group 2: Age 56.8 ± 9.7 54% male 30.8% subcortical, 69.2% brainstem Treatment group 3: Age 56.5 ± 10.1 50% male 58.3% subcortical, 41.7% brainstem Treatment group 4: Age 53.1 ± 10.6 31% male 61.5% subcortical, 38.5% brainstem All data given on participants that finished the trial and follow-up period (n = 52)	Procedure: • 10 rTMS (sham or real) and 10 NMES sessions Mon-Fri during 2 weeks • NMES: 30 min once daily using a battery powered handheld device (HL-08178B; Changsha Huali Biotechnology Co., Ltd., Changsha, China), vertical placement of electrodes. Pulse width of 700 ms, frequency 30–80 Hz, current intensity 7–10 mA. • rTMS delivered by figure-of-eight coil (CCY-IV; YIRUIDE Inc., Wuhan, China) during NMES with a sequence of HF-rTMS over the affected hemisphere followed by LF-rTMS over the unaffected hemisphere (site location method not described). HF-rTMS parameters: 10 Hz, 3 s–s stimulation, 27 s–s interval, 15 min, 900 pulses, and 110% intensity of resting motor threshold (rMT) at the hot spot LF-rTMS parameters: 1 Hz, total of 15 min, 900 pulses, and 80% intensity of rMT at the hot spot Treatment group 1: Sham rTMS + NMES • 10-Hz sham rTMS delivered to the hot spot for the mylohyoid muscle at the ipsilesional hemisphere followed by 1-Hz sham rTMS over the corresponding position of the contralesional hemisphere • Delivered using a vertical coil tilt, generating the same noise as real rTMS without cortical stimulation

Table 2. *Cont.*

Treatment group 2: Ipsilateral rTMS + NMES
10-Hz real rTMS was delivered to the hot spot for the mylohyoid muscle at the ipsilesional hemisphere followed by 1-Hz sham rTMS over the corresponding position of the contralesional hemisphere.

Treatment group 3: Contralateral rTMS + NMES
10-Hz sham rTMS was delivered to the hot spot for the mylohyoid muscle at the ipsilesional hemisphere followed by 1-Hz real rTMS over the corresponding position of the contralesional hemisphere.

Treatment group 4: Bilateral rTMS + NMES
10-Hz real rTMS was delivered to the hot spot for the mylohyoid muscle at the ipsilesional hemisphere followed by 1-Hz real rTMS over the corresponding position of the contralesional hemisphere.

[a] Where information was available on how stimulation site was located and mapped, and whether stimulation was applied ipsilateral or contralateral to the lesion site, it was included. Note. NMES is at motor stimulation level unless explicitly mentioned. Notes. CP—cerebral palsy; CT—computed tomography; DOSS—dysphagia outcome and severity scale; DT—dysphagia therapy; EMG—electromyography; FEES—fiberoptic endoscopic evaluation of swallowing; FOIS—functional oral intake scale; MEP—motor-evoked potentials; MMSE—Mini-Mental State Exam; MRI—magnetic resonance imaging; MS—multiple sclerosis; MT—Motor Threshold; NIHSS—National Institutes of Health Stroke Scale; NMES—neuromuscular electrical stimulation; NR—not reported; NS—not significant; OD—oropharyngeal dysphagia; OST—oral sensorimotor treatment; PAS—penetration—aspiration scale; PES—pharyngeal electrical stimulation; rTMS—repetitive transcranial magnetic stimulation; SLT—Speech and Language Therapist; TBI—traumatic brain injury; tDCS—transcranial direct current stimulation; TOR-BSST—Toronto Bedside Swallowing Screening test; VFSS—videofluoroscopic swallowing study.

Table 3. Outcome of rTMS and tDCS for people with oropharyngeal dysphagia.

Study	Intervention Goal	Outcome Measures	Intervention Outcomes &Conclusions
repetitive Transcranial Magnetic Stimulation (rTMS)—*n* = 11			
Cheng et al. (2017) [46]	To investigate the short-(2-months) and long-term (6 and 12 months) effects of 5 Hz rTMS on chronic post-stroke dysphagia	Primary outcomes: Maximum tongue strength, VFSS (oral transit time, stage transit time, pharyngeal transit time, pharyngeal constriction ratio), and SAPP [52]. Assessed: 1 week pre-, and 2, 6 and 12 months post-intervention.	• No significant differences between groups at any time point post-treatment for any of the VFSS measures nor for tongue strength • No significant different between groups for the SAPP outcome measure
Du et al. (2016) [34]	To investigate the effects of high-frequency versus low-frequency rTMS on poststroke dysphagia during early rehabilitation	Primary outcome: SSA [53]. Secondary outcomes: WST [54], DD [55], NIHSS score [56], BI [57], mRS, measures of mylohyoid MEPs evoked from both hemispheres before and after treatment. Assessed: before treatment, after 5th rTMS session, and at 1-, 2-, and 3-months post-treatment.	Primary outcomes: • SSA scores improved in both 3 Hz and 1 Hz rTMS groups and maintained over 3-month follow-up ($p = 0.001$, compared to Sham) Secondary outcomes: *Both treatment groups compared to sham*. • WST scores significantly better at 5 days ($p = 0.017$), 1 month ($p = 0.002$), 2 months ($p < 0.001$) and 3 months ($p < 0.001$) • DD scores significantly improved at 1 month ($p = 0.001$), 2 months ($p < 0.001$) and 3 months ($p < 0.001$) • BI and mRS improved in all patients • 1 Hz rTMS induced a decrease in the cortical excitability of the unaffected hemisphere, but an increase in that of the affected hemisphere • 3 Hz rTMS enhanced the cortical excitability of the affected hemisphere and slightly affected that of the unaffected hemisphere
Khedr et al. (2009) [47]	To investigate the therapeutic effect of rTMS on post-stroke dysphagia	Primary outcome: Dysphagia rating scale [58] (swallowing questionnaire + bedside examination). Secondary outcomes: Motor power of hand grip, BI [57], measures of oesophageal MEPs from both hemispheres. Assessed: before and immediately after treatment, and at 1- and 2-months post-treatment.	• Dysphagia scores significantly better in the treatment group (no *p* value or CI given), maintained at 2 months post • Hand grip strength and BI improved in both groups. Improvement in BI greater in the treatment group Conclusion: rTMS led to a significantly greater improvement in dysphagia and motor disability that was maintained at 2 months.

Table 3. Cont.

Study	Intervention Goal	Outcome Measures	Intervention Outcomes &Conclusions
Khedr and Abo-Elfetoh (2010) [48]	To assess the effect of rTMS on dysphagia in patients with acute lateral medullary or other brainstem infarction	Primary outcome: DD [55] Secondary outcomes: Hand grip strength, NIHSS [56] and BI [57]. Assessed: before treatment, after 5th rTMS session, and at 1- and 2-months post-treatment.	Results given based on infarction type divided into treatment versus sham. rTMS and lateral medullary infarction • Significant improvement in DD in the treatment group when compared to sham • Barthel Index improved significantly more in the treatment group compared to sham. No significant difference in other secondary outcomes between groups. • Hand grip strength and NIHSS improved in both groups rTMS and other brainstem infarction • Significant improvement in DD in the treatment group when compared to sham • No significant difference in secondary outcomes between groups
Khedr et al. (2019) [30]	To investigate the therapeutic effect of rTMS on dysphagia with Parkinson's Disease	Primary outcomes: Hoen and Yahr staging [59], UPDRS [60] part III, IADL [61], Self-Assessment Scale [62], SDQ [63], Arabic-DHI [64]. VFSS was conducted on 9 rTMS and 6 sham group patients. Assessed: before treatment, post treatment, and at 1-, 2-, and 3-months post-treatment.	• Mean change in UPDRS III was significantly higher in the treatment group ($p = 0.0001$) • Mean reduction in the Arabic-DHI was significantly greater in the treatment group ($p = 0.0001$) • VFSS (n = 15): significant improvement in hyoid bone excursion and pharyngeal transit time for fluid swallows in the treatment group ($p = 0.04$ and 0.03 respectively). No difference in AP scores or residue. • Results for IADL, SDQ or self-assessment scale = NR Conclusion: rTMS improves dysphagia in PD
Kim et al. (2011) [32]	To investigate the effect of rTMS on dysphagia recovery in patients with brain injury	Primary outcomes: FDS [65], PAS [66] and ASHA-NOMS [67] before and after treatment Assessed: before and after treatment, times unspecified.	• FDS and PAS improved significantly in the low intensity group compared to other groups • Significant improvement in ASHA-NOMS Swallow Scale in the sham and low intensity groups
Momosaki et al. (2014) [49]	To assess the effectiveness of a single functional magnetic stimulation session on post-stroke dysphagia	Primary outcomes: Timed WST [54] before and after stimulation Secondary outcome: N/R	• Significant improvement in speed ($p = 0.008$) and capacity ($p = 0.005$) for the treatment group compared to sham • No significant differences in inter-swallow interval between groups. • Within group changes not reported.

Table 3. *Cont.*

Study	Intervention Goal	Outcome Measures	Intervention Outcomes & Conclusions
Park et al. (2013) [50]	To find the therapeutic effect of high-frequency repetitive TMS on a contra-lesional intact pharyngeal motor cortex inpost-stroke dysphagic patients	Primary outcome: VDS [68], PAS [66] (as per VFSS), pre- and post- treatment. 2 and 4 weeks from baseline. Secondary outcomes: Oral and pharyngeal components of VDS	Treatment group: • Significantly improved ($p > 0.05$) VDS scores post-treatment at 2 and 4 weeks. Significantly improved ($p > 0.05$) PAS at 2 and 4 weeks Sham: • NS difference between pre-post measures at 2 or 4 weeks for either VDS or PAS measures
Park et al. (2017) [35]	to investigate the effects of high-frequency rTMS at the bilateral motor cortices over the cortical representation of the mylohyoid muscles in the patients with post-stroke dysphagia.	Primary outcomes: Immediately post-treatment and 3 weeks post-treatment using CDS [69], DOSS [58], PAS [66], and VDS [68]. Secondary outcome: N/R	Significant difference ($p < 0.05$) was found between the bilateral rTMS versus unilateral rTMS and Sham groups across all time-points post-treatment Bilateral treatment group1: • CDS, DOSS, PAS and VDS improved significantly ($p > 0.05$) post-treatment + 3 weeks post-treatment Unilateral treatment group2: • CDS, DOSS, PAS and VDS improved significantly ($p > 0.05$) post-treatment + 3 weeks post-treatment Sham: • DOSS, PAS and VDS improved significantly post-treatment and 3 weeks post-treatment. CDS improved immediately post-treatment only
Tarameshlu et al. (2019) [33]	To compare the effects of standard swallow therapy (DT), rTMS and a combined intervention (CI)on swallowing function in patients with poststroke dysphagia	Primary outcome: MASA [70]. Secondary outcomes: FOIS [71] assessed (a) before treatment, (b) after 5th session and after 10th, 15th and 18th session.	Primary outcome: MASA • No significant difference between groups after 5th treatment session • After 18 sessions: no significant difference between Treatment group 1 and Treatment group 2, nor Treatment group 2 and Treatment group 3 • Significant difference ($p = 0.01$) between Treatment group 3 which improved greater than Treatment group 1 Secondary outcomes: FOIS • No significant difference between groups after 5th treatment session • After 10 and 18 sessions: no significant difference between Treatment group 1 and Treatment group 2 • After 10 and 18 sessions, significant difference between Treatment group 3 (greater improvement) versus Treatment group 1 ($p = 0.03$ and 0.004 for 10 and 18 sessions respectively) and significant improvement for Treatment group 3 versus group 2 ($p = 0.01$ and 0.02 for 10 and 18 months respectively) All groups showed within-group improvements.

Table 3. *Cont.*

Study	Intervention Goal	Outcome Measures	Intervention Outcomes & Conclusions
Ünlüer et al. (2019) [51]	To identify whether applying low-frequency rTMS can enhance the effect of conventional swallowing treatment and quality of life of chronic (2–6 months) stroke patients suffering from dysphagia	Primary outcome: PAS [66], pre-/post treatment, 1 and 3 months post-treatment. Secondary outcomes: VFSS parameters (including oral parameters, tongue retraction, hyolaryngeal elevation, delayed swallow reflex, residue, nutritional status, SWAL-QOL).	• No significant difference between groups at 1 and 3 months post-treatment across any of the outcome measures • Treatment group PAS scores improved ($p = 0.035$) for liquid swallows only at the 1 month post-treatment assessment • Control group PAS scores (for liquids and semi-solids) improved statistically ($p < 0.05$) from baseline to 1 and 3 months post-treatment • Variable improvements in secondary outcome measures across both treatment and control group at different time-points.
transcranial Direct Current Stimulation (tDCS)—*n* = 9			
Ahn et al. (2017) [36]	To investigate the effect of bihemispheric anodal tDCS with conventional dysphagia therapy on chronic post-stroke dysphagia	Primary outcome: DOSS [58] score based on VFSS pre- and post-treatment Secondary outcome: N/R	• No significant difference in DOSS improvement between groups • Significant improvement ($p = 0.02$) of DOSS (from 3.46 pre-Tx to 4.08 post-Tx) in the treatment group • Improvement (NS) in the sham group (from 3.08 to 3.46). • tDCS combined with conventional swallow therapy was not found to be superior to conventional dysphagia therapy with sham treatment
Cosentino et al. (2020) [31]	To investigate the therapeutic potential of tDCS and theta-burst stimulation on primary or secondary presbydysphagia	Primary outcomes: DOSS [58] based on bedside assessment and FEES. Similarity Index based on Electrokinesiographic/electromyographic Study (EES) for Laryngeal-pharyngeal Mechanogram (LPM) and electromyographic activity of the submental/suprahyoid muscles complex (SHEMG). Secondary outcome: N/R Outcomes assessed at baseline, 1 month and 3 months post-treatment	• Both Treatment groups 1 and 2, as well as sham improved post-intervention period Treatment group 1: • tDCS significantly improved DOSS at 1 month post-treatment ($p = 0.014$). tDCS at 3 months and sham groups improved, though NS • tDCS improved Similarity Index at 1 month post-treatment ($p = 0.005$ for SHEMG-Similarity Index and $p = 0.04$ for LPM-Similarity Index) Treatment group 2: • Theta Burst Stimulation improved DOSS score at 1 month ($p = 0.001$) and 3 months post-treatment ($p = 0.005$). Sham improved = NS. • Theta Burst Stimulation improved Similarity Index at 1 month post-treatment only in patients with secondary presbydysphagia ($p = 0.02$)

Table 3. *Cont.*

Study	Intervention Goal	Outcome Measures	Intervention Outcomes &Conclusions
Kumar et al. (2011) [27]	To investigate whether anodal tDCS in combination with swallowing manoeuvres facilitates dysphagia recovery in stroke patients during early stroke convalescence	Primary outcome: DOSS [58]. Secondary outcome: N/R	• Treatment group had significantly improved DOSS scores compared to sham group ($p = 0.019$).
Pingue et al. (2018) [37]	To evaluate whether anodal tDCS over the lesioned hemisphere and cathodal tDCS to the contralateral one during the early stage of rehabilitation can improve poststroke dysphagia	Primary outcome: DOSS [58], PAS [66] post-treatment. Secondary outcome: N/R	• No significant difference between groups for DOSS or PAS post-treatment • Within group: PAS scores improved for both the treatment and sham groups after 6 weeks
Sawan et al. (2020) [29]	To assess the effect of tDCS on improving dysphagia in stroke patients	Primary outcomes: DOSS [58]; Oral Transit Time; laryngeal and hyoid elevation; oesophageal sphincter spasm; aspiration Secondary outcome: N/R	• Significant improvement in all variables when comparing treatment group to sham: DOSS score ($p < 0.001$), oral transit time ($p = 0.004$); laryngeal elevation, hyoid elevation and oesophageal sphincter spasm (all $p < 0.001$) and aspiration ($p = 0.001$) • Significant improvement in all variables post-tDCS in the treatment group • No significant changes in any variables in the sham group
Shigematsu et al. (2013) [38]	To investigate if the application of tDCS to the ipsilateral cortical motor and sensory pharyngeal areas can improve swallowing function in poststroke patients	Primary outcome: DOSS [58] immediately post-treatment and 1 month post-treatment Secondary outcomes: PAS [66], oral intake status.	• Significant difference between groups post-treatment and 1-month post-treatment = not reported. • tDCS: improved significantly from baseline to post-treatment ($p = 0.006$), and 1-month post-treatment ($p = 0.004$) in DOSS measures. PAS and oral intake reported descriptively • Sham: improved significantly from baseline to 1-month post-treatment ($p = 0.026$)
Suntrup-Krueger et al. (2013) [39]	To evaluate the efficacy of a pathophysiologically reasonable tDCS protocol to improve stroke-related OD, via a randomized controlled trial (RCT) in a sufficiently large patient sample with objective measures alongside functional neuroimaging clinical outcome	Primary outcome: Improved FEDSS 4 days post-treatment Secondary outcomes: DSRS [72]; final FEDSS, and FOIS [71] scores prior to discharge; pneumonia rate until discharge; length of stay (in hospital). Activation changes in the swallowing network as measured with MEG.	Primary outcome: • FEDSS = both groups improved, statistically significantly greater improvements with treatment group ($p < 0.001$) Secondary outcomes: • DSRS = statistically significantly greater improvements with treatment group ($p = 0.001$) • FOIS = statistically significantly greater improvements with treatment group compared to sham, at discharge ($p = 0.041$) No other significant differences between groups for other secondary outcomes.

Table 3. Cont.

Study	Intervention Goal	Outcome Measures	Intervention Outcomes & Conclusions
Wang et al. (2020) [40]	To investigate the effects of tDCS combined with conventional swallowing training on the swallowing function in brainstem stroke patients with cricopharyngeal muscle dysfunction.	Primary outcome: FDS [65] (before and immediately after intervention). Secondary outcomes: FOIS [71], MBSImp [73], PESO measurement [74].	Primary outcomes: Statistical difference between the groups at endpoint not reported. • tDCS treatment group improved to a greater extent than the sham group post-treatment for thin fluids (IDDSI-0) and thick fluids (IDDSI-3), $p < 0.001$ and $p = 0.001$, respectively Secondary outcomes: • FOIS and PESO scores improved to a statistically greater extent (both thin and thick fluids) for the tDCS group versus sham. FOIS $p = 0.001$; PESO $p = 0.003$.
Yang et al. (2012) [41]	To investigate the effects of anodal tDCS combined with swallowing training for post-stroke dysphagia.	Primary outcome: FDS [65] immediately post-treatment and at 3 months Secondary outcomes: Oral Transit Time, Pharyngeal Transit Time and total transit time.	• At 1 month: both tDCS and sham group functional dysphagia scale improved immediately post-treatment. NS between groups. • At 3 months: significantly greater FDS improvement ($p = 0.041$) with the tDCS group versus sham group, when adjusted for NIHSS score, baseline FDS score, age, lesion size and time from stroke onset (NB. Between group differences at baseline = NS) • Secondary outcomes showed no significant differences between the groups.

Combined Neurostimulation Interventions—n = 4

Study	Intervention Goal	Outcome Measures	Intervention Outcomes & Conclusions
Cabib et al. (2020) [44]	To investigate the effect of rTMS of the primary sensory cortex (A), oral capsaicin (B) and intra-pharyngeal electrical stimulation (IPES; C) on post-stroke dysphagia	Primary outcomes: Effect size pre-post treatment for neurophysiological variables (pharyngeal and thenar RMT and MEP). Secondary outcomes: Effects on the biomechanics of swallow (PAS [66], impaired efficiency + more) VFSS before and after treatment	• Between group differences (post-treatment) not reported Primary outcomes: · No significant differences in pre-post pharyngeal RMTs with any of the active or sham conditions· Combined analysis (interventions grouped together) showed significantly shorter latency times, increased amplitude, and area of the thenar MEP in the contralesional hemisphereSecondary outcomes: (VFSS) • No significant change/difference in effect size across any of the treatment or sham groups

Table 3. Cont.

Study	Intervention Goal	Outcome Measures	Intervention Outcomes & Conclusions
Lim et al. (2014) [43]	To investigate the effect of low-frequency rTMS and NMES on post-stroke dysphagia.	Primary outcomes: VFSS baseline, 2- + 4-weeks post-treatment (for semi-solids and liquids); FDS [65], PAS [66], Pharyngeal Transit Time. Secondary outcome: N/R	• Difference between groups post-treatment = NR FDS outcome: • For semi-solids all groups improved, no significant difference in pre-post change, between groups • For liquids, the rTMS and NMES improved significantly compared to DT, 2 weeks post-treatment ($p = 0.016$ and $p < 0.001$, respectively) • No significant difference in the change from baseline to the 4th week evaluation among groups ($p = 0.233$) PAS outcome: • For semi-solids all groups improved, no significant difference in pre-post PAS change, between groups • For liquids, the rTMS and NMES improved significantly compared to DT, 2 weeks post-treatment ($p = 0.011$ and $p = 0.014$, respectively) • No significant difference in the change from baseline to the 4th week evaluation among groups ($p = 0.540$)
Michou et al. (2014) [42]	To compare the effects of a single application of one of three neurostimulation techniques (PES, paired stimulation, rTMS) on swallow safety and neurophysiological mechanisms in chronic post-stroke dysphagia.	Primary Outcome: VFSS before and after treatment Secondary outcomes: Percentage change in cortical excitability; Oral Transit Time, pharyngeal response time, Pharyngeal Transit Time, airway closure time and upper oesophageal opening time as per VFSS	Treatment group 1 (PES): significant excitability increase immediately post-Tx in the unaffected hemisphere (real vs. sham $p = 0.043$) and in the affected hemisphere 30 min post-Tx (real vs. sham $p = 0.04$). • With Paired Stimulation, cortical excitability increased 30 min post-Tx in the unaffected side ($p = 0.043$) compared to sham, and immediately post-Tx in the affected hemisphere following contralateral Paired stimulation ($p = 0.027$) Treatment group 2 (paired neurostimulation): an overall increase in corticobulbar excitability in the unaffected hemisphere ($p = 0.005$) with an associated 15% reduction in aspiration ($p = 0.005$) when compared to sham. Pharyngeal response time was significantly shorter post-treatment with real stimulation compared to sham ($p = 0.007$) Treatment group 3 (rTMS): an increase in excitability in the unaffected hemisphere, but no significant difference compared to sham. No change in the affected hemisphere. Corticobulbar excitability of pharyngeal motor cortex was beneficially modulated by PES, Paired Stimulation and to a lesser extent by rTMS.

Table 3. *Cont.*

Study	Intervention Goal	Outcome Measures	Intervention Outcomes &Conclusions
Zhang et al. (2019) [45]	To determine whether rTMS NMES effectively ameliorates dysphagia and how rTMS protocols (bilateral vs. unilateral) combined with NMES can be optimized.	Primary outcome: Cortical excitability(amplitude of the motor evoked potential) Secondary outcomes: SSA [53] and DD [55].	Compared with group 2 or 3 in the affected hemisphere, group 4 displayed a significantly greater percentage change (p.0.017 and p.0.024, respectively). All groups displayed significant improvements in SSA and DD scores after treatment and at 1-month follow-up. The percentage change in cortical excitability increased over time in either the affected or unaffected hemisphere in treatment groups 1, 2 and 4 ($p < 0.05$). In Group 3, the percentage change in cortical excitability in the unaffected hemisphere significantly decreased after the stimulation course ($p < 0.05$). Change in SSA and DD scores in group 4 was markedly higher than that in the other three groups at the end of stimulation (p.0.02, p.0.03, and p.0.005) and still higher than that in group 1 at the 1-month follow-up (p.0.01).

Note. NMES is at motor stimulation level unless explicitly mentioned. Notes. ASHA-NOMS—American speech-language-hearing association national outcome measurement system; BI—Barthel index; CDS—clinical dysphagia scale; CT—computed tomography; DD—degree of dysphagia; DOSS—dysphagia outcome and severity scale; DSRS—dysphagia severity rating scale; DT—dysphagia therapy; EES—electrokinesiographic/electromyographic study of swallowing; EQ-5D—European Quality of Life Five Dimension; FDS—functional dysphagia scale; FEDSS—fiberoptic endoscopic dysphagia severity scale; FEES—fiberoptic endoscopic evaluation of swallowing; FOIS—functional oral intake scale; HNCI—head neck cancer inventory; IADL—instrumental activities of daily living; ICU—intensive care unit; LCD—laryngeal closure duration; LPM—laryngeal-pharyngeal mechanogram; MASA—Mann assessment of swallowing ability; MBS—modified barium swallow; MBSImp—modified barium swallow impairment profile; MDADI—M.D. Anderson dysphagia inventory; MEG—magnetoencephalography; MEP—motor evoked potentials; MMSE—mini-mental state exam; MRI—magnetic resonance imaging; mRS—modified rankin scale; MS—multiple sclerosis; NEDS—neurological examination dysphagia score; NIHSS—National Institutes of Health Stroke Scale; NMES—neuromuscular electrical stimulation; NS—not significant; OD—oropharyngeal dysphagia; OPSE—oropharyngeal swallow efficiency; OST—oral sensorimotor treatment; PAS—penetration—aspiration scale; PES—pharyngeal electrical stimulation; PESO—pharyngoesophageal segment opening; RMT—resting motor thresholdS; rTMS—repetitive transcranial magnetic stimulation; SAPP—swallowing activity and participation profile; SDQ—swallowing disturbance questionnaire; SFS—swallow function score; SHEMG—electromyographic activity of the submental/suprahyoid muscles complex; SLT—speech and language therapist; SSA—standardised swallowing assessment; SWAL-QOL—swallowing quality of life; TBI—traumatic brain injury; tDCS—transcranial direct current stimulation UPDRS—unified Parkinson's disease rating scale; VFSS—videofluoroscopic swallowing study; WST—water swallow test.

3.3. Risk of Bias Assessment and Methodological Quality

The Begg and Mazumdar rank correlation procedure produced a tau of −0.036 (two-tailed $p = 0.902$) and 0.178 (two-tailed $p = 0.536$) for rTMS and tDCS, respectively. The rTMS meta-analysis incorporates data from 8 studies, which yield a z-value of 2.348 (two-tailed p-value = 0.019). The fail-safe N is 4. This means that 4 'null' studies need to be located and included for the combined two-tailed p-value to exceed 0.050. That means there would be need to be 0.5 missing studies for every observed study for the effect to be nullified. The tDCS meta-analysis incorporates data from 8 studies yielding a z-value of 4.857 (two-tailed p-value < 0.001). The fail-safe N is 42 indicating 42 'null' studies need to be located and included for the combined two-tailed p-value to exceed 0.050; there would be need to be 5.3 missing studies for every observed study for the effect to be nullified. Both of these procedures (i.e., Begg and Mazumdar rank correlation and fail-safe N test) indicate the absence of publication bias.

Figures 2 and 3 present, respectively, the risk of bias summary per domain for all included studies combined and for individual studies, assessed using the Revised Cochrane Collaboration tool for assessing risk of bias (RoB 2) [21]. The majority of studies had low risk of bias with very few exceptions.

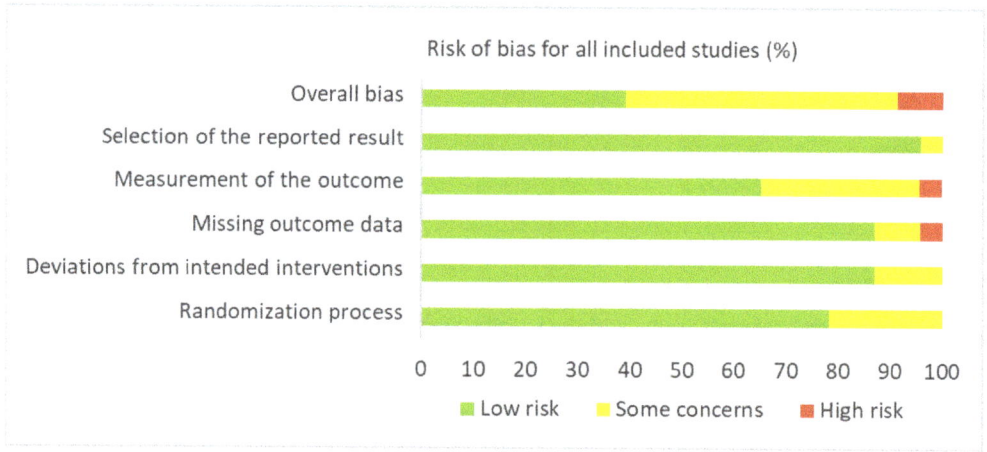

Figure 2. Risk of bias summary for all included studies ($n = 24$) in accordance with RoB 2 [21].

3.4. Meta-Analysis: Effects of interventions

3.4.1. rTMS Meta-Analysis

Eight studies using rTMS [32,33,35,42–44,50,51] were included in the meta-analysis. Of these, three studies provided data for two different interventions groups [32,35,36]. Six studies were excluded as OD was not confirmed by instrumental assessment and one study was excluded as rTMS was combined with NMES.

<u>Overall within-group analysis.</u> Pre-post intervention effect sizes ranged from 0.085 to 2.068 (Figure 4) with seven studies showing large effect sizes (Hedges' $g > 0.8$). Pre-post interventions produced a significant, large effect size (Hedges' $g = 1.038$).

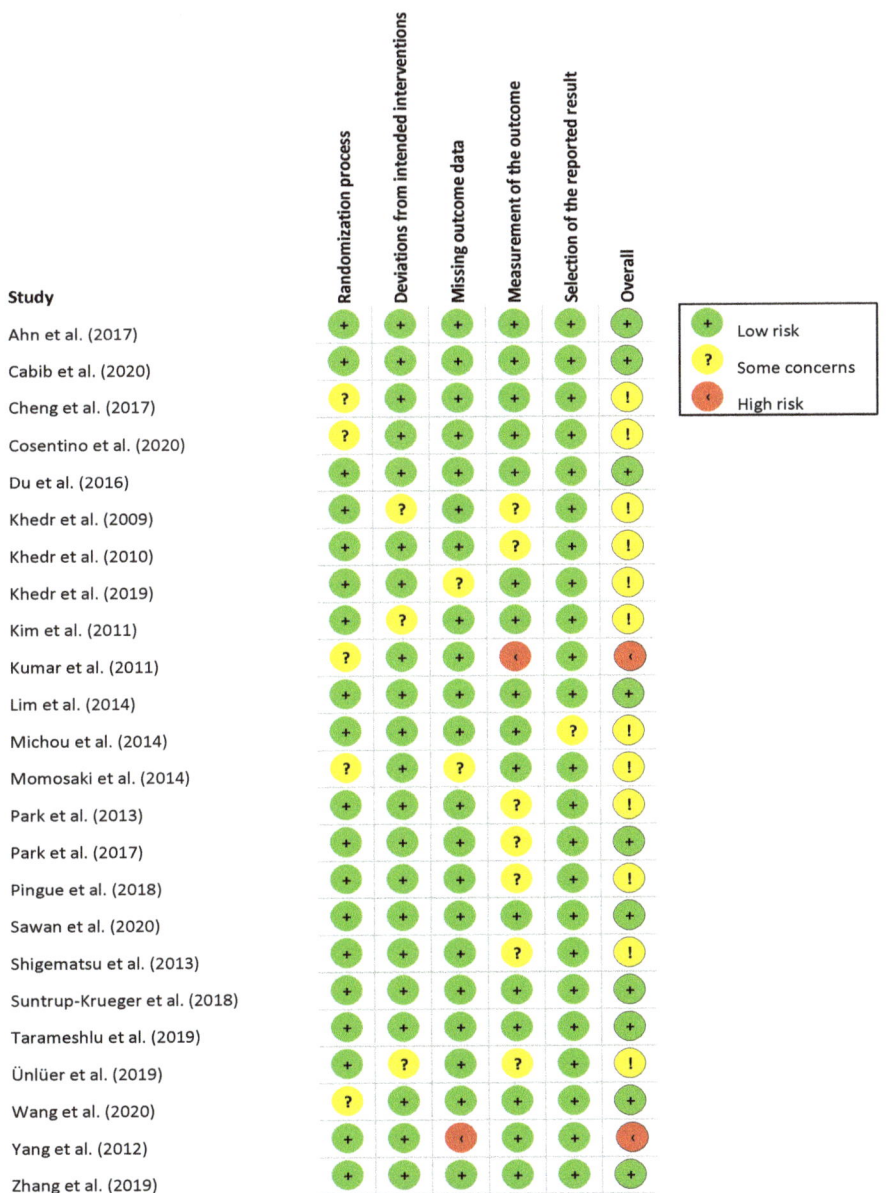

Figure 3. Risk of bias summary for individual studies (n = 24) in accordance with RoB 2 [21,27–34,36–50]. **Note.** If one or more yellow circles (domains) have been identified for a particular study, the Overall score (last column) shows an exclamation mark, indicating that the study shows some concerns (yellow circle with exclamation mark).

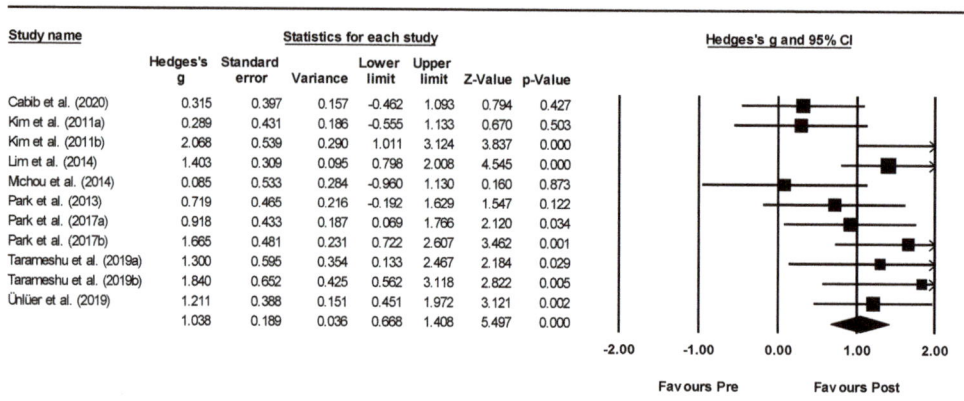

Figure 4. rTMS within intervention group pre-post meta-analysis [32,33,35,42–44,50,51]. *Notes.* Kim et al. (2011a): high frequency, Kim et al. (2011b): low frequency; Park et al. (2017a): unilateral stimulation, Park et al. (2017b): bilateral stimulation; Tarameshu et al. (2019a): rTMS, Tarameshu et al. (2019b): rTMS plus DT.

Overall between-group analysis. A significant, small post-intervention between-group total effect size was calculated in favour of rTMS (random-effects model: $z(7) = 2.338$, $p = 0.019$, Hedges' $g = 0.355$, and 95% CI = 0.057–0.652; Figure 5). Between-study heterogeneity was non-significant ($Q(7) = 6.763$, $p = 0.454$).

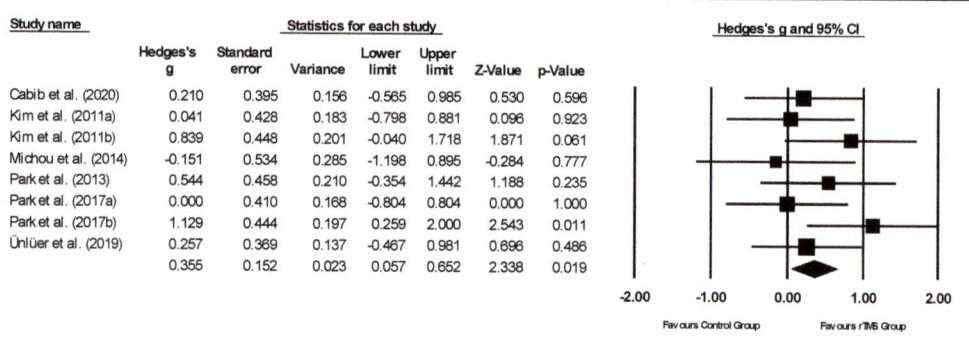

Figure 5. rTMS between group post meta-analysis [32,34,35,37,47,49]. *Notes.* Kim et al. (2011a): high frequency versus sham, Kim et al. (2011b): low frequency versus sham; Park et al. (2017a): unilateral stimulation versus sham, Park et al. (2017b): bilateral stimulation versus sham.

Between-subgroup analyses. Subgroup analyses were conducted to compare time between pre- and post-intervention measurement, stimulation sites (bilateral, contralesional and ipsi-lesional sites), pulse ranges (low: ≤600; medium; >600 and <10,000; high: ≥10,000 pulses), stimulation frequencies (1, 5 and 10 Hz), and optional behavioural training (rTMS versus rTMS + DT; Table 4). No subgroup comparisons for outcome measures were conducted as all but one study used PAS. Studies including a longer time span between pre- and post-interventions (indicating longer stimulation times) showed increased positive effect sizes compared to one-day interventions, which showed negligible effect sizes. When comparing stimulation sites, non-significant, positive effect sizes were obtained for all three stimulation groups with large ranges in effect sizes within groups.

Pulse range comparisons indicated an increased significant, positive effect for higher pulse ranges. Effect sizes were only significant for large numbers of pulses delivered. Sub-analyses comparing stimulation frequencies did not indicate obvious tendencies between groups. rTMS in combination with DT showed non-significant, small positive effect sizes in one study, whereas DT alone showed similar significant, small effects sizes.

Table 4. Between subgroup meta-analyses per type of neurostimulation comparing intervention groups of included studies.

Neurostimulation	Subgroup	Hedges' g	Lower Limit CI	Upper Limit CI	Z-Value	p-Value
rTMS	Time between pre-post (days)					
	1 (n = 2)	0.082	−0.541	0.704	0.257	0.797
	5 (n = 1)	0.257	−0.467	−0.981	0.696	0.486
	14 (n = 5)	0.491	0.054	0.929	2.202	0.028 *
	Stimulation site					
	Bilateral (n = 2)	0.523	−0.730	1.776	0.818	0.413
	Contra-lesional (n = 3)	0.315	−0.141	0.771	1.353	0.176
	Ipsi-lesional (n = 3)	0.272	−0.251	0.795	1.020	0.308
	Pulse range					
	Low [≤ 600] (n = 2)	0.082	−0.541	0.704	0.257	0.797
	Medium [> 600 and < 10000] (n = 3)	0.248	−0.213	0.710	1.054	0.292
	High [≥ 10000] (n = 3)	0.660	0.014	1.306	2.004	0.045 *
	Stimulation frequency (Hz)					
	1 (n = 2)	0.492	−0.067	1.052	1.726	0.084
	5 (n = 4)	0.180	−0.257	0.617	0.809	0.419
	10 (n = 2)	0.552	−0.555	1.658	0.978	0.328
	Behavioural training					
	rTMS + DT (n = 1)	0.257	−0.467	0.981	0.696	0.486
	rTMS (n = 7)	0.375	0.031	0.720	2.135	0.033 *
tDCS	Time between pre-post (days)					
	4 (n = 1)	0.193	−0.312	0.697	0.747	0.455
	5 (n = 1)	0.654	−0.356	1.664	1.269	0.205
	10 (n = 1)	0.432	−0.192	1.037	1.348	0.178
	14 (n = 4)	0.784	0.056	1.512	2.112	0.035 *
	28 (n = 1)	1.024	0.256	1.791	2.614	0.009 *
	Outcome measures					
	DOSS (n = 5)	0.753	0.195	1.311	2.644	0.008 *
	DSRS (n = 1)	0.193	−0.312	0.697	0.747	0.455
	FDS (n = 2)	0.764	0.147	1.381	2.428	0.015 *

Table 4. Cont.

Neurostimulation	Subgroup	Hedges' g	Lower Limit CI	Upper Limit CI	Z-Value	p-Value
	Total stimulation time (min)					
	80 (n = 1)	0.193	−0.312	0.697	0.747	0.455
	150 (n = 1)	0.654	−0.356	1.664	1.269	0.205
	200 (n = 4)	0.419	0.039	0.799	2.161	0.031 *
	300 (n = 1)	1.796	1.072	2.519	4.862	<0.001 *
	400 (n = 1)	1.024	0.256	1.791	2.614	0.009 *
	Stimulation current (mA)					
	1 (n = 6)	0.430	0.148	0.712	2.985	0.003 *
	2 (n = 2)	1.281	0.168	2.395	2.256	0.024 *

Note. * Significant. Notes. CI—confidence interval; DOSS—dysphagia outcome and severity scale; DSRS—dysphagia severity rating scale; DT—dysphagia therapy; FDS—functional dysphagia scale; rTMS—repetitive transcranial magnetic stimulation.

3.4.2. tDCS Meta-Analysis

A total of eight studies using tDCS in stroke patients were included in the meta-analysis [27,29,36–41]. One study was excluded as having too few data for meta-analysis [31].

Overall within-group analysis. The overall pre-post intervention effect size was 1.385, with effect sizes ranging from 0.432 (small effect) to 3.365 (high effect; Figure 6). Studies showed small (n = 2), moderate (n = 1), and high effect sizes (n = 5).

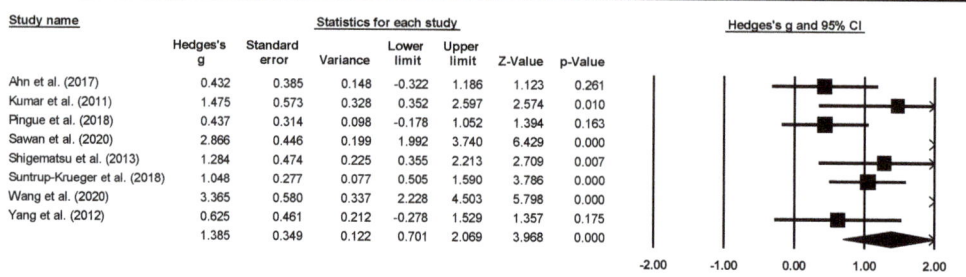

Figure 6. tDCS within intervention group pre-post meta-analysis [27,29,36–41].

Overall between-group analysis. A moderate but significant post-intervention between-group total effect size in favour of tDCS was found using a random-effects model (z(7) = 3.332, p = 0.001, Hedges' g = 0.655, and 95% CI = 0.270–1.040; Figure 7). Between-study heterogeneity was significant (Q(7) = 15.034, and p = 0.036), with I^2 showing that heterogeneity accounted for 53.4% of variation in effect sizes across studies.

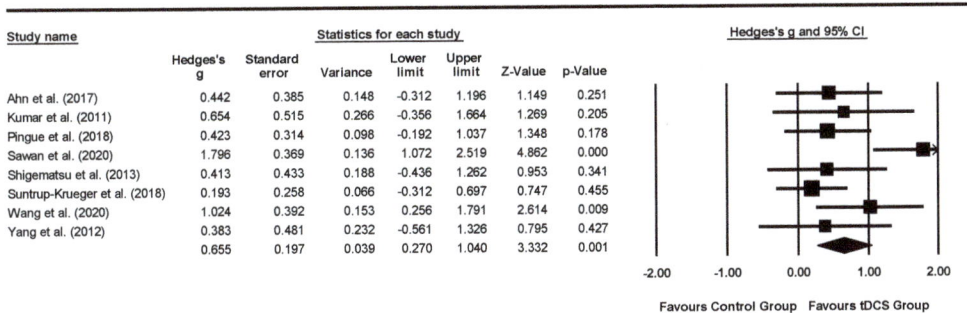

Figure 7. tDCS between group post meta-analysis [27,29,36–41].

Between subgroup analyses. Subgroup analyses were conducted comparing time between pre- and post-intervention measurements, outcome measures, total stimulation times and stimulation current (Table 4). Increasing the number of days between pre- and post-intervention showed a strong tendency towards increased positive effect sizes, with significant effect sizes for two and four-week periods. Comparisons between measures resulted in significant, large positive effect sizes for visuoperceptual evaluation of instrumental assessment, but negligible effects when using an oral intake measure. Effect sizes for comparisons between total stimulation times indicated increased effects when using longer stimulation times. Significant, large effects were demonstrated for stimulation times of 300 min and longer. Additionally, higher stimulation currents resulted in increased significant, large positive effect sizes.

4. Discussion

This systematic review (Part II) aimed to determine the effects of rTMS and tDCS in people with OD. This systematic review and meta-analysis of RCT studies were completed in accordance with PRISMA procedures [19,20]. No populations were excluded based on medical diagnoses.

4.1. Systematic Review Findings

Like the systematic review on effects of NMES and PES in people with OD (Part I) [75], methodological problems were identified relating to unclear definitions of OD and differences in methods of confirming the presence of OD (i.e., using instrumental assessment, patient self-report or clinical assessment). Consequently, to reduce heterogeneity in participant characteristics between RCTs, only studies using instrumental assessment to confirm diagnosis of OD were included in meta-analyses. As most studies included stroke patients only, no meta-analysis could be performed to determine effects per medical diagnosis.

With the exception of one study [33], all rTMS studies included in the meta-analysis used the PAS to evaluate intervention effects. For the tDCS studies, as heterogeneity in outcome measures was larger, data on three different clinical outcome measures were used when conducting the meta-analysis. All rTMS studies used sham stimulation as a comparison group with the exception of one study which included a rTMS plus DT group [33]. For the tDCS studies, all but one study [31] combined neurostimulation with simultaneous DT. When comparing the degree of heterogeneity in study designs between brain neurostimulation (i.e., rTMS and tDCS) and peripheral neurostimulation (i.e., NMES and PES), those in the peripheral neurostimulation group were more diverse, creating greater challenges for conducting meta-analyses. Non-invasive brain stimulation studies tended to recruit smaller sample populations compared to peripheral studies [75].

4.1.1. rTMS

This review prioritised reducing heterogeneity for purposes of meta-analysis. In contrast to previously published reviews that did not confirm OD by instrumental assessment, those studies were excluded from this meta-analysis. With the exception of Bath, Lee [13], earlier reviews identified significant beneficial effects of rTMS. Therefore, even though comparing the current meta-analysis with analyses from previous reviews may be challenging due to the inclusion of different outcome data, the findings from these studies seem in line with each other and this review.

4.1.2. tDCS

Fewer RCTs were identified for tDCS compared with rTMS. Eight out of nine studies were eligible for meta-analysis, with one study excluded due to insufficient data; this was the only study to include non-stroke patients (presbydysphagia) [31]. Again, as previous reviews on tDCS [10,12,13,16–18] applied different criteria for inclusion and study methodology (e.g., differences in selection of electronic databases and publication years), final numbers of studies used for these meta-analyses ranged between two and seven publications, with reviews published before 2020 including four or fewer studies. When comparing the present results with the two most recent reviews [10,18] (both including seven studies), the beneficial effects of tDCS identified by this review were confirmed by significant, small-to-moderate effects in favour of tDCS.

4.1.3. Moderators

Several factors may have had an impact on conducting meta-analyses and results. Comparing previous reviews, different decisions were made concerning criteria for meta-analyses. For example, Bath, Lee [13] excluded comparison groups with active treatment components and Chiang, Lin [12] excluded chronic stroke patients. Chronicity of stroke has shown to influence effect sizes [10,18], but selecting different primary outcomes may also result in deviating findings. For instance, Bath, Lee [13] did not find any positive effects for either rTMS or tDCS on primary outcome measures defined as death or dependency at the end of trials. Additionally, underlying medical diagnoses of OD are expected to affect meta-analyses. However, no conclusions could be drawn as very few studies of non-stroke patients were included in this review, thus no meta-analysis differentiating between diagnoses was conducted.

Similar reasons for hindering comparisons between RCTs are present in the current review, for example, spontaneous recovery and stroke severity, as were identified in the systematic review on effects of NMES and PES in people with OD (Part I) [75]. To account for the possibility of spontaneous recovery in participants, only between-subgroup meta-analyses were conducted using post-intervention data. However, the effects of stroke severity linked to OD severity remains unclear as RCTs usually did not report on the severity of stroke in sufficient detail.

Lastly, brain neurostimulation between RCTs may differ with respect to stimulation protocols (e.g., stimulation site, number and duration of treatment sessions and period) and technical parameters (e.g., frequency or number of pulses). The relatively low numbers of RCTs included in this review meant that meta-analysis could not incorporate all potential moderators. However, many of the included studies lacked sufficient details on technical parameters to allow further comparisons.

4.2. Limitations

Although this review followed PRISMA guidelines and aimed at reducing bias, some limitations may have had an impact on the results as presented. Only RCTs published in English were eligible in this review. Thus, some RCTs may have been excluded based on language criteria when their findings could have contributed to the current meta-analysis. Moreover, the high degree of heterogeneity between included studies hampered meta-analyses. Therefore, the results of meta-analyses and generalisations made should be interpreted with care.

5. Conclusions

The results of this systematic review suggest that both rTMS and tDCS show promising effects in people with OD. Meta-analysis for RCTs identified large pre-post intervention effect sizes for both types of brain neurostimulation. In addition, this analysis found significant, small and moderate post-intervention between-group effects in favour of rTMS and tCDS, respectively. However, comparisons between studies remain uncertain and challenging due to high heterogeneity in stimulation protocols and experimental parameters, potential moderators of stimulation effects, small samples sizes, and inconsistent methodological reporting.

These findings suggest that there is a need for RCTs including larger sample sizes to support future meta-analyses that will be able to adequately account for the presence of moderators. In addition, international consensus on standardised study protocols and reporting guidelines is required to support comparisons between studies.

Supplementary Materials: The following supporting information can be downloaded at: https://www.mdpi.com/article/10.3390/jcm11040993/s1, Table S1: PRISMA 2020 for Abstracts Checklist, Table S2: PRISMA 2020 Checklist.

Author Contributions: Conceptualization: R.S., R.C., A.-L.S., L.B. and S.H., Formal analysis: R.S. and R.C., Methodology: R.S. and R.C., Project administration: R.S. and R.C.; Validation: R.S. and R.C.; Writing—review & editing: R.S., R.C., A.-L.S., L.B., S.H., T.P., M.B. and A.K. All authors have read and agreed to the published version of the manuscript.

Funding: This research received no external funding.

Conflicts of Interest: The authors declare no conflict of interest.

References

1. Melgaard, D.; Westergren, A.; Skrubbeltrang, C.; Smithard, D. Interventions for nursing home residents with dyspaghia—A scoping review. *Geriatrics* **2021**, *6*, 55. [CrossRef]
2. Baijens, L.W.; Clave, P.; Cras, P.; Ekberg, O.; Forster, A.; Kolb, G.F.; Leners, J.C.; Masiero, S.; Mateos-Nozal, J.; Ortego, O.; et al. European Society for Swallowing Disorders—European Union Geriatric Medicine Society white paper: Oropharyngeal dysphagia as a geriatric syndrome. *Clin. Interv. Aging* **2016**, *11*, 1403–1428. [CrossRef] [PubMed]
3. Takizawa, C.; Gemmell, E.; Kenworthy, J.; Speyer, R. A systematic review of the prevalence of oropharyngeal dysphagia in stroke, Parkinson's disease, Alzheimer's disease, head injury, and pneumonia. *Dysphagia* **2016**, *31*, 434–441. [CrossRef] [PubMed]
4. Ciarán, K.; Regan, R.; Balding, L.; Higgins, S.; O'Leary, N.; Kelleher, F.; McDermott, R.; Armstrong, J.; Mihai, A.; Tiernan, E.; et al. Dysphagia prevalence and predictors in cancers outside the head, neck, and upper gastrointestinal tract. *J. Pain Symptom Manag.* **2019**, *58*, 949–958.e942.
5. Seo, Z.W.; Min, J.H.; Huh, S.; Shin, Y.I.; Ko, H.Y.; Ko, S.H. Prevalence and severity of dysphagia using videofluoroscopic swallowing study in patients with aspiration pneumonia. *Lung* **2021**, *199*, 55–61. [CrossRef] [PubMed]
6. Eytan, D.F.; Blackford, A.L.; Eisele, D.W.; Fakhry, C. Prevalence of comorbidities among older head and neck cancer survivors in the United States. *Head Neck Surg.* **2019**, *160*, 85–92. [CrossRef]
7. da Silva, A.F.; Moreira, E.A.M.; Barni, G.C.; Panza, V.S.P.; Furkim, A.M.; Moreno, Y.M.F. Relationships between high comorbidity index and nutritional parameters in patients with oropharyngeal dysphagia. *Clin. Nutr. ESPEN* **2020**, *38*, 218–222. [CrossRef]
8. Jones, E.; Speyer, R.; Kertscher, B.; Swan, K.; Wagg, B.; Cordier, R. Health-related quality of life in oropharyngeal dysphagia. *Dysphagia* **2018**, *33*, 141–172. [CrossRef]
9. Speyer, R. (Ed.) *Behavioural Treatment of Oropharyngeal Dysphagia*; Springer: Berlin/Heidelberg, Germany, 2018.
10. Cheng, I.; Sasegbon, A.; Hamdy, S. Effects of neurostimulation on poststroke dysphagia: A synthesis of current evidence from randomised controlled trials. *Neuromodulation Technol. Neural Interface* **2021**, *24*, 1388–1401. [CrossRef]
11. Cheng, I.; Hamdy, S. Metaplasticity in the human swallowing system: Clinical implications for dysphagia rehabilitation. *Neurol. Sci.* **2021**, 1–11. [CrossRef]
12. Chiang, C.-F.; Lin, M.-T.; Hsiao, M.-Y.; Yeh, Y.-C.; Liang, Y.-C.; Wang, T.-G. Comparative efficacy of noninvasive neurostimulation therapies for acute and subacute poststroke dysphagia: A systematic review and network meta-analysis. *Arch. Phys. Med. Rehabil.* **2019**, *100*, 739–750. [CrossRef] [PubMed]
13. Bath, P.; Lee, H.; Everton, L. Swallowing therapy for dysphagia in acute and subacute stroke (Review). *Cochrane Database Syst. Rev.* **2018**, *10*, CD000323. [CrossRef] [PubMed]

14. Dionísioa, A.; Duartea, I.; Patrícioc, M.; Castelo-Brancoa, M. Transcranial magnetic stimulation as an intervention tool to recover from language, swallowing and attentional deficits after stroke: A systematic review. *Cerebrovasc. Dis.* **2018**, *18*, 176–183. [CrossRef] [PubMed]
15. Liao, X.; Xing, G.; Guo, Z.; Jin, Y.; Tang, Q.; He, B.; McClure, M.; Liu, H.; Chen, H.; Mu, Q. Repetitive transcranial magnetic stimulation as an alternative therapy for dysphagia after stroke: A systematic review and meta-analysis. *Clin. Rehabil.* **2017**, *31*, 289–298. [CrossRef] [PubMed]
16. Momosaki, R.; Kinoshita, S.; Kakuda, W.; Yamada, N.; Abo, M. Noninvasive brain stimulation for dysphagia after acquired brain injury: A systematic review. *J. Med. Investig.* **2016**, *63*, 153–158. [CrossRef]
17. Pisegna, J.; Kaneoka, A.; Pearson, W., Jr.; Kumar, S.; Langmore, S. Effects of non-invasive brain stimulation on post-stroke dysphagia: A systematic review and meta-analysis of randomized controlled trials. *Clin. Neurophysiol.* **2016**, *127*, 956–968. [CrossRef]
18. Marchina, S.; Pisegna, J.; Massaro, J.M.; Langmore, S.E.; McVey, C.; Wang, J.; Kumar, S. Transcranial direct current stimulation for post-stroke dysphagia: A systematic review and meta-analysis of randomized controlled trials. *J. Neurol.* **2021**, *268*, 293–304. [CrossRef]
19. Page, M.J.; McKenzie, J.E.; Bossuyt, P.M.; Boutron, I.; Hoffmann, T.C.; Mulrow, C.D.; Shamseer, L.; Tetzlaff, J.M.; Akl, E.A.; Moher, D.; et al. The PRISMA 2020 statement: An updated guideline for reporting systematic reviews. *Int. J. Surg.* **2021**, *88*, 105906. [CrossRef]
20. Page, M.J.; Moher, D.; Bossuyt, P.M.; Boutron, I.; Hoffmann, T.C.; Mulrow, C.D.; Shamseer, L.; Tetzlaff, J.M.; Akl, E.A.; McKenzie, J.E.; et al. PRISMA 2020 explanation and elaboration: Updated guidance and exemplars for reporting systematic reviews. *BMJ* **2021**, *372*. [CrossRef]
21. Sterne, J.; Savović, J.; Page, M.; Elbers, R.; Blencowe, N.; Boutron, I.; Cates, C.; Cheng, H.-Y.; Corbett, M.; Eldridge, S.; et al. RoB 2: A revised tool for assessing risk of bias in randomised trials. *BMJ* **2019**, *366*. [CrossRef]
22. Borenstein, M.; Hedges, L.; Higgins, J.; Rothstein, H. *Comprehensive Meta-Analysis*; SBiostat, Inc.: Englewood, NJ, USA, 2014; Volume 3.
23. Higgins, J.P.T.; Thompson, S.G.; Deeks, J.J.; Altman, D.G. Measuring inconsistency in meta-analyses. *BMJ* **2003**, *327*. [CrossRef] [PubMed]
24. Cohen, J. *Statistical Power Analysis for the Behavioural Sciences*; Lawrence Erlbaum Associates: Hillsdale, NJ, USA, 1988.
25. Begg, C.B.; Mazumdar, M. Operating characteristics of a rank correlation test for publication bias. *Biometrics* **1994**, *50*, 1088–1101. [CrossRef] [PubMed]
26. Rosenthal, R. The file drawer problem and tolerance for null results. *Psychol. Bull.* **1979**, *86*, 638–664. [CrossRef]
27. Kumar, S.; Wagner, C.W.; Frayne, C.; Zhu, L.; Selim, M.; Feng, W.; Schlaug, G. Noninvasive brain stimulation may improve stroke-related dysphagia: A pilot study. *Stroke* **2011**, *42*, 1035–1040. [CrossRef]
28. Zhang, R.; Ju, X.-M. Clinical improvement of nursing intervention in swallowing dysfunction of elderly stroke patients. *Biomed. Res.* **2018**, *29*, 1099–1102. [CrossRef]
29. Sawan, S.A.E.; Reda, A.M.; Kamel, A.H.; Ali, M.A.M. Transcranial direct current stimulation (tDCS): Its effect on improving dysphagia in stroke patients. *Egypt. J. Neurol. Psychiatry Neurosurg.* **2020**, *56*, 1–7. [CrossRef]
30. Khedr, E.M.; Mohamed, K.O.; Soliman, R.K.; Hassan, A.M.M.; Rothwell, J. The Effect of high-frequency repetitive transcranial magnetic stimulation on advancing Parkinson's Disease with dyspahgia: Double blind randomised clinical trial. *Neurorehabil. Neural Repair* **2019**, *33*, 442–452. [CrossRef]
31. Cosentino, G.; Tassorelli, C.; Preunetti, P.; Bertino, G.; De Icco, R.; Todisco, M.; Di Marco, S.; Brighina, F.; Schindler, A.; Rondanelli, M.; et al. Anodal transcranial direct current stimulation and intermittent theta-burst stimulation deglutition and swallowing reproducibility in elderly patients with dysphagia. *Neurogastroenterol. Motil.* **2020**, *32*, e13791. [CrossRef]
32. Kim, L.; Chun, M.H.; Kim, B.R.; Lee, S.J. Effect of repetitive transcranial magnetic stimulation on patients with brain injury and dysphagia. *Ann. Rehabil. Med.* **2011**, *35*, 765–771. [CrossRef]
33. Tarameshlu, M.; Ansari, N.N.; Ghelichi, L.; Jalaei, S. The effect of repetitive transcranial magnetic stimulation combined with traditional dysphagia therapy on poststroke dysphagia: A pilot double-blinded randomized-controlled trial. *Int. J. Rehabil. Res.* **2019**, *42*, 133–138. [CrossRef]
34. Du, J.; Yang, F.; Liu, L.; Hu, J.; Cai, B.; Liu, W.; Xu, G.; Liu, X. Repetitive transcranial magnetic stimulation for poststroke dysphagia: A randomised, double-blind clinical trial. *Clin. Neurophysiol.* **2016**, *127*, 1907–1913. [CrossRef] [PubMed]
35. Park, E.; Kim, M.S.; Chang, W.H.; Oh, S.M.; Kim, Y.K.; Lee, A.; Kim, Y.-H. Effects of bilateral repetitive transcranial magnetic stimulation on post-stroke dysphagia. *Brain Stimul.* **2017**, *10*, 75–82. [CrossRef] [PubMed]
36. Ahn, Y.H.; Sohn, H.-J.; Park, J.-S.; Ahn, T.G.; Shin, Y.B.; Park, M.; Ko, S.-H.; Shin, Y.-I. Effect of bihemispheric anodal transcranial direct current stimulation for dysphagia in chronic stroke patients: A randomized control trial. *J. Rehabil. Med.* **2017**, *49*, 30–35. [CrossRef] [PubMed]
37. Pingue, V.; Priori, A.; Malovini, A.; Pistarini, C. Dual transcranial direct current stimulation for post-stroke dysphagia: A randomised controlled trial. *Neurorehabil. Neural Repair* **2018**, *32*, 635–644. [CrossRef]
38. Shigematsu, T.; Fujishima, I.; Ohno, K. Transcranial direct current stimulation improves swallowing function in stroke patients. *Neurorehabil. Neural Repair* **2013**, *27*, 363–369. [CrossRef]

39. Suntrup-Krueger, S.; Ringmaier, C.; Muhle, P.; Wollbrink, A.; Kemmling, A.; Hanning, U.; Claus, I.; Warnecke, T.; Teismann, I.; Pantev, C.; et al. Randomized trial of transcranial direct current stimulation for poststroke dysphagia. *Ann. Neurol.* **2018**, *83*, 328–340. [CrossRef]
40. Wang, Z.-Y.; Chen, J.-M.; Lin, Z.-k.; Ni, G.-X. Transcranial direct current stimulation improves the swallowing function in patients with cricopharyngeal muscle dysfunction following a brainstem stroke. *Neurol. Sci.* **2020**, *41*, 569–574. [CrossRef]
41. Yang, E.J.; Baek, S.-R.; Shin, J.; Lim, J.Y.; Jang, H.J.; Kim, Y.K.; Paik, N.-J. Effects of transcranial direct current stimulation (tDCS) on post-stroke dysphagia. *Restor. Neurol. Neurosci.* **2012**, *30*, 303–311. [CrossRef]
42. Michou, E.; Mistry, S.; Jefferson, S.; Tyrrell, P.; Hamdy, S. Characterizing the mechanisms of central and peripheral forms of neurostimulation in chronic dysphagic stroke patients. *Brain Stimul.* **2014**, *7*, 66–73. [CrossRef]
43. Lim, K.-L.; Lee, H.-J.; Yoo, J.; Kwon, Y.-G. Effect of low-frequency rTMS and NMES on subacute unilateral hemispheric stroke with dysphagia. *Ann. Rehabil. Med.* **2014**, *38*, 592–602. [CrossRef]
44. Cabib, C.; Nascimento, W.; Rofes, L.; Arreola, V.; Tomsen, N.; Mundet, L.; Palomeras, E.; Michou, E.; Clavé, P.; Ortega, O. Short-term neurophysiological effects of sensory pathway neurorehabilitation strategies on chronic poststroke oropharyngeal dysphagia. *Neurogastroenterol. Motil.* **2020**, *32*, e13887. [CrossRef] [PubMed]
45. Zhang, C.; Zheng, X.; Lu, R.; Yun, W.; Yun, H.; Zhou, X. Repetitive transcranial magnetic stimulation in combination with neuromuscular electrical stimulation for treatment of post-stroke dysphagia. *J. Int. Med. Res.* **2019**, *47*, 662–672. [CrossRef] [PubMed]
46. Cheng, I.K.Y.; Chan, K.M.K.; Wong, C.S.; Li, L.S.W.; Chiu, K.M.Y.; Cheung, R.T.F.; Yiu, E.M.L. Neronavigated high-frequency repetitive transcranial magnetic stimulation for chronic post-stroke dysphagia: A randomized controlled trial. *J. Rehabil. Med.* **2017**, *49*, 476–481. [CrossRef]
47. Khedr, E.M.; Abo-Elfetoh, N.; Rothwell, J. Treatment of post-stroke dysphagia with repetitive transcranial magnetic stimulation. *Acta Neurol. Scand.* **2009**, *119*, 155–161. [CrossRef] [PubMed]
48. Khedr, E.M.; Abo-Elfetoh, N. Therapeutic role of rTMS on recovery of dysphagia in patients with lateral medullary syndrome and brainstem infarction. *J. Neurol. Neurosurg. Psychiatry* **2010**, *81*, 495–499. [CrossRef] [PubMed]
49. Momosaki, R.; Abo, M.; Watanabe, S.; Kakuda, W.; Yamada, N.; Mochio, K. Functional magnetic stimulation using a parabolic coil for dysphagia after stroke. *Neuromodulation* **2014**, *17*, 637–641. [CrossRef]
50. Park, J.-W.; Oh, J.-C.; Lee, J.-W.; Yeo, J.-S.; Ryu, K.H. The effect of 5Hz high-frequency rTMS over contralesional pharyngeal motor cortex in post-stroke oropharyngeal dysphagia: A randomized controlled study. *Neurogastroenterol. Motil.* **2013**, *25*, 324-e250. [CrossRef]
51. Ünlüer, N.O.; Temuçin, C.M.; Demir, N.; Arslan, S.S.; Karaduman, A. Effects of low-frequency repetitive transcranial magnetic stimulation on swallowing function and quality of life of post-stroke patients. *Dysphagia* **2019**, *34*, 360–371. [CrossRef]
52. Chan, K.; Yiu, E.; Ho, E. The impact of swallowing problems on nursing home residents' quality of life. In Proceedings of the International Symposium on Healthy Aging, ISHA, Hongkong, China, 5–6 March 2011.
53. Perry, L. Screening swallowing function of patients with acute stroke. Part two: Detailed evaluation of the tool used by nurses. *J. Clin. Nurs.* **2001**, *10*, 474–481. [CrossRef]
54. Suiter, D.M.; Leder, S.B. Clinical utility of the 3-ounce water swallow test. *Dysphagia* **2008**, *23*, 244–250. [CrossRef]
55. Ertekin, C.; Aydogdu, I.; Yüceyar, N.; Kiylioglu, N.; Tarlaci, S.; Uludag, B. Pathophysiological mechanisms of oropharyngeal dysphagia in amyotrophic lateral sclerosis. *Brain* **2000**, *123*, 125–140. [CrossRef] [PubMed]
56. Brott, T.; Adams, H.P., Jr.; Olinger, C.P.; Marler, J.R.; Barsan, W.G.; Biller, J.; Spilker, J.; Holleran, R.; Eberle, R.; Hertzberg, V. Measurements of acute cerebral infarction: A clinical examination scale. *Stroke* **1989**, *20*, 864–870. [CrossRef]
57. Mahoney, F.I. Functional evaluation: The Barthel index. *Md. State Med. J.* **1965**, *14*, 61–65.
58. O'Neil, K.H.; Purdy, M.; Falk, J.; Gallo, L. The dysphagia outcome and severity scale. *Dysphagia* **1999**, *14*, 139–145. [CrossRef]
59. Zhao, Y.J.; Wee, H.L.; Chan, Y.H.; Seah, S.H.; Au, W.L.; Lau, P.N.; Pica, E.C.; Li, S.C.; Luo, N.; Tan, L.C. Progression of Parkinson's disease as evaluated by Hoehn and Yahr stage transition times. *Mov. Disord.* **2010**, *25*, 710–716. [CrossRef]
60. Fahn, S.; Elton, R. UPDRS program members. Unified Parkinsons disease rating scale. *Recent Dev. Parkinson's Dis.* **1987**, *2*, 153–163.
61. Lawton, M.; Brody, E.; Médecin, U. Instrumental activities of daily living (IADL). *Gerontologist* **1969**, *9*, 179–186. [CrossRef]
62. Brown, R.G.; MacCarthy, B.; Jahanshahi, M.; Marsden, C.D. Accuracy of self-reported disability in patients with parkinsonism. *Arch. Neurol.* **1989**, *46*, 955–959. [CrossRef]
63. Cohen, J.T.; Manor, Y. Swallowing disturbance questionnaire for detecting dysphagia. *Laryngoscope* **2011**, *121*, 1383–1387. [CrossRef] [PubMed]
64. Farahat, M.; Malki, K.H.; Mesallam, T.A.; Bukhari, M.; Alharethy, S. Development of the arabic version of dysphagia handicap index (dhi). *Dysphagia* **2014**, *29*, 459–467. [CrossRef]
65. Han, T.R.; Paik, N.-J.; Park, J.W. Quantifying swallowing function after stroke: A functional dysphagia scale based on videofluoroscopic studies. *Arch. Phys. Med. Rehabil.* **2001**, *82*, 677–682. [CrossRef] [PubMed]
66. Rosenbek, J.C.; Robbins, J.A.; Roecker, E.B.; Coyle, J.L.; Wood, J.L. A penetration-aspiration scale. *Dysphagia* **1996**, *11*, 93–98. [CrossRef] [PubMed]
67. Mullen, R. Evidence for whom?: ASHA's National outcomes measurement system. *J. Commun. Disord.* **2004**, *37*, 413–417. [CrossRef] [PubMed]

68. Kim, J.; Oh, B.-M.; Kim, J.Y.; Lee, G.J.; Lee, S.A.; Han, T.R. Validation of the videofluoroscopic dysphagia scale in various etiologies. *Dysphagia* **2014**, *29*, 438–443. [CrossRef]
69. Jung, S.H.; Lee, K.J.; Hong, J.B.; Han, T.R. Validation of clinical dysphagia scale: Based on videofluoroscopic swallowing study. *J. Korean Acad. Rehabil. Med.* **2005**, *29*, 343–350.
70. Carnaby-Mann, G.; Lenius, K.; Crary, M.A. Update on assessment and management of dysphagia post stroke. *Northeast Fla. Med.* **2007**, *58*, 31–34.
71. Crary, M.A.; Mann, G.D.C.; Groher, M.E. Initial psychometric assessment of a functional oral intake scale for dysphagia in stroke patients. *Arch. Phys. Med. Rehabil.* **2005**, *86*, 1516–1520. [CrossRef]
72. Scutt, P.; Lee, H.S.; Hamdy, S.; Bath, P.M. Pharyngeal electrical stimulation for treatment of poststroke dysphagia: Individual patient data meta-analysis of randomised controlled trials. *Stroke Res. Treat.* **2015**, *2015*. [CrossRef]
73. Martin-Harris, B.; Brodsky, M.B.; Michel, Y.; Castell, D.O.; Schleicher, M.; Sandidge, J.; Maxwell, R.; Blair, J. MBS measurement tool for swallow impairment—MBSImp: Establishing a standard. *Dysphagia* **2008**, *23*, 392–405. [CrossRef]
74. Ertekin, C.; Turman, B.; Tarlaci, S.; Celik, M.; Aydogdu, I.; Secil, Y.; Kiylioglu, N. Cricopharyngeal sphincter muscle responses to transcranial magnetic stimulation in normal subjects and in patients with dysphagia. *Clin. Neurophysiol.* **2001**, *112*, 86–94. [CrossRef]
75. Speyer, R.; Sutt, A.-l.; Bergström, L.; Hamdy, S.; Heijnen, B.J.; Remijn, L.; Wilkes-Gillan, S.; Cordier, R. Neurostimulation in people with oropharyngeal dysphagia: A systematic review and meta-analyses of randomised controlled trials. Part I: Pharyngeal and neuromuscular electrical stimulation. *J. Clin. Med.* **2022**, *11*, 776. [CrossRef]

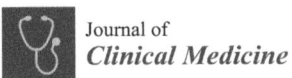

Review

Behavioural Interventions in People with Oropharyngeal Dysphagia: A Systematic Review and Meta-Analysis of Randomised Clinical Trials

Renée Speyer [1,2,3,*], Reinie Cordier [2,4], Anna-Liisa Sutt [5,6], Lianne Remijn [7], Bas Joris Heijnen [3], Mathieu Balaguer [8], Timothy Pommée [8], Michelle McInerney [9] and Liza Bergström [10,11]

1. Department Special Needs Education, Faculty of Educational Sciences, University of Oslo, 0318 Oslo, Norway
2. Curtin School of Allied Health, Faculty of Health Sciences, Curtin University, Perth, WA 6102, Australia; reinie.cordier@northumbria.ac.uk
3. Department of Otorhinolaryngology and Head and Neck Surgery, Leiden University Medical Centre, 2333 ZA Leiden, The Netherlands; b.j.Heijnen@lumc.nl
4. Department of Social Work, Education and Community Wellbeing, Faculty of Health & Life Sciences, Northumbria University, Newcastle upon Tyne NE7 7XA, UK
5. Critical Care Research Group, The Prince Charles Hospital, Brisbane, QLD 4032, Australia; annaliisasp@gmail.com
6. School of Medicine, University of Queensland, Brisbane, QLD 4072, Australia
7. School of Allied Health, HAN University of Applied Sciences, 6525 EN Nijmegen, The Netherlands; lianne.remijn@han.nl
8. IRIT, CNRS, Université Paul Sabatier, 31400 Toulouse, France; mathieu.balaguer@irit.fr (M.B.); timothy.pommee@irit.fr (T.P.)
9. School of Allied Health (SoAH), Australian Catholic University (ACU), Sydney, NSW 2060, Australia; michelle.mcInerney@acu.edu.au
10. Remeo Stockholm, 128 64 Stockholm, Sweden; liza.bergstrom@regionstockholm.se
11. Speech Therapy Clinic, Danderyd University Hospital, 182 88 Stockholm, Sweden
* Correspondence: renee.speyer@isp.uio.no

Abstract: Objective: To determine the effects of behavioural interventions in people with oropharyngeal dysphagia. Methods: Systematic literature searches were conducted to retrieve randomized controlled trials in four different databases (CINAHL, Embase, PsycINFO, and PubMed). The methodological quality of eligible articles was assessed using the Revised Cochrane risk-of-bias tool for randomised trials (RoB 2), after which meta-analyses were performed using a random-effects model. Results: A total of 37 studies were included. Overall, a significant, large pre-post interventions effect size was found. To compare different types of interventions, all behavioural interventions and conventional dysphagia treatment comparison groups were categorised into compensatory, rehabilitative, and combined compensatory and rehabilitative interventions. Overall, significant treatment effects were identified favouring behavioural interventions. In particular, large effect sizes were found when comparing rehabilitative interventions with no dysphagia treatment, and combined interventions with compensatory conventional dysphagia treatment. When comparing selected interventions versus conventional dysphagia treatment, significant, large effect sizes were found in favour of Shaker exercise, chin tuck against resistance exercise, and expiratory muscle strength training. Conclusions: Behavioural interventions show promising effects in people with oropharyngeal dysphagia. However, due to high heterogeneity between studies, generalisations of meta-analyses need to be interpreted with care.

Keywords: deglutition; swallowing disorders; RCT; intervention; compensation; rehabilitation

1. Introduction

Swallowing disorders, or oropharyngeal dysphagia (OD), can be the result of many underlying conditions such as stroke, progressive neurological diseases, and acquired brain injury. They may also be the consequence of treatment side effects; for example, radiation or surgical interventions in patients with head and neck oncological disorders. Prevalence of OD in the general population ranges from 2.3 to 16% [1]. However, depending on underlying disease severity and outcome measures used (e.g., instrumental assessment, screening or patient self-report) [2], prevalence estimates can be as high as 80% in stroke and Parkinson's disease patients, up to 30% in traumatic brain injury patients, and over 90% in patients with community-acquired pneumonia [3]. Also, pooled prevalence estimates for swallowing problems in people with cerebral palsy determined by meta-analyses are as high as 50.4% [4].

OD may have severe effects on a person's health as dysphagia can lead to dehydration, malnutrition, and aspiration pneumonia. OD also has a high disease burden and poses a major societal challenge, which is associated with significant psychological and social burden, resulting in reduced quality-of-life for both patients and caregivers [5].

The treatment of OD may include surgical, pharmacological and behavioural interventions. Behavioural interventions include: bolus modification and management (e.g., adjusting the viscosity, volume, temperature and/or acidity of food and drinks), motor behavioural techniques or oromotor exercises, general body and head postural adjustments, swallowing manoeuvres (e.g., manoeuvres to improve food propulsion into the pharynx and airway protection), and sensory and neurophysiologic stimulation (e.g., neuromuscular electrical stimulation [NMES]) [6].

An increasing number of reviews have been published over the last two decades on the treatment effects of behavioural interventions in people with OD. However, only one systematic review [7] summarised the effects of swallowing therapy as applied by speech and language therapists without restrictions on subject populations or study designs. Furthermore, while most reviews have focussed on selected types of interventions and patient populations, very few reviews use criteria related to study designs (e.g., [8,9] solely including randomised controlled trials [RCTs], ranked as the highest level of evidence [10]).

This systematic review aimed to determine the effects of behavioural interventions in people with OD based on the highest level of evidence (RCTs) only. Behavioural interventions comprised any intervention by a dysphagia expert, excluding surgical and pharmacological interventions. Clinicians being referred to as dysphagia experts include speech therapists, occupational therapists, or physiotherapists, but may incorporate other disciplines depending on national healthcare and education systems. Finally, neurostimulation techniques were considered out of scope of this current review.

2. Methods

The methodology and reporting of this systematic review were based on the Preferred Reporting Items for Systematic Reviews and Meta-Analyses (PRISMA) statement and checklist. The PRISMA 2020 statement and checklist (Supplementary Tables S1 and S2) aim to enhance the essential and transparent reporting of systematic reviews [11,12]. The protocol for this review was registered at PROSPERO, the international prospective register of systematic reviews (registration number: CRD42020179842).

2.1. Information Sources

To identify studies, literature searches were conducted on 6 March 2021, across these four databases: CINAHL, Embase, PsycINFO, and PubMed. Publications dates ranged from 1937–2021, 1902–2021, 1887–2021, and late 1700s–2021, respectively. Additional searches included checking the reference lists of eligible articles.

2.2. Search Strategies

Electronic search strategies were performed in all four databases using subheadings (e.g., MeSH and Thesaurus terms) and free text terms. Two strings of terms were combined: (1) dysphagia and (2) randomised controlled trial. The full electronic search strategies are reported in Table 1.

Table 1. Search strategies.

Database and Search Terms	Number of Records
Cinahl: ((MH "Deglutition") OR (MH "Deglutition Disorders")) AND (MH "Randomized Controlled Trials")	239
Embase: (swallowing/OR dysphagia/) AND (randomization/or randomized controlled trial/OR "randomized controlled trial (topic)"/OR controlled clinical trial/)	4550
PsycINFO: (swallowing/OR dysphagia/) AND (RCT OR (Randomised AND Controlled AND Trial) OR (Randomized AND Clinical AND Trial) OR (Randomised AND Clinical AND Trial) OR (Controlled AND Clinical AND Trial)).af.	231
PubMed: ("Deglutition" [Mesh] OR "Deglutition Disorders" [Mesh]) AND ("Randomized Controlled Trial" [Publication Type] OR "Randomized Controlled Trials as Topic" [Mesh] OR "Controlled Clinical Trial" [Publication Type] OR "Pragmatic Clinical Trials as Topic" [Mesh])	3039

2.3. Inclusion and Exclusion Criteria

The following criteria for inclusion were applied: (1) participants had a diagnosis of OD; (2) behavioural interventions were aimed at reducing swallowing or feeding problems; (3) studies included a comparison group; (4) participants were randomly assigned to one of the study arms or groups; (5) studies were published in English.

Studies focussing on drooling, self-feeding, gastro-oesophageal reflux or oesophageal dysphagia (e.g., dysphagia resulting from oesophageal carcinoma or esophagitis) were excluded. Further excluded studies were those describing drug-induced swallowing problems, temporary swallowing problems caused by oedema post-surgery (e.g., anterior cervical discectomy), or swallowing problems associated with adverse effects of interventions such as inflammation and oedema resulting from recent radiotherapy (≤three months after intervention) or thyroidectomy. Studies reporting solely on feeding tube removal after intervention that did not provide data on swallowing or feeding problems, were also excluded. Studies on behavioural eating problems including bulimia, anorexia, and picky eaters, were out of scope of this review. Finally, only original research was included, thus excluding, for example, conference abstracts, doctoral theses and reviews.

2.4. Systematic Review

Methodological Quality and Risk of Bias. The Revised Cochrane risk-of-bias tool for randomised trials (RoB 2) [13] was used to assess the methodological quality of the included studies. The RoB 2 tool provides a framework for evaluating the risk of bias in the findings of any type of randomised trial. The tool is structured along five domains through which bias might be introduced into the study results: (1) the randomisation process; (2) deviations from intended interventions; (3) missing outcome data; (4) measurement of the outcome; (5) selection of the reported result.

Data Collection Process. A data extraction form was created to extract data from the included studies under the following categories: methodological quality, participant diagnosis, inclusion criteria, sample size, age, gender, intervention goal, intervention agent/delivery/dosage, intervention condition, outcome measures and treatment outcome.

Data, Items and Synthesis of Results. Two independent raters reviewed all titles and abstracts, then original articles, for eligibility. Inclusion of studies was based on consensus between raters. To ensure rating accuracy, two group sessions were held to discuss ratings of one hundred randomly selected records to achieve consensus before rating the remaining abstracts. Where consensus could not be reached between the first two raters, a third party was consulted for resolution. Methodological quality assessment was also rated by two independent researchers, after which consensus was reached with involvement of a third reviewer, when necessary. No evident bias in article selection or methodological study quality rating was present as none of the reviewers had formal or informal affiliations with any of the authors of the included studies. At this stage reviewers did not exclude studies based on type of intervention (e.g., behavioural intervention, neurostimulation).

During data collection, data points across all studies were extracted using comprehensive data extraction forms. Risk of bias was assessed per individual study using RoB 2 [13]. The main summary measures for assessing treatment outcome were effect sizes and significance of findings.

2.5. Meta-Analysis

Data was extracted from relevant studies to compare the effect sizes for the following: (1) pre-post outcome measures of OD and (2) mean difference in outcome measures from pre to post between different types of behavioural interventions. All interventions were categorised into compensatory (e.g., body and postural adjustments, or bolus modification), rehabilitative (e.g., oromotor exercises or Shaker exercise), combined compensatory and rehabilitative interventions, and no dysphagia intervention. Only studies using instrumental assessment (videofluoroscopic swallow study [VFSS] or fiberoptic endoscopic evaluation of swallowing [FEES]) to confirm OD were included. Outcome measures based on visuoperceptual evaluation of instrumental assessment and clinical non-instrumental assessments, were eligible for inclusion in meta-analyses. However, if both types of data were available, instrumental assessment was preferred over non-instrumental assessment outcome data. Oral intake measures, screening tools and patient self-report measures were excluded from meta-analyses. Measures other than the authors' primary outcomes may have been selected if these measures helped to reduce heterogeneity between studies.

To compare effect sizes, group means, standard deviations, and sample sizes for pre- and post-measurements were entered into Comprehensive Meta-Analysis Version 3.3.070 [14]. If only non-parametric data were available (i.e., medians, interquartile ranges), then data were converted into parametric data for meta-analyses. Participants in studies of multiple intervention groups were analysed separately. Where studies used the same participants, only one study was included in the meta-analysis. If studies provided insufficient data for meta-analyses, authors were contacted by e-mail for additional data.

Effect sizes were calculated in Comprehensive Meta-Analysis using a random-effects model. Due to variations in participant characteristics, intervention approaches, and outcome measurements, studies were unlikely to have similar true effects. Heterogeneity was estimated using the Q statistic to determine the spread of effect sizes about the mean and I^2 was used to estimate the ratio of true variance to total variance. I^2-values of less than 50%, 50% to 74%, and higher than 75% indicate low, moderate, and high heterogeneity, respectively [15]. Using the Hedges g formula for standardized mean difference with a confidence interval of 95%, effect sizes were calculated and interpreted using Cohen's d convention: $g \leq 0.2$ as no or negligible effect; $0.2 < g \leq 0.5$ as minor effect; $0.5 < g \leq 0.8$ as moderate effect; and $g > 0.8$ as large effect [16].

Forest plots of effect sizes for OD outcome scores were generated for pre-post behavioural interventions. Due to blended configurations of intervention groupings across studies it was not possible to compare a homogenous behavioural intervention group against a comparison group that did not have a behavioural component. For this reason, only a subgroup between group analysis was conducted (and not an overall between group analysis) to explore effect sizes as a function of various moderators. Behavioural interventions (compensatory, rehabilitative, or combined compensatory and rehabilitative interventions) were compared with conventional dysphagia treatment (CDT), or no dysphagia therapy groups. Other subgroup analyses were conducted to compare effect sizes between selected interventions (i.e., Shaker exercise, Chin Tuck Against Resistance exercise [CTAR], and Expiratory Muscle Strength Training [EMST]), medical diagnoses, and outcome measures. Only between-subgroup meta-analyses were conducted using post-intervention data, to account for possible spontaneous recovery during the period of intervention.

Using Comprehensive Data Analysis software, publication bias was assessed following the Begg and Muzumdar's rank correlation test and the fail-safe N test. The Begg and Muzumdar's rank correlation test reports the rank correlation between the standardised effect size and the variances of these effects [17]. This statistical procedure produces tau as well as a two tailed p value; values of zero indicate no relationship, whereas deviations away from zero indicate a relationship. High standard error would be associated with larger effect sizes if asymmetry is caused by publication bias. Tau would be positive if larger effects are presented by low values, while tau would be negative if larger effects are represented by high values.

The fail-safe N test calculates how many studies with effect size zero could be added to the meta-analysis before the result lost statistical significance. That is, the number of missing studies that would be required to nullify the effect [18]. If this number is relatively small, then there is cause for concern. However, if this number is large, it can be stated with confidence that the treatment effect, while possibly inflated by the exclusion of some studies, is not nil.

3. Results

3.1. Study Selection

A total of 8059 studies were retrieved across four databases: CINAHL (n = 239), Embase (n = 4550), PsycINFO (n = 231), and PubMed (n = 3039). After removal of duplicate titles and abstracts (n = 1113), a total of 6946 records remained. After assessing titles and abstracts, 261 original articles were identified. Full-text records were accessed to verify all inclusion criteria. During full-text assessment, articles were divided into different types of interventions, as this systematic review reports on behavioural interventions only. Based on the inclusion criteria, 36 articles were included, after which one study was identified through reference checking of the included articles. Figure 1 presents the flow diagram of the article selection process according to PRISMA.

3.2. Description of Studies

All 37 included studies are described in detail in Tables 2 and 3. Table 2 reports on study characteristics, definitions and methods of diagnosing oropharyngeal dysphagia, and details on participant groups. Information such as medical diagnosis, sample size, age and gender, is provided on all study groups. Table 3 presents intervention goals, intervention components, outcome measures and treatment outcome of each included study.

Participants (Table 2). The 37 studies included a total of 2656 participants (mean = 72; SD = 124.5), with the sample sizes across studies ranging from 10 [30] to 742 participants [38]. All but two studies reported the mean age of participants [38,49], which was 65.6 years (SD = 8.8). Participant age range was only reported in five studies, ranging between 55 [36] and 95 [38] years. The mean percentage of male participants across all studies was 55.8% (SD = 13.7).

Most studies included stroke patients (n = 24). Other diagnoses included: patients with Parkinson's disease [19,39,52], acquired brain injury [30], multiple sclerosis [51] and nasopharyngeal cancer [50]. Two studies included a mixed patient population with Parkinson's disease or dementia [38], and stroke or head and neck cancer patients after chemoradiation [40]. Five studies did not provide further details on diagnoses [28,38,49,54,55]. The most frequent method for confirming OD was VFSS (n = 17), with only four studies using FEES (n = 4) [20,31,38,40]. Seven studies used non-instrumental clinical assessments, five studies used a screening tool [28,29,39,48,56], and four studies used patient self-reported dysphagia [49,52,54,55]. The included studies were conducted across fifteen countries, with studies most frequently conducted in Korea (n = 13), USA (n = 6), China (n = 3) and Japan (n = 3).

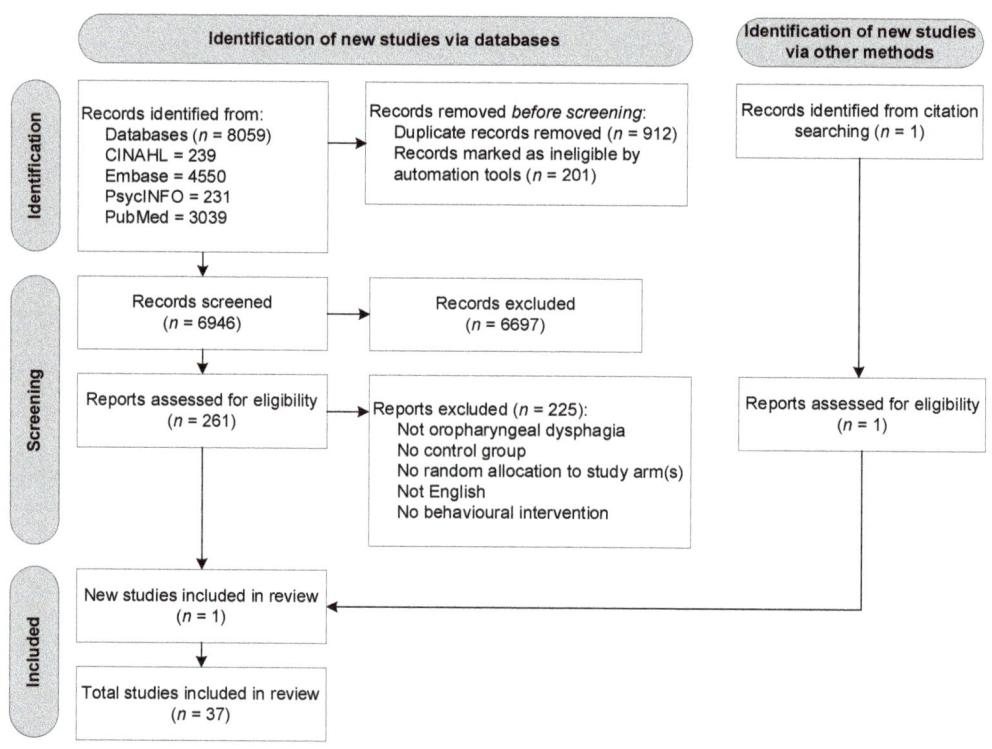

Figure 1. Flow diagram of the reviewing process according to PRISMA.

Outcome measures (Table 3). Many different outcome measures were used across the included studies targeting different domains within the area of OD. The most frequently used measures were the Penetration Aspiration Scale (PAS; 15 studies), the Functional Oral Intake Scale (FOIS; 8 studies), various water swallow tests (4 studies), and the Mann Assessment of Swallowing Ability (MASA; 3 studies). All other outcome measures were used in one or two studies only, confirming the substantial heterogeneity in outcome measures.

Interventions (Table 3). The included 37 studies comprised a range of behavioural interventions, delivered by various health professionals. The interventions were most frequently implemented by single allied health disciplines: occupational therapists in ten studies, speech pathologists in eight studies, physical therapists in two studies [36,48], and nursing staff in one study [55]. In five studies, more than one discipline was involved [23,27,28,33,48], and two studies reported caregivers as the intervention agent either as a single agent [24] or in addition to occupational therapists [22]. Nine studies did not specify disciplines involved in providing the interventions. The intervention dosage varied greatly, ranging from one training session [54] to exercise 3 times daily, 7 days per week for 42 days [25].

Behavioural intervention groups (Table 3). Of the 37 included studies, seven studies comprised three participant groups [19–21,23,25,26,38], whereas all other studies included two groups. Based on authors' description of therapy contents, all intervention groups were categorised into compensatory, rehabilitative, and combined compensatory and rehabilitative interventions. Ten studies included different types of intervention groups (i.e., compensatory, rehabilitative and/or combined compensatory and rehabilitative intervention groups). Five studies included only compensatory groups [20,24,38,39,55], ten studies included only rehabilitative groups, and thirteen studies included only groups combining compensatory and rehabilitative interventions.

Table 2. Study characteristics of studies on behavioural interventions for people with oropharyngeal dysphagia.

Study • Country	OD (Definition/Terminology; Diagnostic Measure/Method) • Diagnosis • Main Inclusion/Exclusion Criteria	Sample (N) • Groups (n) [a]	Group Descriptive (Mean ± SD) (Age, Gender, Relevant Medical Diagnoses)
Ayres, et al. [19] • Brazil	OD: Oropharyngeal dysphagia determined by FEES Diagnosis: PD Inclusion: PD and oro-pharyngeal dysphagia. Exclusion: Presenting language and/or hearing disorders that could complicate the understanding of intervention; diagnosis of dementia, or other neurological illnesses.	n = 32: - Experimental group: Chin-down manoeuvre and swallowing orientation (n = 11) - Orientation group: Swallowing orientation only (n = 7) - Control group: No intervention (n = 14)	Experimental group/Orientation group/control group Age years: 62 (11.5)/64.5 (5.6)/62.8 (6.2) Male: 80%/66.7%/75% Schooling: 5.9 (4.1)/12 (9.1)/10.3 (8.4) Time of disease: 10.7 (4.7)/11.8 (8)/8.8 (6) H & Y disability score: 2.8 (0.8)/2.5 (0.7)/2.5 (0.8) MOCA: 21.9 (4.9)/20.5 (7.7)/21.2 (8.4) PDQ-39: 41.4 (13.8)/38.7 (16.7)/36.5 (17.1) BDI: 13.8 (7.7)/17.1 (9.2)/14.7 (9.3) FOIS: 5.9 (1.3)/6.8 (0.5)/6.8 (0.4)
Carnaby, et al. [20] • USA	OD: Diagnosis of swallowing difficulty by speech pathologist, <85 on Hospital's dysphagia assessment Diagnosis: Clinician diagnosed Stroke, WHO definition Inclusion: Stroke < 7 days Exclusion: NR	n = 306: - UC (n = 102) - Low intensity (n = 102) - High intensity (n = 102)	High intensity/low intensity/UC: mean (SD) Age yr: 69.8 (12.5)/72 (12.4)/71.4 (12.7) Male: 59%/58%/58% Severity Barthel index <15: 78%/78%/79% Rankin score >3: 85%/79%/83% Length hospital stay, days: 19.1/19.2/21.4
Carnaby, et al. [21] • USA	OD: Dysphagia on admission- score < 178 on MASA, no history of swallowing disability, head/neck surgery. Diagnosis: Sub-acute stroke confirmed by attending neurologist according to the WHO definition Inclusion: Able to adhere to behavioural treatment regimens Exclusion: NR	n = 53: - MDTP + NMES (NMES; n = 18). - MDTP + sham NMES (MDTP; n = 18) [Denoted as 'Carnaby et al. (2020a)' in Figure 4.] - UC (n = 17) [Denoted as 'Carnaby et al. (2020b)' in Figure 4.]	NMES/MDTP/UC: mean (SD) Age yr: 62.7 (12.2)/70.6 (11.8)/64.3 (14.7) Male: 55%/44%/41% Modified Rankin: 4.5 (0.6)/4.46 (0.5)/4.56 (0.5) Modified Barthel: 5.3 (3.4)/5.5 (2.8)/5.6 (2.6) Days post stroke: 7.83 (3.9)/8.47 (7.17)/6.7 (5.1) MASA score: 157.8 (16.5)/154.62 (18.87)/158.4 FOIS score: 3.72 (1.44)/3.25 (1.61)/4.35 (1.8)
Choi, et al. [22] • Korea	OD: Dysphagia after stroke confirmed by VFSS Diagnosis: Stroke (method NR) Inclusion: No major cognitive deficit (MMSE >20), >fair grade on neck muscle testing, symmetric neck posture Exclusion: neck pain or neck surgery; poor general condition, severe communication problem, unstable medical condition, presence of a tracheostomy tube	n = 32: - Experimental-Shaker exercise (SE) + CDT/ conventional dysphagia therapy (CDT; n = 16) [Denoted as 'Choi et al. (2017a)' in Figure 4.] - Control-CDT (n = 16) [Denoted as 'Choi et al. (2017b)' in Figure 4.]	Experimental SE + CDT/control (CDT): mean (SD) Age yr: 60.8 (10.9)/60.4 (10.5) Gender (male/female): 10/6//9/6 Time since stroke onset months: 3.4 (1.6)/4.1 (1.0) PAS: 4.6 (0.8)/4.9 (0.1) FOIS: 3.1 (1.0)/3.2 (0.68)
DePippo, et al. [23] • USA	OD: MBS, BDST, VFSS, speech pathologists determined dysphagia Diagnosis: Stroke by clinical history, neurologic examination CT/MRI Inclusion: 20–90 yrs, no history of oral or pharyngeal anomaly Exclusion: aspirated >50% of all consistencies,	n = 115, allocated to graded therapist treatment levels: - Group A (n = 38) - Group B (n = 38) - Group C (n = 39)	Group A/Group B/Group C Age yr: 76/74.5/73 Male/Female: 22/16/19/19/27/12 Mini-Mental State score: 16 (12)/17 (10)/18 (10) Barthel-ADL Mobility: 37 (23)/48 (20)/46 (38) Weeks post stroke: 4.6/4.5/4.9
Eom, et al. [24] • Korea	OD: Dysphagia caused by a stroke, confirmed by VFSS Diagnosis: Stroke Inclusion: Age > 65, onset duration < 3 months, score ≥ 24 on MMSE. Exclusion: Presence of severe orofacial pain, significant malocclusion or facial asymmetry, unstable breathing or pulse, tracheostomy, aphasia or apraxia, inadequate lip closure	n = 30: - Experimental- resistance expiratory muscle strength training (n = 15) - Placebo group (n = 15).	Experimental/Placebo Age yr: 69.2 (4.1)/70.2 (3.6) Male/Female: 5/8/6/7 PAS baseline: 5.1 (0.8)/4.9 (0.6)

Table 2. Cont.

Study • Country	OD (Definition/Terminology; Diagnostic Measure/Method) • Diagnosis • Main Inclusion/Exclusion Criteria	Sample (N) • Groups (n) [a]	Group Descriptive (Mean ± SD) (Age, Gender, Relevant Medical Diagnoses)
Gao and Zhang [25] • China	OD: VFSS evaluation Diagnosis: Chinese diagnosis guidelines for acute ischemic stroke, CT or MRI Inclusion: >60 yrs, positive Neill screening test, first-time cerebral infarction. Exclusion: unstable conditions, previous abnormality in mouth, throat or neck, multiple organ dysfunction syndromes, uncooperative patients, severe mental illness, complete or sensory aphasia	n = 90: - Control (n = 30) [Denoted as 'Goa & Zhang (2017c)' in Figure 4.] - Shaker exercise (n = 30 [Denoted as 'Goa & Zhang (2017a)' in Figure 4.] - Chin tuck against resistance (CTAR; n = 30) [Denoted as 'Goa & Zhang (2017b)' in Figure 4.] [Figure 5: Shaker-Control denoted as 'Goa & Zhang (2017b)'; CTAR-Control: denoted as 'Goa & Zhang (2017a)']	Control/Shaker/CTAR Age yr: 71.1 (6.4)/71.1 (7.1)/70.9 (6.6) Male: 14/15/13 Therapeutic course (day): 12.2 (1.4)/13.0 (1.4)/13.0 (1.6)
Guillén-Solà, et al. [26] • Spain	OD: Dysphagia confirmed by VFSS score ≥ 3 in 8-point PAS Diagnosis: Subacute ischemic stroke Inclusion: Stroke within 1–3 wks. Exclusion: Cognitive impairment and/or history of previous neurological diseases associated with dysphagia	n = 62: - Group 1: control standard swallow therapy (SST) (n = 21), - Group 2: SST + IEMT (n = 21) - Group 3: SST + sham IEMT+ NMES (n = 20).	Control/IEMT/NMES Age yrs: 68.9 (7.0)/67.9 (10.6)/70.3 (8.4) Male: 12 (57.1%)/16 (76.2%)/10 (47.6%) Modified Rankin: 3.7 (0.8)/3.9 (0.5)/3.6 (0.8) Barthel Index: 44.0 (18.5)/42.7 (14.6)/41.8 (12.2) Stroke onset (days): 9.3 (5.1)/10.8 (8.7)/11.0 (5.5) FOIS: 4.3 (0.6)/4.5 (0.5)/4.4 (1.0) PAS: 5.4 (2.3)/5 (2.7)/5.5 (2.2)
Hägglund, et al. [27] • Sweden	OD: Swallowing function assessed with timed water swallow test; diagnosed dysfunction when swallowing rate did not exceed 10 mL/s. Diagnosis: NR Inclusion: ≥65 yrs, No cognitive impairment, ≥3 days intermediate care. Exclusion: Patients receiving end of life care, moderate or severe cognitive impairment	n = 116: - Intervention: Oral neuromuscular training (n = 49) - Control: Usual care (n = 67)	Control/Intervention Age yr: 85/83 Male: 29 (43.3)/27 (55.1) Dysphagia risk condition: 32 (47.8)/25 (52.1) Care moderate dependence: 27 (40.9)/18 (36.7) Swallowing rate (mL/s): 4.10/5.31
Hägglund, et al. [28] • Sweden	OD: Swallowing dysfunction (pathological TWST test 4-weeks post-stroke) Diagnosis: Stroke Inclusion: First-time stroke and a pathological timed water swallow test. Exclusion: Inability to cooperate; neurological diseases other than stroke, known history of dysphagia prior to the stroke, prominent horizontal overbite (contra-indication due to the oral device's design), or hypersensitivity to the acrylate	n = 40: - Control group: 5 weeks of continued of oro-facial sensory stimulation (n = 20) [Denoted as 'Hägglund et al. (2020b)' in Figure 4.] - Intervention group: Oral neuromuscular training using oral device (Muppy®) for 5 weeks + oro-facial sensory vibration stimulation (n = 20) [Denoted as 'Hägglund et al. (2020a)' in Figure 4.]	Control/Intervention Age years: 75 (56–90) yrs./75 (60–85) Male = 14/11; Female: 6/9. Stroke type: Ischemic (16 16); ICH= 3/4: ischemic and ICH = 1/0; left hemisphere = −6/7; right hemisphere = 10/10; supratentorial = 15/16; infratentorial = 3/4; supra-and infratentorial = 1/0. Lowered consciousness at hospital admission: 6/6
Hwang, et al. [29] • Korea	OD: OD confirmed by VFSS Diagnosis: Stroke Inclusion: Dysphagia <3 months, swallow voluntarily. Exclusion: trigeminal neuropathy, tongue deviation, facial asymmetry, communication disorders.	n = 25: - Experimental, tongue stretching exercises (TSE) (n = 13) [Denoted as 'Hwang et al. (2019a)' in Figure 4.] - Control group (n = 12) [Denoted as 'Hwang et al. (2019b)' in Figure 4.]	Experimental/Control Age (yrs): 60.5 (12.5)/62.2 (10.3) Male: 6/5 Time since stroke, weeks: 8.2 (2.9)/9.1 (2.7) Type of stroke (n) Haemorrhage: 7/6 Type of stroke (n) Infarction: 4/4

Table 2. Cont.

Study • Country	OD (Definition/Terminology; Diagnostic Measure/Method) • Diagnosis • Main Inclusion/Exclusion Criteria	Sample (N) • Groups (n) [a]	Group Descriptive (Mean ± SD) (Age, Gender, Relevant Medical Diagnoses)
Jakobsen, et al. [30] • Denmark	OD: Clinical signs of dysphagia; score ≥3 on PAS, FEES. Diagnosis: Severe ABI, non-sedated GCS <9, <24 hrs of injury Inclusion: 18–65 yrs Exclusion: formerly acquired or congenital brain damage, psychiatric diagnosis, history of treatment for head and neck cancer, need for a tracheostomy tube, agitated behaviour	n = 10: - Intervention facilitation of swallowing (n = 5) [Denoted as 'Jakobsen et al. (2019a)' in Figure 4.] - Control basic care + usual treatment (n = 5) [Denoted as 'Jakobsen et al. (2019b)' in Figure 4.]	Control/Intervention Age yrs: 45.6 (37.5–57.8)/53.8 (41.8–61.4) Male: 4/2 Days from injury: 70.4 (43.0)/76.4 (21.8) GCS at injury (3–15 points): 6.8 (4.4)/6.0 (5.2)
Jang, et al. [31] • Korea	OD: Swallowing difficulty VFSS-patients who showed velopharyngeal incompetence (VPI) on VFSS were enrolled Diagnosis: Subacute stroke Inclusion: Diagnosis of subacute stroke Exclusion: Previous stroke, pharyngeal structural abnormalities, unable to cooperate	n = 36: - Study-conventional therapy + mechanical inspiration, expiration exercise (n = 18) [Denoted as 'Jang et al. (2019a)' in Figure 4.] - Control-conventional therapy only (n = 18) [Denoted as 'Jang et al. (2019b)' in Figure 4.]	Study/Control Age yrs: 67.3 (9.5)/71.15 (8.6) Male, n: 10/9 Stroke type, n Haemorrhage: 8/6 Days from stroke onset: 20.5 (13.6)/18.4 (12.5)
Jan, et al. [32] • Korea	OD: Swallowing dysfunction/dysphagia as determined by VDS and PAS scores on VFSS Diagnosis: Stroke disease Inclusion: MMSE-K score ≥19 points; stroke disease duration ≥6 mths and <2 years Exclusion: Altered neck posture. VitalStim contraindications or cardiopulmonary disease.	n = 34: - Experimental group: NMES + upper cervical spine mobilisation (n = 17) - Control group: NMES and sham mobilization (n = 17)	Experimental/Control Age yrs: 63.12 (13.5)/64.47 (8.43) Male: 11/6; 11/6 Side of stroke (left/right): 6/11; 7/10 Haemorrhage/infarction: 14/3; 12/5 Weight: 69.11 (11.95); 65.55 (12.66) K-MMSE (point): 24.53 (2.62)/24.2 (2.91) K-NIHSS (point): 10.41 (3.06)/10.76 (3.75)
Kim, et al. [33] • Korea	OD: Dysphagia defined as a disorder that causes difficulty with chewing and swallowing food Diagnosis: Stroke Inclusion: Diagnosed with dysphagia between May and July 2014; Symptoms of dysphagia for 6 months prior to treatment; 24 points or higher on MMSE- K; fair grade of manual muscle testing of neck flexors. Exclusion: Heart/internal/musculoskeletal disease	n = 26: - Experimental group: PNF short-flexion neck exercises (n = 13) - Control group: Shaker exercise (n = 13)	Experimental/Control Age yrs: 63.2 (10.2)/63.6 (8.1) Male: 8/5; 7/8 Side of stroke (right/left): 7/6; 7/6
Kim and Park [34] • Korea	OD: Dysphagia confirmed by VFSS Diagnosis: Diagnosed as having had stroke within 6 months post-onset Inclusion: Liquid aspiration or penetration on VFSS, nasogastric tube able to communicate, no cognitive deficit Exclusion: Secondary stroke, gastronomy tube, tracheostomy, neck or shoulder pain, cervical herniated nucleus, cervical spine orthosis or brainstem stroke	n = 30: - Experimental group, mCTAR exercise and traditional dysphagia treatment (n = 12) - Control group, only traditional (n = 13)	Experimental/Control Age yrs: 63.5 (5.5)/65.2 (6.2) Male: 6/6 Type of stroke–haemorrhage: 5/7 Side of stroke (right/left): 5/7/4/9 Facial palsy: 1/1 Dysarthria: 1/0
Koyama, et al. [35] • Japan	OD: Stroke related dysphagia, hypopharyngeal residue found by VFSS Diagnosis: Stroke Inclusion: able to perform real or sham exercise Exclusion: Level 1 to 4 on FOIS, pulmonary aspiration with 2 mL of barium water in VFSS, past or present temporomandibular joint disease and/or tumor in head or neck, past or present progressive disease	n = 12: - Intervention, modified jaw opening exercise (MJOE; n = 6) - Control, isometric jaw closing exercise (n = 6)	Intervention/control Age yrs: 66.0 (9.3)/71.8 (7.6) Male: 5/5 Post-onset weeks, mean (SD): 6.7 (2.1)/9.2 (4.0) FOIS, n, Level 5/Level 6: 3/3/4/2

Table 2. Cont.

Study • Country	OD (Definition/Terminology; Diagnostic Measure/Method) • Diagnosis • Main Inclusion/Exclusion Criteria	Sample (N) • Groups (n) a	Group Descriptive (Mean ± SD) (Age, Gender, Relevant Medical Diagnoses)
Krajczy, et al. [36] • Poland	OD: Level 1–3 or 5–7 on SRS *Diagnosis:* Ischaemic stroke- using the National Institutes of Health Stroke Scale *Inclusion:* Early post-stroke (first stroke) period (<30 days) *Exclusion:* 2nd or 3rd stroke, level 1–3 dysphagia or level 5–7 dysphagia according to SRS, cognitive function disorders, total aphasia, anarthria, bilateral facial nerve paralysis, tracheostomy	n = 60: - Study, original dysphagia treatment (n = 30) - Control (n = 30)	Study/Control *Age yrs:* 55–65 (3.3)/55–65 (1.5) *Male:* 12/14 *Paresis, right side:* 15/12
Kyodo, et al. [37] • Japan	OD: Dysphagia determined by endoscopic swallowing evaluation *Diagnosis:* Elderly patients with moderate-to-severe dysphagia. Diagnosis: NR *Inclusion:* Patients hospitalized between May 2017 and Sept 2018 who underwent endoscopic swallowing evaluation *Exclusion:* Patients ≥65 years old; the presence of an acute infection; patients who developed cerebrovascular disease, myocardial infarction, aspiration pneumonia within 2 weeks	n = 62 (randomized crossover trial): - Control group: Pureed diet without gelling agent - Intervention group: Pureed diet with gelling agent	Total sample *Age years:* 83 (9) *Male/female:* 36/26 *Height (cm):* 153.4 (6) *Weight (kg):* 51.8 (5) Concurrent medical conditions: - Aspiration pneumonia: 22 (35%) - CVA: 19 (31%) - Other: 21 (34%) *Hyodo-Komagane Score* Mild 0-3: 8 (13%) Moderate 4-7: 35 (56%) Severe 8-9: 19 (31%)
Logemann, et al. [38] • USA	OD: Speech pathologist referral after swallow screening, patient aspirating thin liquids. *Diagnosis:* Physician's diagnosis of dementia or PD. Bedford Alzheimer Nursing Severity Scale; neurologist rated PD using Hoehn and Yahr scale. *Inclusion:* 50–95 yrs *Exclusion:* Inability to perform chin down intervention	n = 742 All patients received all 3 interventions (random order): - Chin-down intervention - Nectar - Honey-thickened liquids	*Age range:* 50–79, 41% *Age range:* 80–95, 59% *Male:* 70% PD–No dementia: 32% PD–Dementia: 19% Dementia–Other: 19% Dementia–Single or multistroke: 15% Dementia–Alzheimer's: 15%
Manor, et al. [39] • UK	OD: Referred to speech pathologist for evaluation of swallowing disturbances, confirmed via FEES. *Diagnosis:* PD had been diagnosed according to the UK Brain Bank criteria *Inclusion:* Diagnosis as above *Exclusion:* History of other uncontrolled neurological or medical disorders interfering with swallowing	n = 42: - Experimental group –received video-assisted swallowing therapy (VAST; n = 21) - Control group-conventional therapy (n = 21)	Vast/Conventional therapy *Age yrs:* 67.7 (8.3)/69.9 (9.7) *Disease duration (years)* 7.4 (4.7)/8.8 (5.7) *Disease severity (H&Y 1–5)* 2.2 (0.8)/2.2 (0.8) *MMSE score (range 0–30)* 28.1 (1.6)/27.8 (1.5) *Swallowing disturbances questionnaire:* 14.7 (5.8)/14.3 (7.2) *Fiberoptic endoscopic evaluation of swallowing:* 0.7 (0.4)/0.6 (0.4)
Mepani, et al. [40] • USA	OD: Post deglutitive dysphagia, pharyngeal phase dysphagia, VFSS to confirm *Diagnosis:* Stroke or chemoradiation for head and neck cancer *Inclusion:* Pharyngeal phase dysphagia, incomplete UES opening and postdeglutitive aspiration, hypopharyngeal residue, able to comply with protocol, dysphagia with aspiration of at least 3 month duration *Exclusion:* History of pharyngeal surgical procedures excluded.	n = 11: - Traditional swallowing therapy (n = 6) [Denoted as 'Mepani et al. (2009a)' in Figure 4.] - Shaker Exercise (n = 5) [Denoted as 'Mepani et al. (2009b)' in Figure 4.]	Traditional/Shaker *Age years:* 70.5 (9.5)/64 (22.8) *Males:* 5 (83%)/3 (60%) Etiology of dysphagia: - CVA: 4 (67%) 2 (40%) - Cancer: 2 (33%) 3 (60%)

Table 2. Cont.

Study · Country	OD (Definition/Terminology; Diagnostic Measure/Method) · Diagnosis · Main Inclusion/Exclusion Criteria	Sample (N) · Groups (n) [a]	Group Descriptive (Mean ± SD) (Age, Gender, Relevant Medical Diagnoses)
Moon, et al. [41] · Korea	OD: Aspiration or penetration, oropharyngeal residue, confirmed VFSS. Diagnosis: Subacute stage 3–12 weeks after the onset of stroke Inclusion: Diagnosis as above, could follow instructions provided, score of > 21 on Mini Mental State Exam, decreased lingual pressures with either anterior or posterior tongue as 40 kPa Exclusion: Nonstroke patients with dysphagia.	n = 16: - TPSAT plus traditional dysphagia therapy (n = 8) [Denoted as 'Moon et al. (2018a)' in Figure 4.] - Control, traditional dysphagia therapy (n = 8). [Denoted as 'Moon et al. (2018b)' in Figure 4.]	TPSAT/Control *Age years*: 62.0 (4.2)/63.5 (6.1) *Male*: 3/4 *Stroke type (ischemic/hemorrhagic)*: 6/2/6/2 *Poststroke duration days*: 56.0 (17.4)/59.9 (20.0) *MMSE*: 22.87 ± 2.47 23.50 ± 2.00
Park, et al. [42] · Korea	OD: Dysphagia confirmed by VFSS Diagnosis: Stroke Inclusion: Onset within 6 months; score ≥24 on the MMSE Exclusion: Stroke prior to that resulting in dysphagia, severe orofacial pain, significant malocclusion or facial asymmetry, unstable breathing or pulse, tracheostomy, severe communication disorder, inadequate lip closure	n = 27: - Experimental group, Expiratory muscle strength training (EMST) (n = 14) - Placebo sham (n = 13)	Experimental/Placebo *Age years*: 64.3 (10.77)/65.8 (11.3) *Male n*: 6/6 *Time since onset weeks*: 27.4 (6.3)/26.6 (6.8)
Park, et al. [43] · Korea	OD: Dysphagia following stroke was confirmed by VFSS Diagnosis: Stroke Inclusion: Onset duration was <12 months, swallow voluntarily, MMSE score ≥20 Exclusion: Secondary stroke, severe communication disorder, pain in the neck region, unstable medical conditions, head and neck cancer	n = 22: - Experimental, chin tuck against resistance exercise (CTAR; n = 11) [Denoted as 'Park et al. (2018a)' in Figure 4.] - Control group, only conventional dysphagia treatment (n = 11). [Denoted as 'Park et al. (2018b)' in Figure 4.]	Experimental/Control *Age years*: 62.2 (17.3)/58.4 (12.5) *Male*: 6/4 *Infarction*: 7/6 *Time after stroke (weeks)*: 37.2 (54.3)/14 (14.4) *Oral feeding*: 4/5 *Tube feeding*: 7/6
Park, et al. [44] · Korea	OD: OD after stroke by VFSS Diagnosis: Stroke based on computed tomography or MRI Inclusion: Inpatient, no significant cognitive problems (MMSE score > 24) Exclusion: Secondary stroke, trigeminal neuropathy, significant malocclusion or facial asymmetry, parafunctional oral habits, tongue strength could not be measured, severe communication disorders, neck pain or neck surgery, presence of tracheostomy tube	n = 24: - Experimental, effortful swallowing training (EST; n = 12) [Denoted as 'Park, Oh et al. (2019a)' in Figure 4.] - Control, saliva swallowing (n = 12). [Denoted as 'Park, Oh et al. (2019b)' in Figure 4.]	Experimental/Control *Age years*: 66.5 (9.5)/64.8 (11.2) *Male*: 6/5 *Stroke lesion middle cerebral artery*: 6/6 *Time since stroke onset, wks*: 24.4 (8.6)/25.7 (6.3)
Park, et al. [45] · Korea	OD: pharyngeal dysphagia confirmed through VFSS Diagnosis: Diagnosed as having stroke Inclusion: Within 6 months post-onset, nasogastric tube; absence of cognitive deficits. Exclusion: Secondary stroke, presence of other neurological, pain in the disc and cervical spine, cervical spine orthosis, presence of gastronomy tube, problems with the oesophageal phase of dysphagia	n = 37 patients: - Experimental, game-based chin tuck against resistance exercise (n = 19) [Denoted as 'Park, Lee et al. (2019a)' in Figure 4.] - Control, traditional head-lift exercise (n = 18) [Denoted as 'Park, Lee et al. (2019b)' in Figure 4.]	Experimental/Control *Age years*: 60.9 (11.2)/59.5 (9.3) *Male n*: 13/10 *Type of stroke, haemorrhage, n*: 12/14 *Paretic side, right, n*: 11/13 *Time since stroke, months*: 3.60 (1.19)/3.85 (1.18)
Park, et al. [46] · Korea	OD: Dysphagia after stroke, by VFSS Diagnosis: Stroke due to hemorrhage or infarction Inclusion: <6 months of onset, liquid aspiration or penetration on VFSS; nasogastric tube; voluntary swallowing; coughing after water swallow test. Exclusion: Secondary stroke, difficulty in using both upper limbs, significant malocclusion or facial asymmetry, pain in the disc and cervical spine, limitations in opening jaw, use of cervical spine orthosis, tracheostomy, severe communication difficulties associated with dementia or aphasia, presence of gastronomy tube, problems with the oesophageal phase of dysphagia	n = 40: - Experimental, resistive jaw opening exercise (RJOE (n = 20) [Denoted as 'Park et al. (2020a)' in Figure 4.] - Placebo group (n = 20) [Denoted as 'Park et al. (2020a)' in Figure 4.]	Experimental/Placebo *Age years*: 62.1 (10.1)/61.8 (12.1) *Male*: 9/8 *Infarction*: 7/8

Table 2. Cont.

Study · Country	OD (Definition/Terminology; Diagnostic Measure/Method) · Diagnosis · Main Inclusion/Exclusion Criteria	Sample (N) · Groups (n) [a]	Group Descriptive (Mean ± SD) (Age, Gender, Relevant Medical Diagnoses)
Ploumis, et al. [47] · Greece	OD: Dysphagia screening-at least one severe symptom, validated in Greek Ohkuma questionnaire Diagnosis: Hemiparesis following stroke Inclusion: Hemiparesis following stroke, at least one severe symptom of the validated Greek Ohkuma questionnaire Exclusion: Exclusion-Barthel Index >20, Motor Function Hemispheric Stroke Scale <25, history of OD.	n = 70: - Experimental group cervical isometric exercises (n = 37) - Control (n = 33)	Experimental/Control Age years (all participants): 52 (15) Barthel Index: 22.8 (2.4)/23.4 (2.7) Motor function, Stroke Scale: 22.8 (2.4)/23.4 (2.7) Sagittal C2-C7 Cobb angle: 16.9 (18.5)/14.0 (16.2) Coronal C2-C7 Cobb angle: 6.9 ± 5.3/6.2 ± 5.0 VFSS Score: 1.0 (0)/1.0 (1.0)
Sayaca, et al. [48] · Turkey	OD: 'Swallowing difficulties' determined with Turkish version of the eating assessment tool (T-EAT-10) Diagnosis: No neurological problems after neurologist's examination Inclusion: Over 65 yrs, adequate cognitive status. Exclusion: Head/neck conditions affecting swallowing	n = 50: - Proprioceptive neuromuscular facilitation (PNF; n = 25) - Shaker exercises (n = 25)	Shaker/PNF Age years: 69 (4.9)/67 (2.1) Male: 10/10 T-EAT-10 scores: 3.5 (1.8)/3.6 (1.3) Peak amplitude (µV): 425.1 (170.7)/417.9 (143.0) Swallow speed (secs): 1.3 (0.3)/1.3 (0.3) Swallow capacity (mL/sec): 1.2 (0.1)/1.2 (0.1) Swallow volume (mL/sec): 1.3 (0.1)/1.3 (0.1)
Steele, et al. [49] · Canada	OD: Dysphagia post stroke (VFSS) Diagnosis: Recent stroke (4–20 wks) Inclusion: Recent stroke, one repetition maximum posterior maximum isometric tongue-palate pressure measure <40 kPa at intake, stage transition duration if < 350 ms on at least one liquid barium swallow at intake VFSS Exclusion: Severe dysphagia with no functional opening of upper esophageal sphincter; pre-existing dysphagia or diagnoses of head and neck.	n = 14: - Experimental TPPT treatment arm (n = 7) [Denoted as 'Steele et al. (2016a)' in Figure 4.] - Comparison TPSAT treatment arm (n = 7) [Denoted as 'Steele et al. (2016b)' in Figure 4.]	TPPT/TPSAT Age years, range: 56–84/49–89 Male: 4/5 Days post onset, range: 28–126/33–150
Tang, et al. [50] · China	OD: Radiation-induced dysphagia and trismus by non-instrumental clinical assessment Diagnosis: Nasopharyngeal carcinoma (NPC) patients after radiotherapy Inclusion: Diagnosed as above Exclusion: Dysphagia or trismus as initial symptoms of NPC excluded	n = 43: - Rehabilitation group, routine treatment + 3 months rehabilitation therapy (n = 22) - Control group, routine treatment (n = 21)	Rehabilitation group/Control group Age years (total sample): 49.3 (11) Male (total sample), n: 32 Postradiotherapy, years: 4.6 (1.8)/4.8 (1.6) Interincisor distance (IID), cm: 1.9 (0.7)/1.8 (0.6)
Tarameshlu, et al. [51] · Iran	OD: Dysphagia based on DYMUS questionnaire (patient self-report) Diagnosis: Established diagnosis of MS according to McDonald's criteria Inclusion: 20–60 years, lack of acute relapse in past two months, no other conditions such as stroke Exclusion: severe reflux, dysphagia due to drug toxicity, pregnancy	n = 20: - Experimental (TDT), sensorimotor exercises and swallowing manoeuvres (n = 10) [Denoted as 'Tarameshlu et al. (2019a)' in Figure 4.] - Usual Care (UC), diet prescription and postural changes (n = 10) [Denoted as 'Tarameshlu et al. (2019b)' in Figure 4.]	TDT/UC Age years: 47.5 (12.9)/39.9 (9.7) Male: 2/5 Disease Duration (years): 6.8 (2.9)/6.1 (2.7) Expanded Disability Status Scale: 3.6(2.1)/3.2(2.5) MS Type-Relapse-Remitting: 4/7 MS Type-Primary Progressive: 4/1 MS Type-Secondary Progressive: 2/2
Troche, et al. [52] · USA	OD: Swallowing disturbance (screening followed by VFSS) Diagnosis: PD-diagnostic criteria of the UK Brain Bank Inclusion: 55–85 yrs, same PD medication, >24 MMSE. Exclusion: other neurologic disorders; head/neck cancer	n = 60: - Expiratory muscle strength training (EMST; n = 30) - Sham (n = 30)	EMST/Sham Age years: 66.7 (8.9)/68.5 (10.3) Male: 25/22 Hoehn & Yahr stage 2.5: 8/13, stage 3: 14/8 Unified Parkinson's Disease Rating Scale III motor total: 39.4 (9.2)/40.0 (8.5)

Table 2. Cont.

Study • Country	OD (Definition/Terminology; Diagnostic Measure/Method) • Diagnosis • Main Inclusion/Exclusion Criteria	Sample (N) • Groups (n) [a]	Group Descriptive (Mean ± SD) (Age, Gender, Relevant Medical Diagnoses)
Wakabayashi, et al. [53] • Japan	OD: Dysphagia, Eating Assessment Tool (EAT-10) score ≥3 points Diagnosis: NR (Community-dwelling, ≥65 yrs) Inclusion: Receiving long-term care via day-service or day-care program, mild cognitive impairment/dementia Exclusion: Severe or moderate dementia, inability to perform training	n = 91: - Intervention group, resistance training of swallowing muscles (n = 43) - Control group (n = 48)	Intervention/Control Age, years: 80 (7)/79 (7) Male: 19/28 Tongue pressure (kPa): 23.3 (8.3)/23.3 (10.0) EAT-10, median (IQR): 7 (5–13)/8 (4–11) Barthel Index: 81 (9)/81 (21)
Woisard, et al. [54] • France	OD: Dysphagia- by Deglutition Handicap Index (DHI) Diagnosis: NR. (Sitting abnormality- by seated postural control measure, SPCM) Inclusion: >18 years; DHI score >11, score >0 on 1 item SPCM, chronic dysphagia. Exclusion: NR	n = 56: - Group without device (D−) (n = 30) [Denoted as 'Woisard et al. (2020b)' in Figure 4.] - Group with the device (D+) (n = 26) [Denoted as 'Woisard et al. (2020a)' in Figure 4.]	D−/D+ Age, years (total sample): 61.5 (11.8) Male, n (total sample): 35 Degenerative dysphagia, N (total sample): 24 NIHSS: 1.3 (1.4)/1.3 (1.6) PAS: 1.7 (1.3)/1.9 (1.9) FOIS: 6.0 (0.9)/5.8 (1.1)
Zhang and Ju [55] • China	OD: Swallowing dysfunction (water swallow test upon inclusion) Diagnosis: Stroke Inclusion: Swallowing dysfunction exclusion: NR (admitted patients with dysphagia)	n = 120: - Intervention, nursing intervention (n = 60) - Control, conventional nursing service (n = 60)	Control/intervention Age, years: 70.6 (7.4)/70.3 (7.4) Males: 33/32

[a] Terminology as used by author(s). Notes. ABI = Acquired brain injury; BDI = Beck Depression Inventory; BDST = Burke Dysphagia Screening Test; CVA = cerebrovascular accident; DOSS = Dysphagia Outcome and Severity scale; FEES = Fiberoptic Endoscopic Evaluation of Swallowing; FOIS = Functional Oral Intake Scale; GCS = Glasgow Coma Scale; H&Y disability score = Hoehn and Yahr disability score; K-MMSE or MMSE-K = Mini-mental examination Korean version; K- NIHSS = Korean version of National Institute of Health Stroke Scale; MASA = Mann Assessment of Swallowing Ability; MBS = Modified Barium Swallow; MIE = Minimally Invasive Oesophagectomy; MDTP = McNeill Dysphagia Therapy Program; MMSE = Mini-Mental State Examination; MOCA = Montreal Cognitive Assessment; NIHSS = National Institute of Health Stroke Scale; NMES = Neuromuscular Electrical stimulation; NR = Not reported; OD = Oropharyngeal dysphagia; PAS = Penetration-Aspiration Scale; PD = Parkinson's disease; P-DHI = Persian Dysphagia Handicap Index; PDQ-39: Parkinson's Disease Questionnaire-39; PNF = proprioceptive neuromuscular facilitation; RCT = Randomised Controlled Trial; SLP = Speech-Language Pathology; SRS = Swallowing Rating Scale; SSA = Standardized Swallowing Assessment; SIS-6 = Swallowing Impairment Score; SWAL-QOL = Swallow Quality-of-Life Questionnaire; tDCS = transcranial Direct Current Stimulation; UC = Usual Care; VDS = Video-fluoroscopic Dysphagia Scale; VFSS = Video-Fluoroscopic Swallowing Study; WHO = World Health Organisation; WST = Water Swallow Test; TWST = Timed Water-Swallow Test.

Table 3. Outcome of behavioural interventions for people with oropharyngeal dysphagia.

Study	Intervention Goal	Intervention Agent, Delivery and Dosage [a]	Materials and Procedures [a]	Outcome Measures	Treatment Outcome [a]
Ayres et al. [19]	To verify the effectiveness of a manoeuvre application in swallowing therapy in patients with PD.	*Intervention agent*: NR *Dosage*: Experimental group: chin-down manoeuvre and swallowing orientation: 4 sessions per week (30 min each). Orientation group: Swallowing orientation only: 4 sessions per week (30 min each).	Three groups: Experimental group: Chin-down posture manoeuvre (patient instructed to swallow lowering the head until chin touches in the neck'). Patients performed manoeuvre twice a day, swallowing saliva, during meals, throughout the week, at home. Patients were given a form to record the number of times the manoeuvre was performed at home. Patients also given instructions for optimal feeding and swallowing related to 'swallowing orientations': (1) environment during feeding (2) posture (3) meal-time (4) oral hygiene. Written instructions given. Orientation group: Patients also given instructions for optimal feeding and swallowing related to 'swallowing orientations': (1) environment during feeding (2) posture (3) meal-time (4) oral hygiene. Written instructions given. Control group: No intervention received during 4-week period. Written instructions given.	*Primary outcomes*: FEES; Clinical evaluation (checking 21 signs and symptoms of oropharyngeal dysphagia and rating these as present or absent); FOIS; SWAL-QOL.	Experimental group showed significant improvement in clinical evaluation of dysphagia compared to two other groups regarding solid ($p = < 0.001$) and liquid ($p = 0.022$). Analysis of FEES did not show differences between groups. Experimental group presented with significant improvement in scores of domains frequency of symptoms ($p = 0.029$) and mental health ($p = 0.004$) on the SWAL-QOL when compared with the groups that did not receive intervention.
Carnaby et al. [20]	Compare standard low-intensity and high-intensity behavioural interventions with usual care (UC) for dysphagia	*Intervention agent*: Speech pathologist (Low/high intensity); physician and speech pathologist when referred (UC) *Dosage (average)*: Swallowing sessions = 8.1, treatment days = 15.3, duration of session = 21.6 min	UC (control): Physician management. Patient referred to hospital speech pathology if needed. Treatment- feeding supervision, safe swallowing. If prescribed–VFSS. Standard low-intensity: Swallowing techniques, environmental modifications (upright for feeding); safe swallowing advice (eating rate); dietary modification (speech pathologist, 3 times per wk for 1 month. Strategies VFSS. Standard high-intensity: Direct swallowing exercises (effortful swallow, supraglottic swallow technique), dietary modification (from speech pathologist, daily for 1 month. Swallowing exercises established by examination and VFSS.	*Primary outcomes*: return to pre stroke diet < 6 months *Secondary outcomes*: time to return to normal diet, proportion recovered, functional swallowing, dysphagia-related complications, died, were institutionalised, or dependent in daily living 6 months post stroke.	Compared with usual care and low-intensity therapy, high-intensity therapy was associated with an increased proportion of patients who returned to a normal diet ($p = 0.04$) and recovered swallowing ($p = 0.02$) by 6 months.
Carnaby et al. [21]	Effectiveness and safety of exercise based swallowing therapy and neuromuscular electrical stimulation for dysphagia	*Intervention agent*: NMES & MDTP-Speech pathologists, >5 years dysphagia experience. UC-experienced therapist *Dosage*: 1 h/day × 3 wks (15 sessions)	McNeill Dysphagia Therapy Program (MDTP): Exercise-based swallowing–criteria for initial oral bolus materials for therapy and advancement on 11-step "food hierarchy". Simple swallowing. Clinicians monitor each swallow. Neuromuscular Electrical stimulation (NMES): VitalStim®. Active NMES/sham, common single electrode placement-midline above hyoid bone to superior to cricoid cartilage/-ascending amplitude until amplitude reached. Usual care treatment control (UC): Behavioural swallowing treatment strategies common in dysphagia treatment.	*Primary outcomes*: Ability to swallow (MASA), oral intake (FOIS). *Secondary outcomes*: Barium swallow outcomes, self-perceived swallowing, weight, time to pre-stroke diet, complications.	Post treatment dysphagia severity significant between groups ($p \leq 0.01$), MDTP greater change vs. NMES or UC for increased oral intake ($p \leq 0.02$), functional outcomes at 3-mnths (RR = 1.7, 1.0–2.8), earlier time for "return to pre-stroke diet" ($p < 03$).
Choi et al. [22]	Effects of Shaker exercise on aspiration and oral diet	*Intervention agent*: Caregiver (SE), occupational therapist (CDT) *Dosage*: 30 min/day, 5 days/wk × 4 wks	Shaker Exercise (SE): Isometric and isokinetic movements. 3 head lifts held for 60 s in supine; 60 s rest. 30 reps head lifts observe toes without raising shoulders–without hold. Conventional Dysphagia Therapy (CDT): Orofacial muscle exercises, thermal tactile stimulation, therapeutic/compensatory manoeuvres.	*Primary outcomes*: PAS from VFSS. *Oral diet level* by FOIS.	Experimental group greater improvement on PAS ($p < 0.05$) and FOIS ($p < 0.05$) vs. control group.

Table 3. Cont.

Study	Intervention Goal	Intervention Agent, Delivery and Dosage [a]	Materials and Procedures [a]	Outcome Measures	Treatment Outcome [a]
DePippo et al. [23]	Effect of graded intervention on occurrence of dysphagia related complications	Intervention agent: Dysphagia therapist (SLP?) Dosage: Bi-weekly session monitoring for all groups	Group A–Patient-managed diet. One session-therapist recommended diet based on MBS results and compensatory swallowing techniques. Patient chose diet (regular vs. graded). Group B–Therapist-prescribed diet (MBS) and swallowing techniques, evaluated every other week. Group C–Therapist prescribed diet and daily reinforcement of swallowing techniques through mealtime dysphagia group.	Primary outcomes: Dysphagia related complications: Pneumonia, dehydration, calorie-nitrogen deficit, recurrent upper airway obstruction, and death.	No significance between groups for time until end inpatient stay or to 1-year post. Only significance was patients in group B developed pneumonia sooner than group A.
Eom et al. [24]	Effect of resistance Expiratory Muscle Strength Training (EMST) on swallowing function	Intervention agent: NR Dosage: 5 days p/wk × 4 wks, 5 sets of 5 breaths on device × 25 p/day. Both groups treatment 30 min × 5 days/wk × 4 wk	Experimental group (EMST + Conventional treatment): Portal Expiratory Muscle Strength Trainer (EMST150). Patients opened mouth after inhalation, EMST mouthpiece between lips. Blew strongly and rapidly until pressure release valve within EMST device opens. Pressure release set to open if pressure target exceeded. <1-min break after each session, for muscle fatigue and dizziness. Placebo group (Sham EMST + Conventional treatment): Trained using a sham non-functional EMST device with no loading device. Conventional treatment.	Primary outcomes: VDS and PAS based on a VFSS to analyse oropharyngeal swallowing function.	Experimental significant in VDS pharyngeal phase ($p = 0.02$ and 0.01) and PAS vs. placebo ($p = 0.01$). Both significant VDS all phases (all $p < 0.05$). Experimental only significant in PAS ($p = 0.01$ vs. 0.102).
Gao and Zhang [25]	Effects of rehabilitation training on dysphagia and psychological state	Intervention agent: NR Dosage: 3 sessions/actions performed morning, midday and evening. 7 days p/wk × 42 days	All patients received routine treatment including internal medicine, traditional rehabilitation and routine nursing. Control: Traditional tongue and mouth exercises. Each movement repeated 10 times as one session. Shaker exercise: Supine position, single action raised head to look at feet. 30 reps = set of actions. Perform 3 sets of actions-continuously or with 1-min relaxation until complete. (Denoted as 'Goa & Zhang, 2017a' in Figure 5.) Chin Tuck Against Resistance (CTAR) exercise: Patients seated tucking chin to compress inflatable rubber ball for 30 reps = set of actions. Perform 3 sets, continuously or with relaxation. (Denoted as 'Goa & Zhang, 2017b' in Figure 5.)	Primary outcomes: Dysphagia: VFSS at baseline, 2, 4, 6 wks post. Swallowing function, PAS Psychological state: Self-Rating Depression Scale (SDS) baseline, 6 wks post.	Degrees of dysphagia improvement, between 2–4 wks in CTAR and Shaker. Significantly higher in CTAR (87%) and Shaker (77%) vs. control (43%) (all $p < 0.05$). Significantly lower SDS in CTAR vs. Shaker/control 6 wks post (all $p < 0.05$).
Guillén-Solà et al. [26]	Effectiveness of inspiratory/expiratory muscle training (IEMT) and neuromuscular electrical stimulation (NMES)	Intervention agent: Occupational, speech, physical therapist Dosage: Control- 3 hrs p/day × 5 days wk × 3 wks. Group 2-2 × p/day, 5 days × 3 wks. Group 3-40-min daily sessions (5 days per wk × 3 wks)	Control/SST: Multidisciplinary inpatient rehabilitation for mobility, activities of daily living, swallowing and communication. Education self-management of dysphagia, oral exercises and compensatory techniques based on VFSS. EMST + SST: Inspiratory/Expiratory Muscle Training (EMST)-respiratory training, 5 sets of 10 respirations, 1 min unloaded recovery breathing, with therapist. Pressure 30% of maximal expiratory pressures increased weekly. NMES + Sham EMST + SST: Sham respiratory muscle training, fixed at 10 cmH2O. Neuromuscular electrical stimulation using VitalStim device. Supervision by speech therapist, electrodes on suprahyoid muscles 80 Hz of transcutaneous electrical stimulus, patients to swallow when felt muscle contraction.	Primary outcomes: Dysphagia severity by PAS. Respiratory muscle strength (maximal inspiratory and expiratory pressures). Post- and 3-month follow-up.	Maximal respiratory pressures most improved Group 2: treatment effect 12.9 (CI 4.5–21.2) and 19.3 (CI 8.5–30.3) for maximal inspiratory and expiratory pressures. Swallowing security improved in Groups 2 and 3. PAS and complications-no between group difference 3-months.

Table 3. Cont.

Study	Intervention Goal	Intervention Agent, Delivery and Dosage [a]	Materials and Procedures [a]	Outcome Measures	Treatment Outcome [a]
Hägglund et al. [27]	Effect of oral neuromuscular training among older people in intermediate care with impaired swallowing	*Intervention agent*: Dental hygienists and speech pathologist *Dosage*: NR	*Intervention (IQoro® + Usual care)*: The device IQoro® was used for oral neuromuscular training. The device is designed to stimulate sensory input and strengthen the facial, oral, and pharyngeal muscles. Professionals provided training instructions. If participants had difficulties performing training, staff or family members were instructed on how to assist. *Control (Usual care)*: Usual care with adjustments in food consistencies and posture instructions.	Primary outcomes: Swallowing rate (timed water swallow test) Secondary outcomes: Signs of aspiration during water swallow, swallowing related quality of life (QOL).	Swallowing rate significant improvement, intervention vs. controls post ($p = 0.01$), 6 months following ($p = 0.03$). Aspiration significantly reduced in intervention vs. controls ($p = 0.01$). QoL: no between-group differences
Hägglund et al. [28]	To determine the effects of neuromuscular training on swallowing function in patients with stroke and dysphagia.	*Intervention agent*: Discipline NR *Dosage*: Neuromuscular training = 3 times per session and 3 times daily before eating Orofacial sensory vibration stimulation was performed 3 times daily before meals. 5 weeks of training in total.	Group A-Orofacial sensory-vibration stimulation: Patients received 5 weeks of continued oro-facial sensory vibration stimulation using an Oral B® electric toothbrush. Instructions given on how to stimulate the buccinator mechanism, lips, external floor, tongue. Group B-Orofacial sensory-vibration stimulation + oral neuromuscular training (Muppy®): Patients received oral neuromuscular training for 5 weeks + oro-facial sensory vibration stimulation 1) Oral device (Muppy®) was used for oral neuromuscular training that aims to stimulate sensory input and strengthen facial, oral, pharyngeal muscles. Muppy® is placed pre-dentally behind closed lips and pt sits in horizontal position. Patients hold device against a gradually increasing horizontal pulling force for 5–10 s whilst trying to resist the force by tightening the lips (2) oro-facial sensory stimulation of buccinator using electric toothbrush. Verbal, practical and written instructions about training given. Patient/caregiver reported training in a log-book. All patients in both groups self-administered or were assisted by relatives or ward staff in oro-facial sensory vibratory stim.	*Primary outcome*: Changes in swallowing rate measured by the Timed Water Swallow Test (TWST). *Secondary outcomes*: changes in lip force measured by lip-force test + swallowing dysfunction as measured by VFS (in lateral projection).	Swallowing rate: After intervention, both groups had improved significantly (Group B, $p < 0.001$; Group A, $p = 0.0001$) in TWST, but no significant between-group difference in swallowing rate. At 12 month follow-up, Group2 had improved significantly in swallowing rate compared to Group A ($p = <0.032$) Lip force: Significant improvement in lip force in Group 2 ($p < 0.001$) compared to non-significant improvement in Group 1 ($p = 0.079$). Improvement in Group 2 maintained at 12 month follow up.
Hwang et al. [29]	Effect of tongue stretching exercises (TSE) on tongue motility and oromotor function in patients with dysphagia after stroke.	*Intervention agent*: TDT/TSE by occupational therapists. *Dosage*: TSE-5 × p/wk × 4 wks. Stretching 20 × p/day.	*Control group*: Traditional Dysphagia Treatment (TDT)– oral facial massage, thermal-tactile stimulation, compensatory skill straining. Both groups received TDT. *Experimental group*: +Tongue Stretching Exercise (TSE); dynamic/static stretching exercises (20 reps each). Dynamic-therapist pulled patient's tongue to end feel point of ROM and held for 2–3 s before guiding back to mouth. Static-therapist pulled tongue to end feel point, held 20 s.	Primary outcomes: *Oromotor function*-Oral phase events of VDS, VFSS *Tongue motility*-Distance from lower lip to tip of tongue during maximum protrusion of the tongue.	Experimental significant differences in tongue motility, bolus formation, tongue to palate, bolus loss, oral transit time-oral VDS phase ($p < 0.05$ for all). Control significant for lip closure only ($p < 0.05$).
Jakobsen et al. [30]	Effect of the intensification of the nonverbal facilitation of swallowing on dysphagia.	*Intervention agent*: Occupational therapist *Dosage*: 30 sessions (10-min rest, 20-min session, 10-min rest), 3 wks (2 × /day).	*Experimental treatment*: Facial Oral Tract Therapy (F.O.T.T.) concept-rehabilitation intervention using structured tactile input and nonverbal facilitation techniques (to allow for effective function in meaningful daily life activities). *Control group*: Treatment comprised stimulating activities in the facial oral tract similar to those of the intervention group but without facilitation of swallowing or verbal request to swallow.	Primary outcomes: FOIS, PAS, and electrophysiological swallowing specific parameters (EMBI).	Intervention feasible. PAS and FOIS improved in both groups, no group differences. Swallowing specific parameters reflected clinically observed changes.

Table 3. Cont.

Study	Intervention Goal	Intervention Agent, Delivery and Dosage [a]	Materials and Procedures [a]	Outcome Measures	Treatment Outcome [a]
Jang et al. [31]	Effects of Mechanical Inspiration and Expiration (MIE) exercise using mechanical cough assist on velopharyngeal incompetence	Intervention agent: NR Dosage: 20 sessions Both groups, 30 min 2 × day, 5 × wk × 2 wks.	Study group MIE exercise: CNS-100 Cough Assist® and conventional swallowing rehabilitation. Inspiration- positive pressure 15–20 cm H2O, increased to 40 cm H2O for 2 s. Expiration–similar pressure 10–20 cm H2O above positive pressure; held 3–6 s, simulating airflow during cough. Patient coordinated respiratory rhythm to cough assist machine. Control: Conventional dysphagia rehabilitation of oral motor and sensory stimulation, NMES, oral exercises for safe swallow.	Primary outcomes: Swallowing function American Speech-Language-Hearing association scale, functional dysphagia score, and PAS, VFSS. Coughing function-peak cough flow.	Study group significant improvement in functional dysphagia score- nasal penetration degree. Nasal penetration degree and peak cough flow showed greater improvement in study vs. control group.
Jeon et al. [32]	To investigate the effects of NMES plus upper spine cervical mobilisation on forward head posture, and swallowing in stroke patients with dysphagia.	Intervention agent: Joint mobilisation was performed by a physical therapist (with over 160 h of manual therapy education. NMES was delivered by 3 experienced OTs. Dosage: once a day, 3 × times a week, for 4 weeks; both groups received NMES for 30 min; experimental group received 10 min of upper cervical spine mobilisation; control group received 10 min of sham mobilisation.	All interventions were performed in sitting position. NMES: Intervention group received upper cervical spine (C1–2) mobilisation with NMES. Mobilisation: Therapist used one hand to hold the subject's C1 (atlas); other hand placed on subject's occiput. Mobilisation force could not be standardised. NMES was applied to the suprahyoid using VitalStim®. Electrodes attached to the motor point of the suprahyoid muscles (digastric) to induce anterior excursion and vertical elevation movements of hyoid bone during normal swallowing. Stimulation was applied by gradually increasing the intensity to the level that patients felt a grabbing sensation in the neck without pain or laryngospasm. Control group: Patients received upper cervical spine sham mobilisation combined with NMES.	Primary outcome: Forward head posture measured by CCFT (Stabilizer ™ Pressure Biofeedback) and craniovertebral angle (CVA). Swallowing function measured by VFS and PAS.	The intervention group showed significantly better scores in CCFT ($p = 0.05$) and in CVA ($p = 0.05$) than in control group. PAS scores were significantly better in the intervention group compared to control group ($p = < 0.05$). Significant increase in VFS total score and PAS than in the control group ($p = < 0.05$)
Kim et al. [33]	The effects of Proprioceptive Neuromuscular Facilitation (PNF) on swallowing function of stroke pts with dysphagia	Intervention agent: NR Dosage: PNF-based short neck exercises 3 times a week for 30 min each time for 6 weeks	Experimental group: PNF 1. Patients started by lying on a bed with head and neck positioned off the bed (tester supported left laryngeal region with his right hand and placed left fingertips below patient's jaw) 2. Patient instructed to look at target object in a direction 15 degrees diagonally to the right side 3. Tester then initiated given exercises by moving the patient's neck in a diagonal direction opposite to the direction specified 4. Patient instructed to 'draw your jaw inward' and tester applied a level of resistance to the patients jaw to fully activate neck flexor below jaw (rotation to the right) 5. Same exercises applied in opposite direction. Control group: Shaker exercise 1. Isometric exercises: Patients lay on bed and raised their heads without moving shoulders off the bed, looked at ends of their feet for 60 s, and then lowered heads back on the bed. If patient had difficulty raising his/her head, they were asked to perform same exercise for 3 times for as long as they could. Isotonic exercises: Patients raised their head in same posture and looked at the ends of their feet 30 consecutive times.	Primary outcome: New VFSS and ASHA NOMS Scales.	Statistically significant improvements in: premature bolus loss, residue in the valleculae, laryngeal evaluation, epiglottic closure, residue in pyriform sinuses, coating of pharyngeal wall after swallowing, pharyngeal transit time and aspiration on both new VFSS scale and ASHA NOMS scale ($p < 0.05$). Control group also demonstrated statistically significant improvements in premature bolus loss, residue in the valleculae, laryngeal evaluation, epiglottic closure, residue in pyriform sinuses, pharyngeal transit time and aspiration ($p < 0.05$). No statistically significant differences between the groups were found in new VFSS scale and ASHA NOMS scale.

Table 3. Cont.

Study	Intervention Goal	Intervention Agent, Delivery and Dosage [a]	Materials and Procedures [a]	Outcome Measures	Treatment Outcome [a]
Kim and Park [34]	Effect of modified chin tuck against resistance (mCTAR) exercise on patients with post-stroke dysphagia.	*Intervention agent:* Occupational therapist *Dosage:* 30 min × 5 days a week, for 6 weeks	*Experimental group mCTAR exercise:* PhagiaFLEX-HF device. Subject seated, fixed part of device to desk, firmly attach chin surface under chin. Exercise performed in isotonic/isometric. Isometric- holding chin down for 10 s against resistance. Isotonic-30 × reps chin-down against resistance. (10 s, 3 times). *Traditional dysphagia treatment (TDT):* Oral facial massage, thermal-tactile stimulation and compensatory training.	*Primary outcomes: Aspiration and oral diet* -PAS and FOIS. *Secondary outcomes:* Rate of *nasogastric tube removal* was analysed.	Experimental statistically significant improvement in PAS and FOIS vs. control ($p < 0.001$). Rates of nasogastric tube removal were 25% (experimental) vs. 15% (control).
Koyama et al. [35]	Feasibility and effectiveness newly developed Modified Jaw Opening Exercise (MJOE) in poststroke patients with pharyngeal residue.	*Intervention agent:* Speech pathologist/physician *Dosage:* 4 × sets daily, 5 × p/wk × 6 wks. (6 s × 5 reps = 1 set)	*Intervention MJOE:* Surface electrodes mandibular midline. Participants closed mouth, sitting position, pressed tongue against hard palate. Trainer hand under participant's chin and applied upward vertical resistance. Visual feedback given. Maintained 80% Maximum Voluntary Contraction (MVC). *Control sham exercise isometric jaw closing exercise:* Surface electrodes to masseter, visual feedback, 20% MVC.	*Primary outcomes:* VFSS was performed before and after exercise. The distance between the mental spine and the hyoid bone (DMH) and hyoid displacement (HD) were measured.	No temporomandibular joint or neck pain. Intervention group, DMH decrease where anterior HD ended and an increase in anterior HD were seen. Control, no changes.
Krajczy et al. [36]	Effects of dysphagia therapy in patients in the early post-stroke period.	*Intervention agent:* Physiotherapist *Dosage:* Physiotherapy program average 60 min × day, × 15 days	*Control/both groups:* Safe food education and neurological physiotherapy depending on patient dysfunction. Therapy included passive, assisted, supported and respiration exercises, erect posture, walking re-education, and training on NDT Bobath and PNF methods. *Study group:* +original dysphagia treatment, restoring chewing and swallowing functionality–Strengthening and breathing exercises and thermal stimulation.	*Primary outcomes: Swallowing function* - Timed test of swallowing *Swallowing reflux* – Controlled swallowing after swallowing blended food. Reflex categorised as good or delayed.	*Swallowing reflux, Cough and voice quality and swallowing time, number of swallows* and SpO2 All Statistically significant differences between groups after therapy ($p = <0.01$).
Kyodo et al. [37]	To evaluate the effectiveness of puree diets containing a gelling agent for the prevention of aspiration pneumonia in elderly patients with moderate to severe dysphagia.	*Intervention agent:* Gastroenterologists experienced in transnasal endoscopy along with a speech therapist evaluated swallowing. Discipline who created gelling agent (intervention) NR. *Dosage (average):* NR	Patients underwent endoscopic swallowing evaluation while sitting in a chair/sitting up in bed. Images of oropharynx and larynx were displayed on a monitor and recorded on digital video recorder. Pureed diet *without* gelling agent was made by mixing 100 g of white rice and 50 mL of water with a blender for one minute. Texture characteristics (IDDSI Level 4) were: hardness, 1760 ± 125 N/m²; cohesiveness, 0.59 ± 0.03; adhesiveness, 224 ± 56 J/m³. Pureed diet *with* gelling agent was made by mixing 100 g of rice porridge at > 70 degrees with 0.5 g of the gelling agent with a blender for one minute. Texture characteristics (IDDSI Level 4) were: hardness, 312 ± 11.3 N/m²; cohesiveness, 0.81 ± 0.02; adhesiveness, 108 ± 5.8 J/m³.	*Primary outcome:* Presence of material in throat using endoscopic cyclic ingestion score (0 to 4) *Secondary outcomes:* Sense of material remaining in the throat after swallowing of pureed rice and/or test jelly; degree of dysphagia using Hyodo-Komagane score (0 to 12: mild 0–3; moderate 4–7; severe 8–9)	Residuals in throat were significantly less likely with pureed rice than without the gelling agent (median cyclic ingestion score (range); 1 (0–4) vs. 2 (0–4); $p = 0.001$. Irrespective of presence or absence of the gelling agent, the sense of materials in the throat was significantly less frequent in older patients ($p = <0.01$). No adverse events occurred.
Logemann et al. [38]	3 treatments for aspiration on thin liquids—chin-down posture, nectar-thickened liquids, or honey-thickened Liquids.	*Intervention agent:* Speech pathologist *Dosage:* NR	*Chin-down intervention:* chin to the front of the neck, three swallows of 3 mL of thin liquid from a spoon and three swallows of the same liquid from an 8-oz cup filled with 6 oz of liquid. *Nectar* or *Honey-thickened liquids:* on the two thickened liquid interventions, three swallows of 3 mL of thickened liquid from a spoon and three self-regulated swallows, performed as separate swallows, each from an 8-oz cup filled with 6 oz of the thickened liquid.	*Primary outcomes: Swallowing function*-VFSS	49% aspirated all interventions, 25% not any. More on thin liquids despite chin-down posturing vs. using nectar-($p < 0.01$) or honey-thickened ($p < 0.01$). More on nectar- vs. honey thickened ($p < 0.01$).

Table 3. Cont.

Study	Intervention Goal	Intervention Agent, Delivery and Dosage [a]	Materials and Procedures [a]	Outcome Measures	Treatment Outcome [a]
Manor et al. [39]	Effectiveness of visual information while treating swallowing disturbances in patients with PD.	*Intervention agent:* Speech and swallowing therapist. *Dosage:* Each group 5 × 30 min sessions, during 2-wk period and a 6th session 4 wks after the 5th one.	*Control—conventional therapy:* Both interventions swallowing exercises and compensatory therapy based on FEES. Compensatory strategies carried out with different food and liquid consistencies in clinic, patient practiced at home. *VAST:* video-assisted tool during each session, for educating and assisting understanding structure of swallowing. Patients observed a normal swallowing process and their distorted one. After learning compensatory technique, patient practiced it during drinking and eating in the clinic after observing video then at home. During next four sessions patients observed video with suitable compensatory swallowing technique while eating and drinking focusing on the new swallowing behaviour.	*Primary outcomes:* Swallowing function—by fiberoptic endoscopic evaluation of swallowing (FEES). Quality of life—quality of care and degree of pleasure from eating assessed by questioners.	Significant improvement in swallowing functions both groups. FEES significantly greater reduction in food residues in pharynx in VAST vs. conventional treatment group. SWAL-QOL scores significant between groups favour of VAST: burden, eating desire, social functioning, mental health, symptom frequency ($p < 0.01$).
Mepani et al. [40]	Effect of the Shaker exercise on thyrohyoid muscle Shortening improve pharyngeal dysphagia	*Intervention agent:* Speech pathologist *Dosage:* Biweekly 45-min therapy sessions for 6 weeks.	*Traditional therapy:* 5 times daily. Laryngeal and tongue ROM exercises and swallowing manoeuvres (Super-Supraglottic Swallow, Mendelsohn Manoeuvre, Effortful Swallow). Shaker Exercise: 3 times per day for 6 weeks. Isometric and isokinetic head-lift in supine position. Patients raised head high and forward to observe toes. Isokinetic–3 times head lifts held 60 s, 60-s rest period. Isometric–30 head lifts at constant velocity, performed without holding or rest periods.	*Primary outcomes:* Change in thyrohyoid muscle shortening by Videofluoroscopy	After therapy, the percent change in thyrohyoid distance in the Shaker Exercise group was significantly greater vs. traditional therapy ($p = 0.034$).
Moon et al. [41]	Effects of Tongue pressure strength and accuracy training (TPSAT) on tongue pressure strength, swallowing function, and quality of life in stroke patients with dysphagia.	*Intervention agent:* Occupational therapist *Dosage:* TPSAT and traditional dysphagia therapy 30 min × day; Only traditional therapy performed 30 min × twice daily. Both groups, daily 5 × times wk × 8 wks.	Both groups received standardized physical/occupational therapies. *Traditional dysphagia therapy:* thermal tactile stimulation, Mendelsohn manoeuvre, effortful swallow, diet modification. *TPSAT with traditional dysphagia treatment:* TPSAT consisted of an anterior and posterior isometric tongue strength exercise and an isometric tongue accuracy exercise. The protocol involved five sets of tongue-to-palate presses, 6 reps per set for each session. Isometric tongue accuracy exercise, amplitudes were set at 50, 75, 100% of maximum pressure from first isometric strength. Participants generated precise pressures within 10 kPa error for each amplitude.	*Primary outcomes:* Tongue pressure strength—maximum isometric tongue pressures (MIPs) of anterior, posterior tongue using Iowa Oral Performance Instrument. Swallowing function—MASA; QoL-SWAL-QOL	TPSAT with traditional dysphagia significantly improved MASA, SWAL-QOL, and MIPs. Traditional dysphagia significantly increased MASA, SWAL-QOL, and MIPs anteriorly ($p < 0.05$). TPSAT significant in anterior, posterior MIPs, tongue movement MASA, vs. controls ($p < 0.05$).
Park et al. [42]	Effects of EMST on the activity of suprahyoid muscles, aspiration and dietary stages in stroke patients with dysphagia.	*Intervention agent:* Occupational therapist *Dosage:* 5 days × wk × 4 wks. 5 sets × 5 breaths on device, 25 breaths per day.	*Experimental group:* resistance set at 70% range of MEP (Maximal Expiratory Pressure). Subjects open mouth following maximum inhalation, and fast until pressure release valve in EMST device opens-strong and fast and fast EMST mouthpiece between lips, close mouth. Blow strong and fast until pressure release valve in EMST device opens-expiratory pressure exceeded set target. *Placebo group:* training using sham device-non-functional device, little effect of physiologic load on targeted muscles.	*Primary outcomes:* Activity in the suprahyoid muscle group -using surface electromyography (sEMG). PAS used to assess VFSS results. Dietary stages-FOIS.	Experimental significantly more in suprahyoid muscle activity ($p = 0.01$), liquid PAS ($p = 0.03$) and FOIS ($p = 0.06$), but not semisolid type PAS ($p = 0.32$), vs. placebo.
Park et al. [43]	Effect of chin tuck against resistance exercise (CTAR) on the swallowing function in patients with dysphagia following subacute stroke.	*Intervention agent:* Occupational therapist *Dosage:* 30 min × day, × 5/wk, × 4 wks	*CTAR:* Isometric CTAR, patients chin tuck against device 3 × 60 s no repetition. Isotonic CTAR, patient 30 reps by strongly pressing against resistance of the device and releasing it. Therapist demonstrated exercise methods. *Conventional dysphagia treatment:* Both groups -orofacial muscle exercises, thermal tactile stimulation, and therapeutic or compensatory manoeuvres.	*Primary outcomes:* Swallowing function—Functional Dysphagia Scale (FDS) and PAS, based on VFSS	Experimental more improvement in oral cavity, laryngeal elevation/epiglottic closure, residue in valleculae, and residue in pyriform sinuses of FDS and PAS compared vs. controls ($p < 0.05$, all).

Table 3. Cont.

Study	Intervention Goal	Intervention Agent, Delivery and Dosage [a]	Materials and Procedures [a]	Outcome Measures	Treatment Outcome [a]
Park et al. [44]	Effects of Effortful Swallowing Training (EST) on tongue strength and swallowing function in patients with stroke.	*Intervention agent:* Occupational therapist *Dosage:* Training 30 min, 5× days per wk × 4 wks. Both groups conventional dysphagia treatment 30 min/day, 5 days/wk × 4 wks.	*Experimental EST:* Patients pushed tongue onto palate, squeezing neck muscles, swallow forcefully. Performed 10 times p/session, 3 sessions p/day. Effortful swallowing confirmed by therapist through visual observation and palpation. *Control group:* Swallow naturally without intentional force. Patients given small spray of water to induce swallowing, and rest. Both groups received conventional dysphagia therapy (compensatory techniques -chin tuck, head tilting, rotation; therapeutic techniques -orofacial muscle exercises, thermal tactile stimulation using ice sticks, expiratory training).	*Primary outcomes:* Tongue strength-Iowa Oral Performance Instrument. Oropharyngeal swallowing function VDS, based on VFSS.	Experimental group greater improvements in anterior and posterior tongue strength vs. control ($p = 0.05$ and 0.04), and greater improvement in oral phases of VDS ($p = 0.02$).
Park et al. [45]	Effects of game-based Chin Tuck against resistance exercise (gbCTAR) and head-lift exercise on swallowing function and compliance in dysphagia post-stroke	*Intervention agent:* Occupational therapist *Dosage:* 5 × wk × 4 weeks. Traditional dysphagia treatment (TDT) 30 min per day	*Experimental group:* performed gbCTAR exercise LES 100 device. Before gbCTAR exercise, 1-RM measured for resistance values. 1-RM, resistance bar placed directly beneath jaw, and chin tuck directed against resistance. gbCTAR exercise at threshold of 70% 1-RM, divided into isometric and isotonic exercises, combined with the game. *Control group:* head lift exercises in supine (isometric and isotonic). Both groups TDT- oral facial massage, thermal-tactile stimulation and compensatory training.	*Primary outcomes:* Swallowing function-VDS and PAS. Dietary assessment-FOIS Compliance with the 2 exercises-(motivation, interest, physical effort, fatigue), numerical rating self-report scale.	No significant between group difference in VDS, PAS, FOIS. Compliance, motivation and interest Scores significantly higher, and scores for physical effort needed and fatigue significantly lower, in experimental vs. control.
Park et al. [46]	Effect of Resistive Jaw Opening Exercise (RJOE) on hyoid bone movement, aspiration, and oral intake level in stroke patients.	*Intervention agent:* Occupational therapist *Dosage:* 30 min × 5 times wk × 4 wks.	*Experimental group:* RJOE device to provide resistance to suprahyoid muscles. Isometric exercise, 30 s with device resistors pressed downward (3 times, 30–60 s of rest). Isotonic exercise repeatedly depressed by RJOE by holding device resistance down for 2–3 s then returned to original state (10 reps, 3 sets) with 30 s rest. *Placebo group:* RJOE using 1-mm thick device with almost no resistance to suprahyoid muscles. Exercise type and frequency of RJOE same as experimental group. Both groups received conventional dysphagia therapy after intervention, which involved orofacial muscle exercises, thermal tactile stimulation and therapeutic or compensatory manoeuvres.	*Primary outcomes:* Hyoid bone movement - by two-dimensional analysis of anterior and superior motion on VFSS. Aspiration-PAS Oral intake level-FOIS.	Both groups significant differences in hyoid movement, PAS, FOIS ($p < 0.05$). No significant difference between groups except for liquid type, PAS. Effect sizes (Cohen's d) 0.6–1.1 for anterior, superior movement of hyoid bone, semisolid and liquid type of PAS, and FOIS respectively.
Ploumis et al. [47]	Evaluate cervical isometric exercises in dysphagic patients with cervical spine alignment disorders due to hemiparesis after stroke.	*Intervention agent:* Allied health *Dosage:* inpatient 12 wks, speech 30 min daily. Experimental-4× reps 10 min, 3× day, 12 wks.	All patients -inpatient program including physiotherapy, occupational and speech therapy. Speech included deglutition muscle strengthening, compensatory techniques. *Experimental group:* +plus cervical isometric strengthening exercises contract neck muscles under resistance forward-backward-sidewards). *Control group:* Regular speech therapy plus sitting balance.	*Primary outcomes:* Cervical spine radiographs in erect (sitting/standing) position coronal, sagittal C2-C7 Cobb angle, VFSS to evaluate deglutition.	Experimental group- more pronounced correction ($p < 0.01$) of cervical alignment in both planes and greater improvement ($p < 0.05$) of deglutition too, than control group.

Table 3. Cont.

Study	Intervention Goal	Intervention Agent, Delivery and Dosage [a]	Materials and Procedures [a]	Outcome Measures	Treatment Outcome [a]
Sayaca et al. [48]	Whether combined isotonic technique of Proprioceptive Neuromuscular Facilitation (PNF) is superior to Shaker exercises in improving function of swallowing muscles.	Intervention agent: Shaker 'CS' (?). PNF physiotherapist Dosage: Each exercise set 1 × per day, 3× wk × 6 wks.	Shaker exercises: isometric (3 reps) and isotonic contractions (30 reps) neck flexor muscles. Patients raised head to observe toes without raising shoulders. Isometric- lifted head, held for 1-min 3 times, 1-min rest. Isotonic- lifted head 30 reps, no holding. PNF: Combined isotonic technique– concentric, stabilizing and eccentric contraction without relaxation. Stabilizing contractions to improve control, force, coordination, and eccentric contraction. Moved head against resistance with open mouth- kept position for 6 s against resistance in seated position; kept position while physiotherapist moved back to initial position. 30 reps per day.	*Primary outcomes:* *Swallowing difficulties* Turkish Eating Assessment Tool (T-EAT-10); *Capacity, volume, and speed of swallowing*-100 mL-water swallow test. *Contraction amplitude changes*–motor unit activity by superficial electromyography.	T-EAT-10 decreased both groups ($p < 0.001$). Water swallowing capacity and volume improved both groups ($p < 0.001$). No change in swallowing speed both groups ($p > 0.05$). Maximal voluntary contraction of suprahyoid muscles higher in PNF vs. Shaker ($p < 0.05$).
Steele et al. [49]	Compare outcomes of two tongue resistance training protocols	Intervention agent: Speech pathologist Dosage: 24 sessions (TPPT or TPSAT), 2–3× wk, 8–12 wks. 60 tongue-pressure tasks per session.	*Tongue-pressure profile training (TPPT):* emphasized pressure-timing patterns that are typically seen in healthy swallows by focusing on gradual pressure release and saliva swallowing tasks. *Tongue- pressure strength and accuracy training (TPSAT):* emphasized strength and accuracy in tongue-palate pressure generation and did not include swallowing tasks.	*Primary outcomes:* Posterior tongue strength, oral bolus control, penetration– aspiration and vallecular residue- VFS, PAS	Both groups significant tongue strength and post-swallow vallecular residue with thin liquids. Stage transition duration (bolus control), PAS no significant differences.
Tang et al. [50]	Effect of rehabilitation therapy on radiation-induced dysphagia and trismus in nasopharyngeal carcinoma (NPC) patients after radiotherapy.	Intervention agent: Therapists, assistants Dosage: Rehabilitation group, exercises 3× per day, each 15 cycles, 45 cycles per day.	Both groups routine treatment. *Rehabilitation group:* training by therapists at hospital, continued at home post-discharge by exercise booklet, guardian oversight and calendar *Exercises: Tongue*-range of motion exercises included passive and active movement exercises. *Pharynx and Larynx*-exercises changing body position to maximize swallow function and minimize aspiration. Swallow manoeuvres included effortful swallow and Mendelsohn manoeuvre. Sensory procedures utilizing pharyngeal cold stimulation performed by therapists. *Exercise for Trismus*– Active jaw movements- opening/closing mouth repeatedly, opening mouth slightly, moving lower mandible to left and right, stretched chin downward and forward and a range of passive jaw movements. *Control group:* No rehabilitation exercises Both groups received routine treatment (e.g., anti inflammatory treatment for aspiration pneumonia)	*Primary outcomes:* *Severity of dysphagia*- water swallow test *Trismus*-LENT/SOMA score and the interincisor distance (IID).	Rehabilitation group only significant improvement in swallowing function. Percentage of patients with effective results in rehabilitation higher than control ($p = 0.02$). Control IID significantly decreased at Post ($p = 0.001$), both groups decreased at 3 months, rehabilitation group less than controls ($p = 0.004$). Trismus in rehabilitation higher vs. control ($p = 0.02$).
Tarameshlu et al. [51]	Effects of Traditional Dysphagia Therapy (TDT) on swallowing function in Multiple Sclerosis (MS) patients with dysphagia.	Intervention agent: Therapist Dosage: both groups 6 weeks, 18 sessions, 3 × per week, every other day.	*Traditional Dysphagia Therapy (TDT):* Includes oral motor control, range of motion exercises, swallowing manoeuvres, strategies to heighten sensory input. *Usual care (UC):* postural changes, modifying volume and speed of food presentation, changing food consistency and viscosity, and improving sensory oral awareness.	*Primary outcomes:* *Swallowing ability*- Mann Assessment of Swallowing Ability (MASA) *Secondary outcomes:* PAS and PRRS.	Groups improved MASA, PAS and PRRS ($p < 0.001$). All significantly greater in TDT vs. UC group. Large effect size MASA in TDT ($d = 3.9$) and UC ($d = 1.1$).

Table 3. Cont.

Study	Intervention Goal	Intervention Agent, Delivery and Dosage [a]	Materials and Procedures [a]	Outcome Measures	Treatment Outcome [a]
Troche et al. [52]	Treatment outcome of device-driven EMST on swallow safety, physiologic measures of swallow timing and hyoid displacement.	*Intervention agent:* Clinician *Dosage:* EMST, 4 weeks, 5 days per week, for 20 min per day, using a calibrated or sham, handheld device.	*Expiratory muscle strength training (EMST):* device set to 75% of participant's average MEP. Visited weekly by clinician-instructed to wear nose clips, deep breath, hold cheeks lightly, blow hard into device, identify air was flowing freely through device (once reached threshold pressure). *Sham:* Sham device identical to EMST device, pressure release valve non-functional and to 75% of participants' average MEP-no physiologic load to muscles.	*Primary outcomes: Swallow function*-judgments of swallow safety, PAS scores, swallow timing, and hyoid movement from VFS images.	EMST improved swallow safety. PA scores vs. sham. EMST improvement of hyolaryngeal function during swallowing, findings not evident for sham group.
Wakabayashi et al. [53]	Effects of resistance training of swallowing muscles in community dwelling older individuals with dysphagia.	*Intervention agent:* Research co-workers *Dosage: intervention* exercises for 10 s; 1 set = 10 reps. 2 sets per day 3× per wk × 3 months	*Control/both groups:* dysphagia brochure (about oral hygiene, tongue resistance exercise, head flexion exercise against manual resistance, nutrition, and food modifications). *Intervention:* resistance exercises for swallowing muscles involving tongue resistance exercise and head flexion against manual resistance. Research co-workers instructed participants once to perform resistance training.	*Primary outcomes:* Improvement in dysphagia -Eating Assessment Tool (EAT-10) score. *Secondary outcomes:* Tongue pressure	Percentage of participants with EAT-10 scores <3 not statistically significantly different between groups $p = 0.6$). Post intervention EAT-10 ($p = 0.7$) and mean tongue pressure ($p = 0.4$).
Boisard et al. [54]	Effect of a personalised transportable folding device for seating on dysphagia	*Intervention agent:* Occupational therapy *Dosage:* 1 × training session with device (D+ group) and without device (D- group).	*D-/All groups:* All patients training session: evaluation of needs, impact of head positioning on swallowing, adapted position of head through body positioning, practice using occupational therapy cushions or personalised transportable folding device for seating (DATP) according to randomisation. *D+ group:* In charge to determine characteristics of the device required so they could have them during the training session. Instruction for patients was to put the personalised instructions into practice by using the device.	*Primary outcomes: quality of swallowing Secondary outcomes: posture, device acceptability, QoL.* Measurement of hyoid bone movement during swallowing. VFSE and questionnaire.	Significantly better posture both groups ($p < 0.001$), more hyoid bone motion in D+ group. Significant mean difference for D+ group vs. D- group. for horizontal and vertical movement. Other swallowing markers not significant.
Zhang and Ju [55]	Clinical improvement of nursing intervention in swallowing dysfunction of elderly stroke patients.	*Intervention agent:* Nursing staff *Dosage:* NR	*Control group:* conventional nursing service that strictly conforms to the doctor's advice. *Nursing intervention:* (1) Psychological intervention, nurses communication with patients/family, evaluates psychological state, encourages and comforts. (2) Health education, nurse introduces knowledge about swallowing dysfunction and effects through videos and images. (3) Rehabilitation exercises, pronunciation training, muscle training, mouth opening exercises, ingestion training, (4) Diet intervention, appropriate foods should be chosen according to specific conditions.	*Primary outcomes: Swallowing dysfunction*–30 mL water drink test *Living quality*-assessment questionnaire of living quality (GQOL-74), includes physical, psychological and social functions, and material life. *Pulmonary infection*–rate *Nursing satisfaction*–self-made questionnaire.	Improved swallowing dysfunction higher in intervention vs. control ($p < 0.05$). Scores of physical, psychological and social functions, and material life and nursing satisfaction higher in intervention vs. control ($p < 0.05$). Pulmonary infection lower in intervention vs. control $p < 0.05$).

[a] Terminology as by authors. *Notes.* CVA = cerebrovascular accident; EMST = Expiratory Muscle Strength Training; FEES = Fiberoptic Endoscopic Evaluation of Swallowing; FOIS = Functional Oral Intake Scale; MASA = Mann Assessment of Swallowing Ability; MBS = Modified Barium Swallow; MIE = Minimally Invasive Oesophagectomy; MDTP = McNeill Dysphagia Therapy Program; MEP = Maximum Expiratory Pressure; NMES = Neuromuscular Electrical stimulation; NR = Not reported; OD = Oropharyngeal dysphagia; PAS = Penetration-Aspiration Scale; PD = Parkinson's disease; P-DHI = Persian Dysphagia Handicap Index; PNF= Proprioceptive Neuromuscular Facilitation; PRRS = Pharyngeal Residue Rating Scale; QoL = Quality of life; RCT = Randomised Controlled Trial; SIS-6 = Swallowing Impairment Score; SWAL-QOL= Swallow Quality-of-Life Questionnaire; VDS= Video-fluoroscopic dysphagia scale; VFSS = Video-Fluoroscopic Swallowing Study; TWST = Timed Water-Swallow Test; VDS = Videofluoroscopic Dysphagia Scale; VFSE = Videofluoroscopic Examination.

Most studies (n = 23) included a comparison group that received a type of dysphagia treatment often referred to as traditional therapy, standard swallow therapy, or conventional dysphagia treatment (CDT). Some studies also used the term usual care for CDT groups. CDT treatment could include counselling and the provision of information about swallowing and dysphagia, compensatory strategies (e.g., bolus modification and adjusted head positioning), rehabilitation, oromotor exercises and/or thermal stimulation. Three studies included a comparison group receiving medical standard care without dysphagia treatment [20,51,56]. In three studies, patients underwent sham dysphagia training [36,43,53]. Several studies compared two or three behavioural interventions without having a CDT or medical standard care group included [33,34,46,49,50,55].

3.3. Risk of Bias Assessment

The Begg and Mazumdar rank correlation procedure produced a tau of 0.305 (two-tailed p = 0.113), indicating there is no evidence of publication bias. This meta-analysis incorporates data from 15 studies, which yield a z-value of 7.528 (two-tailed $p < 0.001$). The fail-safe N is 207. This means that 207 'null' studies need to be located and included for the combined two-tailed p-value to exceed 0.050. That is, there would need to be 13.8 missing studies for every observed study for the effect to be nullified. Both of these procedures (i.e., Begg and Mazumdar rank correlation and fail-safe N) indicate the absence of publication bias.

3.4. Methodological Quality

Risk of bias of the included RCTs was assessed using the RoB 2 tool. Figures 2 and 3 present the risk of bias summary per domain for individual studies and for all included studies. Most studies showed low risk of bias per domain, but more than half of the included studies (19/37) scored overall as having some concerns, with three studies identified as being at high risk.

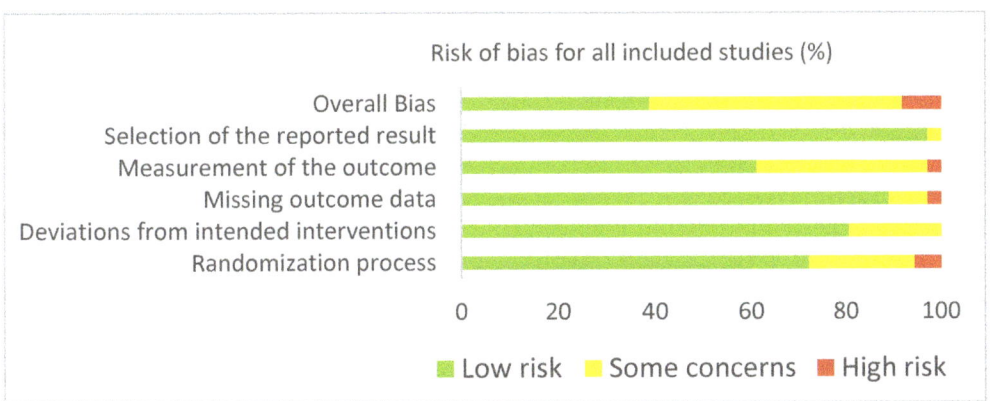

Figure 2. Risk of bias summary for all included studies (n = 37) in accordance with RoB2.

3.5. Meta—Analysis: Effect of Interventions

Twenty-one studies were included in the meta-analyses [21,22,24,25,28–31,34,35,40–46,49,51,52,54]. All study groups were categorised into compensatory interventions, rehabilitative interventions, combined compensatory and rehabilitative interventions, and no dysphagia intervention. Seventeen studies were excluded from meta-analyses: one study included patients with self-reported swallowing difficulties without confirmed OD diagnosis by instrumental assessment (VFSS or FEES) [48], four studies did not report on instrumental or clinical non-instrumental outcome data [20,28,37,40], ten studies provided insufficient data for meta-analysis [21,24,27,34,38,39,48,51,56,57], and two studies were excluded to reduce heterogeneity between studies [32,53].

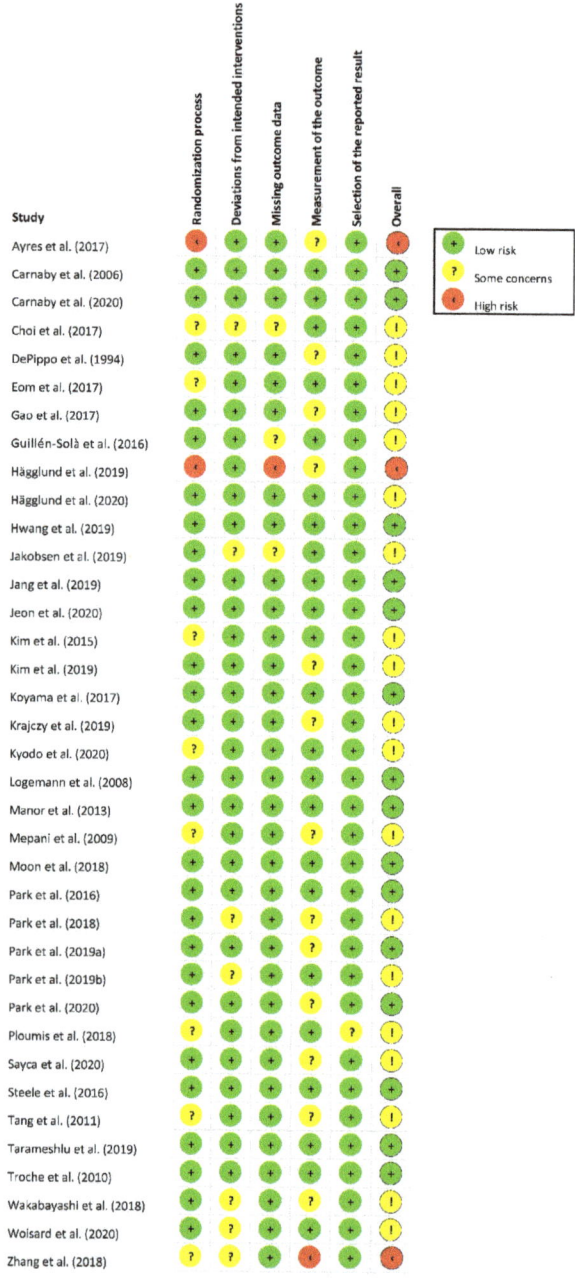

Figure 3. Risk of bias summary for individual studies (n = 37) in accordance with RoB2 [19–55]. *Note.* If one or more yellow or red circles (domains) have been identified for a particular study, the Overall score (last column) shows an exclamation mark, indicating that either the study shows some concerns (yellow circle with exclamation mark) or is at high risk (red circle with exclamation mark).

Overall, within group analysis. (Figure 4). A significant, large pre-post intervention effect size was calculated using a random-effects model ($z(35)$ = 8.047, $p < 0.001$, Hedges' g = 1.139, and 95% CI = 0.862–1.416). Pre-post intervention effects varied greatly between studies, ranging from 0.058 to 5.732. Of the 36 intervention groups included in the meta-analysis, 19 groups showed large effect sizes (Hedges' $g > 0.8$), six groups showed moderate effects sizes ($0.5 <$ Hedges' $g \leq 0.8$), seven groups showed minor effect sizes ($0.2 <$ Hedges' $g \leq 0.5$), and four groups showed negligible effect sizes (Hedges' $g \leq 0.2$). Between-study heterogeneity was significant ($Q(35)$ = 152.938, and $p < 0.001$), with I^2 showing heterogeneity accounted for 77.115% of variation in effect sizes across studies.

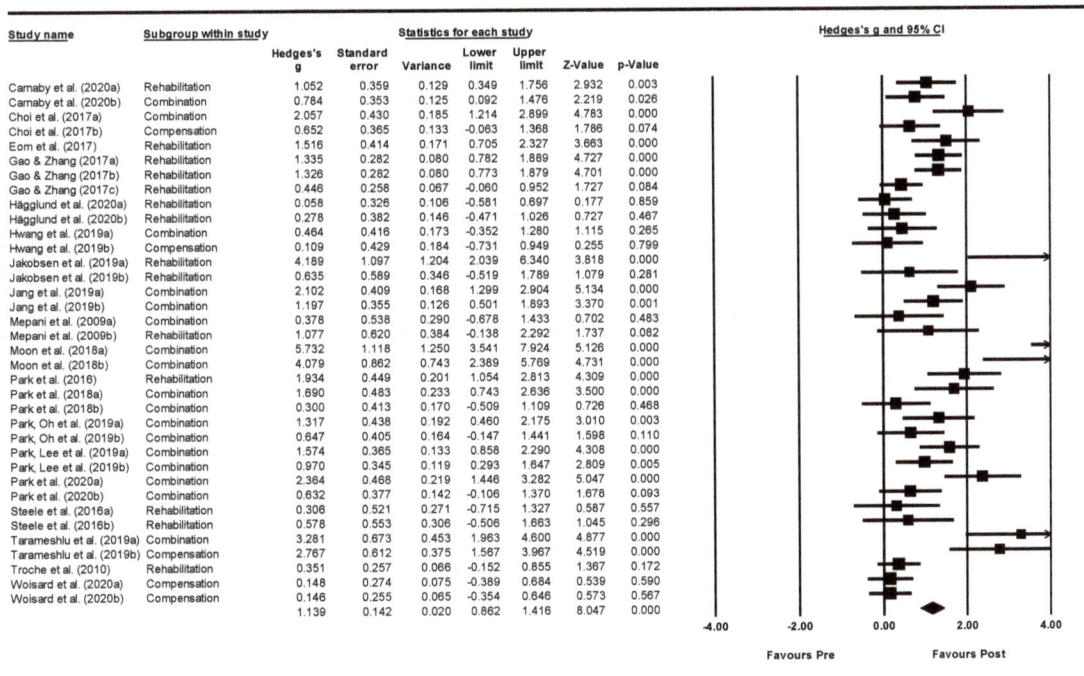

Figure 4. Within intervention group pre-post meta-analysis [21,22,24,25,28–31,40–46,49,51,52,54,56]. *Note.* Refer to Table 2 for explanation of the subgroups.

Between subgroup analyses. Subgroup analyses (Table 4) were conducted comparing different types of interventions: behavioural interventions were compared with conventional dysphagia treatment (CDT), or no dysphagia therapy groups (Figure 5). Both behavioural interventions and CDT were categorised into mainly compensatory, rehabilitative, and combined compensatory and rehabilitative interventions. Overall, significant treatment effects were identified favouring behavioural interventions. In particular, large effect sizes were found when comparing rehabilitative interventions with no CDT, and combined interventions with compensatory CDT. When comparing selected interventions based on commonalities across studies against CDT, significant, large effect sizes were found in favour of Shaker exercise, chin tuck against resistance exercise (CTAR), and expiratory muscle strength training (EMST). Most studies were conducted in stroke populations and showed significant, moderate effect sizes. Comparisons between outcome measures indicated at significant effects for PAS only.

Table 4. Between subgroup meta-analyses comparing intervention groups of included studies.

Subgroup	Hedge's g	Lower Limit CI	Upper Limit CI	Z-Value	p-Value
Intervention type					
Combined vs. CDT (Combined) (n = 5)	0.610	0.263	0.957	3.446	0.001 *
Combined vs. CDT (Compensation) (n = 3)	1.180	0.362	1.998	2.828	0.005 *
Rehabilitation vs. CDT (Combined) (n = 1)	0.019	−0.656	0.659	0.057	0.955
Rehabilitation vs. CDT (Rehabilitation) (n = 3)	0.178	0.304	1.133	3.395	0.001 *
Rehabilitation vs. No CDT (n = 3)	0.842	0.440	1.244	4.110	<0.001 *
Selected interventions					
Shaker vs. CDT (n = 2)	1.038	0.300	1.776	2.756	0.006 *
CTAR vs. CDT (n = 3)	1.045	0.427	1.663	3.316	0.001 *
EMST vs. no CDT (n = 2)	0.819	0.389	1.250	3.733	<0.001 *
Diagnostic groups					
Acquired Brain Injury (n = 1)	0.947	−0.247	2.141	1.554	0.120
Parkinson's disease (n = 1)	0.792	0.273	1.311	2.898	0.003 *
Stroke (n = 13)	0.731	0.474	0.988	5.573	<0.001 *
Outcome measures					
Superior hyoid displacement (n = 1)	0.994	−0.124	2.112	1.743	0.081
MASA (n = 2)	0.512	−0.574	1.599	0.925	0.355
PAS (n = 11)	0.804	0.572	1.036	6.789	<0.001 *
Tongue motility oromotor function (n = 1)	0.359	−0.470	1.189	0.849	0.396

Notes. * Significant.

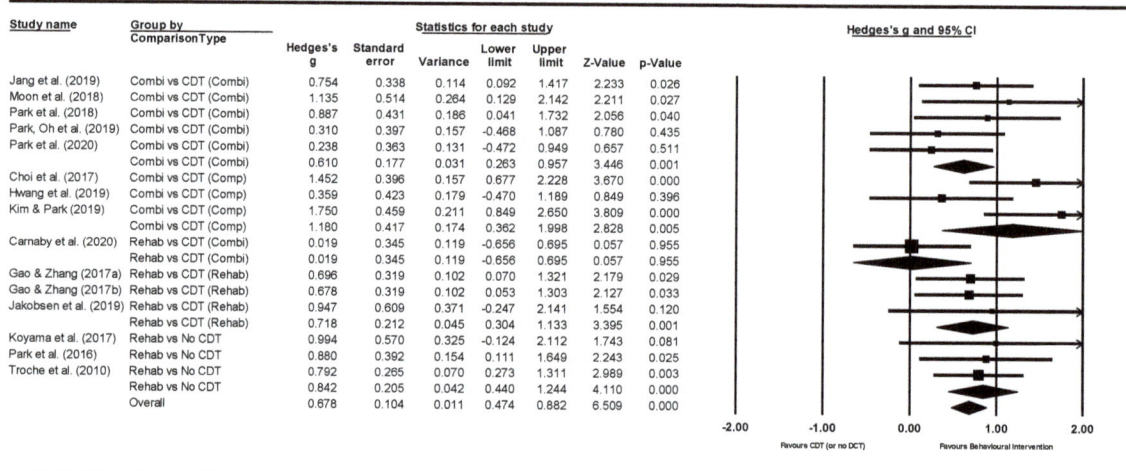

Figure 5. Between subgroup meta-analysis for different types of interventions: behavioural interventions compared with conventional dysphagia treatment (CDT) or no dysphagia therapy [21,22,25,29–31,34,35,41–44,46,52]. Note. Refer to Table 2 for explanation of the subgroups.

4. Discussion

This systematic review aimed to determine the effects of behavioural interventions in people with OD based on the highest level of evidence (RCTs) only. Findings from the literature were reported using PRISMA and meta-analysis procedures.

4.1. Systematic Review Findings

In total, 37 behavioural RCTs in OD were identified. Considering the high prevalence [3] and severe impact of OD on health [57], quality of life [5,58], and health-economics [59], the limited number of high-level evidence studies is concerning. RCTs are costly and usually require extensive funding [60]. Possibly, the general lack of awareness of OD [61] might place funding applications in this research area at a disadvantage when competing with well-known, life-threatening diseases such as cancer or stroke. Although OD is a symptom of these diseases, and many other underlying conditions, limited public knowledge persists, resulting in reduced understanding and recognition of the devastating consequences of OD, in both health-care and non-health-care practitioners [61].

Further, although RCTs are characterised by random allocation and allocation concealment, few of the included studies included sufficient reporting on the processes of randomization and blinding. These finding are in line with current literature on quality assessments of RCTs [62,63], confirming that the risk of selection bias [63] and the success of blinding methods in RCTs [62] can often not be ascertained due to frequent poor reporting.

When comparing behavioural RCTs in OD, several methodological challenges arise. Authors may use different definitions for OD or fail to provide sufficient details when reporting on the swallowing problems of the included patient populations. Also, several studies used non-instrumental assessments (i.e., patient self-report or a screening tool) to identify or confirm OD, making the comparison between studies precarious. The use of a screening tool is especially problematic in identifying OD and cannot act as confirmation of OD. A screening tool's purpose is merely to identify patients at *risk* of OD, after which further assessment may confirm or refute the diagnosis [2]. Additionally, although instrumental assessment is considered the optimal tool for confirming OD diagnosis, VFSS and FEES protocols may differ (e.g., using different numbers of swallow trials, viscosities, and volumes).

Studies used a wide range of outcome measures to evaluate treatment effects. Since OD is a multidimensional phenomenon [64], different dimensions of OD may result in different therapy outcomes. For example, changes in dysphagia-related quality of life or oral intake do not necessarily correlate with findings from instrumental assessment. As such, to reduce heterogeneity in meta-analyses, patient self-report and oral intake measures were excluded. Also, some studies included outcome measures with poor or unknown psychometric properties, which in turn undermines the interpretation of treatment effects as data may not be valid or reliable. In addition, measures with weak responsiveness characteristics are not sensitive to treatment changes and should therefore be avoided as outcome measures aiming to determine intervention effects [2].

Most studies included a combined rehabilitative and compensatory intervention group or a rehabilitative intervention group, with only a few studies including exclusively compensatory groups. As the interventions classified as CDT comparison groups showed large variation as well, CDT comparison groups were categorised into similar group types (compensatory and/or rehabilitative CDT). Overall, terminology in the literature referring to CDT comparison groups was varied and complex. This was especially pertinent when interventions were not described in sufficient detail and descriptive terms such as "usual care" or "traditional therapy" did not provide further clarity on the type or content of CDT provided. Despite using categories to group different types of interventions, some degree of heterogeneity was inevitable. Interventions used different types of exercises or care, in distinct dosages, and were applied by different health care professionals. Therefore, it is challenging to identify the "active" ingredients of individual interventions, especially as most studies combined the use of different treatment strategies.

4.2. Meta-Analysis Findings

When considering meta-analyses for behavioural interventions, overall significant treatment effects were identified as favouring behavioural interventions over CDT and withholding dysphagia therapy. Most promising intervention approaches were rehabilitative interventions, which were associated with large effect sizes. Additionally, rehabilitative interventions such as Shaker exercise, CTAR exercise, and EMST showed significant, large effect sizes. However, since most studies included in the meta-analysis provided data on stroke patients only, future research still needs to confirm these findings in other diagnostic populations such as Parkinson's disease, acquired brain injury or patients with head and neck oncology. As stated above, patient self-report and oral intake measures were excluded from meta-analyses to increase homogeneity between studies. Though self-report and oral intake data might be interesting for future meta-analyses, this would require additional RCTs to be published, as currently there is limited data available in the literature. Finally, future studies should report on treatment dosage and duration in more detail. Due to high heterogeneity between studies and incomplete reporting, no subgroup meta-analyses could be conducted for these variables.

4.3. Limitations

Although reporting of this review followed the PRISMA guidelines to reduce bias, some limitations are inherent to this study. As only RCTs published in English were included, some RCTs may have been excluded based on language criteria. In addition, meta-analyses were restricted because of heterogeneity of the included studies. As such, comparisons across studies are challenging and, generalisations and meta-analyses results should be interpreted with caution.

5. Conclusions

Meta-analyses for behavioural studies in oropharyngeal dysphagia identified an overall, significant, large pre-post interventions effect size. Significant treatment effects were identified favouring behavioural interventions over conventional dysphagia treatment. Notably, large effect sizes were found when comparing rehabilitative interventions with no dysphagia treatment and combined interventions with compensatory conventional dysphagia treatment. Selected interventions compared with conventional dysphagia treatment showed significant, large effect sizes in favour of Shaker exercise, CTAR, and EMST.

Behavioural interventions show promising effects in people with oropharyngeal dysphagia. Still, generalisations from this meta-analysis need to be interpreted with care due to high heterogeneity across studies.

Supplementary Materials: The following supporting information can be downloaded at: https://www.mdpi.com/article/10.3390/jcm11030685/s1, Table S1: PRISMA 2020 for Abstracts Checklist; Table S2: PRISMA 2020 Checklist.

Author Contributions: Conceptualization: R.S., R.C., A.-L.S., L.B. Formal analysis: R.S., R.C. Methodology: R.S., R.C. Project administration: R.S., R.C. Validation: R.S., R.C. Writing–review & editing: R.S., R.C., A.-L.S., L.R., B.J.H., M.B., T.P., M.M., L.B. All authors have read and agreed to the published version of the manuscript.

Funding: This research received no external funding.

Conflicts of Interest: The authors declare no conflict of interest.

References

1. Kertscher, B.; Speyer, R.; Fong, E.; Georgiou, A.; Smith, M. Prevalence of oropharyngeal dysphagia in the Netherlands: A telephone survey. *Dysphagia* **2015**, *30*, 114–120. [CrossRef] [PubMed]
2. Speyer, R.; Cordier, R.; Farneti, D.; Nascimento, W.; Pilz, W.; Verin, E.; Walshe, M.; Woisard, V. White paper by the European society for Swallowing Disorders: Screening and non-instrumental assessment for dysphagia in adults. *Dysphagia* **2021**. [CrossRef] [PubMed]
3. Takizawa, C.; Gemmell, E.; Kenworthy, J.; Speyer, R. A systematic review of the prevalence of oropharyngeal dysphagia in stroke, Parkinson's disease, Alzheimer's disease, head injury, and pneumonia. *Dysphagia* **2016**, *31*, 434–441. [CrossRef] [PubMed]
4. Speyer, R.; Cordier, R.; Kim, J.-H.; Cock, N.; Michou, E.; Wilkes-Gillan, S. Prevalence of drooling, feeding and swallowing problems in cerebral palsy across the lifespan: Systematic review and meta-analysis. *Dev. Med. Child Neurol.* **2019**, *61*, 1249–1258. [CrossRef] [PubMed]

5. Jones, E.; Speyer, R.; Kertscher, B.; Swan, K.; Wagg, B.; Cordier, R. Health-related quality of life in oropharyngeal dysphagia. *Dysphagia* **2018**, *33*, 141–172. [CrossRef] [PubMed]
6. Speyer, R. (Ed.) *Behavioural Treatment of Oropharyngeal Dysphagia*; Springer: Berlin/Heidelberg, Germany, 2018.
7. Speyer, R.; Baijens, L.; Heijnen, M.; Zwijnenberg, I. The effects of therapy in oropharyngeal dysphagia by speech therapists: A systematic review. *Dysphagia* **2010**, *25*, 40–65. [CrossRef] [PubMed]
8. Foley, N.; Teasell, R.; Salter, K.; Kruger, E.; Martino, R. Dysphagia treatment post stroke: A systematic review of randomised controlled trials. *Age Ageing* **2008**, *37*, 258–264. [CrossRef]
9. Cheng, I.; Sasegbon, A.; Hamdy, S. Effects of neurostimulation on poststroke dysphagia: A synthesis of current evidence from randomised controlled trials. *Neuromodulation Technol. Neural Interface* **2021**, *24*, 1388–1401. [CrossRef]
10. National Health and Medical Research Council. *Guidelines for the Development and Implementation of Clinical Guidelines*, 1st ed.; Australian Government Publishing Service: Canberra, Australia, 1995.
11. Page, M.J.; McKenzie, J.E.; Bossuyt, P.M.; Boutron, I.; Hoffmann, T.C.; Mulrow, C.D.; Shamseer, L.; Tetzlaff, J.M.; Aki, E.A.; Brennan, S.E.; et al. The PRISMA 2020 statement: An updated guideline for reporting systematic reviews. *Brittish Med. J.* **2021**, *372*, n71. [CrossRef]
12. Page, M.J.; Moher, D.; Bossuyt, P.M.; Boutron, I.; Hoffmann, T.C.; Mulrow, C.D.; Shamseer, L.; Tetzlaff, J.M.; Akl, E.A.; Brennan, S.E.; et al. PRISMA 2020 explanation and elaboration: Updated guidance and exemplars for reporting systematic reviews. *Brittish Med. J.* **2021**, *372*, n160. [CrossRef]
13. Sterne, J.; Savović, J.; Page, M.; Elbers, R.; Blencowe, N.; Boutron, I.; Cates, C.; Cheng, H.-Y.; Corbett, M.; Eldridge, S.; et al. RoB 2: A revised tool for assessing risk of bias in randomised trials. *Brittish Med. J.* **2019**, *366*, 14898. [CrossRef] [PubMed]
14. Borenstein, M.; Hedges, L.; Higgins, J.; Rothstein, H. *Comprehensive Meta-Analysis*; Biostat: Englewood, NJ, USA, 2014; Volume 3.
15. Higgins, J.P.T.; Thompson, S.G.; Deeks, J.J.; Altman, D.G. Measuring inconsistency in meta-analyses. *Brittish Med. J.* **2003**, *327*, 557–560. [CrossRef] [PubMed]
16. Cohen, J. *Statistical Power Analysis for the Behavioural Sciences*; Lawrence Erlbaum Associates: Hillsdale, NJ, USA, 1988.
17. Begg, C.B.; Mazumdar, M. Operating characteristics of a rank correlation test for publication bias. *Biometrics* **1994**, *50*, 1088–1101. [CrossRef] [PubMed]
18. Rosenthal, R. The file drawer problem and tolerance for null results. *Psychol. Bull.* **1979**, *86*, 638–664. [CrossRef]
19. Ayres, A.; Jotz, G.P.; Rieder, C.R.M.; Olchik, M.R. Benefit from the Chin-Down Maneuver in the swallowing performance and self-perception of Parkinson's Disease patients. *Parkinson's Dis.* **2017**, *8*. [CrossRef]
20. Carnaby, G.; Hankey, G.J.; Pizzi, J. Behavioural intervention for dysphagia in acute stroke: A randomised controlled trial. *Lancet Neurol.* **2006**, *5*, 31–37. [CrossRef]
21. Carnaby, G.; LaGorio, L.; Silliman, S.; Crary, M. Exercise-based swallowing intervention (McNeill Dysphagia Therapy) with adjunctive NMES to treat dysphagia post stroke: A double blind placebo-controlled trial. *J. Oral Rehabil.* **2020**, *47*, 501–510. [CrossRef] [PubMed]
22. Choi, J.-B.; Shim, S.-H.; Yang, J.-E.; Kim, H.-D.; Lee, D.-H.; Park, J.-S. Effects of Shaker exercise in stroke survivors with orophagyngeal dysphagia. *Neurorehabilitation* **2017**, *41*, 753–757. [CrossRef]
23. DePippo, K.L.; Holas, M.A.; Reding, M.J.; Mandel, F.S.; Lesser, M.L. Dysphagia therapy following stroke: A controlled trial. *Neurology* **1994**, *44*, 1655–1660. [CrossRef]
24. Eom, M.-J.; Chang, M.-Y.; Oh, D.-H.; Kim, H.-D.; Han, N.-M.; Park, J.-S. Effects of resistance expiratory muscle strength training in elderly patients with dysphagic stroke. *Neurorehabilitation* **2017**, *41*, 747–752. [CrossRef]
25. Gao, J.; Zhang, H.-J. Effects of chin tuck against resistance exercise versus Shaker exercise on dysphagia and psychological state after cerebral infarction. *Eur. J. Phys. Rehabil. Med.* **2017**, *53*, 426–432. [CrossRef] [PubMed]
26. Guillén-Solà, A.; Sartor, M.M.; Soler, N.B.; Duarte, E.; Barrera, M.C.; Marco, E. Respiratory muscle strength training and neuromuscular electrical stimulation in subacute dysphagic stroke patients: A randomized controlled trial. *Clin. Rehabil.* **2016**, *31*, 761–771. [CrossRef] [PubMed]
27. Hägglund, P.; Hägg, M.; Wester, P.; Jäghagen, E.L. Effects of oral neuromuscular training on swallowing dysfunction among older people in intermediate care—A cluster randomised, controlled trial. *Age Aging* **2019**, *48*, 533–540. [CrossRef] [PubMed]
28. Hägglund, P.; Hägg, M.; Jäghagen, E.L.; Larsson, B.; Wester, P. Oral neuromuscular training in patients with dysphagia after stroke: A prospective, randomized, open-label study with blinded evaluators. *BMC Neurol.* **2020**, *20*, 1–10. [CrossRef] [PubMed]
29. Hwang, N.-K.; Kim, H.-H.; Shim, J.-M.; Park, J.-S. Tongue stretching exercises improve tongue motility and oromotor function in patients with dysphagia after stroke: A preliminary randomized controlled trial. *Arch. Oral Biol.* **2019**, *108*, 104521. [CrossRef] [PubMed]
30. Jakobsen, D.; Poulson, I.; Schultheiss, C.; Riberholt, C.G.; Curtis, D.J.; Peterson, T.H.; Seidl, R.O. The effect of intensified nonverbal facilitation of swallowing on dysphagia after severe acquired brain injury: A randomised controlled pilot study. *Neurorehabilitation* **2019**, *45*, 525–536. [CrossRef] [PubMed]
31. Jang, K.W.; Lee, S.J.; Kim, S.B.; Lee, K.W.; Lee, J.H.; Park, J.G. Effects of mechanical inspiration and expiration exercise on velopharyngeal incompetence in subacute stroke patients. *J. Rehabil. Med.* **2019**, *51*, 97–102. [CrossRef] [PubMed]
32. Jeon, Y.H.; Cho, K.H.; Park, S.J. Effects of Neuromuscular Electrical Stimulation (NMES) plus upper cervical spine mobilization on forward head posture and swallowing function in stroke patients with dysphagia. *Brain Sci.* **2020**, *10*, 478. [CrossRef]

33. Kim, K.D.; Lee, H.J.; Lee, M.H.; Ruy, H.J. Effects of neck exercises on swallowing function of patients with stroke. *J. Phys. Ther. Sci.* **2015**, *27*, 1005–1008.
34. Kim, H.-H.; Park, J.-S. Efficacy of modified chin tuck against resistance exercise using hand-free device for dysphagia in stroke survivors: A randomised controlled trial. *J. Oral Rehabil.* **2019**, *46*, 1042–1046. [CrossRef]
35. Koyama, Y.; Sugimoto, A.; Hamano, T.; Kasahara, T.; Toyojura, M.; Masakado, Y. Proposal for a modified jaw opening exercise for dysphagia: A randomized, controlled Trial. *Tokai J. Exp. Clin. Med.* **2017**, *42*, 71–78. [PubMed]
36. Krajczy, E.; Krajczy, M.; Luniewski, J.; Bogacz, K.; Szczegielniak, J. Assessment of the effects of dysphagia therapy in patients in the early post-stroke period: A randomised controlled trial. *Neurol. I Neurochir. Pol.* **2019**, *53*, 428–434. [CrossRef] [PubMed]
37. Kyodo, R.; Kudo, T.; Horiuchi, A.; Sakamoto, T.; Shimizu, T. Pureed diets containing a gelling agent to reduce the risk of aspiration in elderly patients with moderate to severe dysphagia. *Medicine* **2020**, *99*, e21165. [CrossRef] [PubMed]
38. Logemann, J.A.; Gensler, G.; Robbins, J.; Lindbland, A.S.; Brandt, D.; Hind, J.A.; Kosek, S.; Dikeman, K.; Kazandjian, M.; Gramigna, G.D.; et al. A randomized study of three interventions for aspiration of thin liquids in patients with dementia or Parkinson's Disease. *J. Speech Lang. Hear. Res.* **2008**, *51*, 173–183. [CrossRef]
39. Manor, Y.; Mootanah, R.; Freud, D.; Giladi, M.; Cohen, J.T. Video-assisted swallowing therapy for patients with Parkinson's disease. *Parkinsonism Relat. Disord.* **2013**, *19*, 207–211. [CrossRef]
40. Mepani, R.; Antonik, S.; Massey, B.; Kern, M.; Logemann, J.A.; Pauloski, B.R.; Rademaker, A.; Easterling, C.; Shaker, R. Augmentation of deglutitive thyrohyoid muscle shortening by the Shaker Exercise. *Dysphagia* **2009**, *24*, 26–31. [CrossRef]
41. Moon, J.-H.; Hahm, S.-C.; Won, Y.S.; Cho, H.-Y. The effects of tongue pressure strength and accuracy training on tongue pressure strength, swallowing function, and quality of life in subacute stroke patients with dysphagia: A preliminary randomized clinical trial. *Int. J. Rehabil. Res.* **2018**, *41*, 204–210. [CrossRef] [PubMed]
42. Park, J.-S.; Oh, D.-H.; Chang, M.-Y.; Kim, K.M. Effects of expiratory muscle strength training on oropharyngeal dysphagia in subacute stroke patients: A randomised controlled trial. *J. Oral Rehabil.* **2016**, *43*, 364–372. [CrossRef]
43. Park, J.-S.; An, D.-H.; Oh, D.-H.; Chang, M.-Y. Effect of chin tuck against resistance exercise on patients with dysphagia following stroke: A randomized pilot study. *Neurorehabilitation* **2018**, *42*, 191–197. [CrossRef]
44. Park, H.-S.; Oh, D.-H.; Yoon, T.; Park, J.-S. Effect of effortful swallowing training on tongue strength and oropharyngeal swallowing function in stroke patients with dysphagia: A double-blind, randomized controlled trial. *Int. J. Lang. Commun. Disord.* **2019**, *54*, 479–484. [CrossRef]
45. Park, J.-S.; Lee, G.; Jung, Y.-J. Effects of game-based chin tuck against resistance exercise vs head-lift exercise in patients with dysphagia after stroke: An assessor-blind, randomized controlled. *J. Rehabil. Med.* **2019**, *51*, 749–754. [CrossRef] [PubMed]
46. Park, J.-S.; An, D.-H.; Kam, K.-Y.; Yoon, T.; Kim, T.; Chang, M.-Y. Effects of resistive jaw opening exercise in stroke patients with dysphagia: A doubleblind, randomized controlled study. *J. Back Musculoskelet. Rehabil.* **2020**, *33*, 507–513. [CrossRef] [PubMed]
47. Ploumis, A.; Papadopoulou, S.L.; Theodorou, S.J.; Exarchakos, G.; Givissis, P.; Beris, A. Cervical isometric exercises improve dysphagia and cervical spine malalignment following stroke with hemiparesis: A randomized controlled trial. *Eur. J. Phys. Rehabil. Med.* **2018**, *54*, 845–852. [CrossRef] [PubMed]
48. Sayaca, C.; Serel-Arslan, S.; Sayaca, N.; Demir, N.; Somay, G.; Kaya, D.; Karaduman, A. Is the proprioceptive neuromuscular facilitation technique superior to Shaker exercises in swallowing rehabilitation? *Eur. Arch. Oto-Rhino-Laryngology* **2020**, *277*, 497–504. [CrossRef] [PubMed]
49. Steele, C.M.; Bayley, M.T.; Peladeau-Pigeon, M.; Nagy, A.; Namasivayam, A.M.; Stokely, S.L.; Wolkin, T. A randomized trial comparing two tongue-pressure resistance training protocols for post-stroke dysphagia. *Dysphagia* **2016**, *31*, 452–461. [CrossRef] [PubMed]
50. Tang, Y.; Shen, Q.; Wang, Y.; Lu, K.; Wang, Y.; Peng, Y. A randomized prospective study of rehabilitation therapy in the treatment of radiation-induced dysphagia and trismus. *Strahlenther. Onkol.* **2011**, *187*, 39–44. [CrossRef] [PubMed]
51. Tarameshlu, M.; Ghelichi, L.; Azimi, A.R.; Ansari, N.N.; Khatoonabadi, A.R. The effect of traditional dysphagia therapy on the swallowing function in patients with Multiple Sclerosis: A pilot double-blinded randomized controlled trial. *J. Bodyw. Mov. Ther.* **2019**, *23*, 171–176. [CrossRef]
52. Troche, M.S.; Okun, M.S.; Rosenbek, J.C.; Musson, N.; Fernandez, H.H.; Rodriguez, R.; Romrell, J.; Pitts, T.; Wheeler-Hegland, K.M.; Sapienza, C.M. Aspiration and swallowing in Parkinson disease and rehabilitation with EMST: A randomized trial. *Neurology* **2010**, *75*, 1912–1919. [CrossRef]
53. Wakabayashi, H.; Matsushima, M.; Momosaki, R.; Yoshida, S.; Mutai, R.; Yodoshi, T.; Murayama, S.; Hayashi, T.; Horiguchi, R.; Ichikawa, H. The effects of resistance training of swallowing muscles on dysphagia in older people: A cluster, randomized, controlled trial. *Nutrition* **2018**, *48*, 111–116. [CrossRef]
54. Woisard, V.; Costes, M.; Colineaux, H.; Lepage, B. How a personalised transportable folding device for seating impacts dysphagia. *Eur. Arch. Oto-Rhino-Laryngology* **2020**, *277*, 179–188. [CrossRef]
55. Zhang, R.; Ju, X.-M. Clinical improvement of nursing intervention in swallowing dysfunction of elderly stroke patients. *Biomed. Res.* **2018**, *29*, 1099–1102. [CrossRef]
56. Ahn, Y.H.; Sohn, H.-J.; Park, J.-S.; Ahn, T.G.; Shin, Y.B.; Park, M.; Ko, S.-H.; Shin, Y.-I. Effect of bihemispheric anodal transcranial direct current stimulation for dysphagia in chronic stroke patients: A randomized control trial. *J. Rehabil. Med.* **2017**, *49*, 30–35. [CrossRef] [PubMed]

57. Eltringham, S.A.; Kilner, K.; Gee, M.; Sage, K.; Bray, B.D.; Smith, C.J.; Pownall, S. Factors associated with risk of stroke-associated pneumonia in patients with dysphagia: A systematic review. *Dysphagia* **2020**, *35*, 735–744. [CrossRef] [PubMed]
58. Ninfa, A.; Crispiatico, V.; Pizzorni, N.; Bassi, M.; Casazza, G.; Schindler, A.; Delle Fave, A. The care needs of persons with oropharyngeal dysphagia and their informal caregivers: A scoping review. *PLoS ONE* **2021**, *9*, e0257683. [CrossRef]
59. Attrill, S.; White, S.; Murray, J.; Hammond, S.; Doeltgen, S. Impact of oropharyngeal dysphagia on healthcare cost and length of stay in hospital: A systematic review. *BMC Health Serv. Res.* **2018**, *18*, 594. [CrossRef]
60. Speich, B.; von Niederhäusern, B.; Schur, N.; Hemkens, L.G.; Fürst, T.; Bhatnagar, N.; Alturki, R.; Agarwal, A.; Kasenda, B.; Pauli-Magnus, C.; et al. Systematic review on costs and resource use of randomized clinical trials shows a lack of transparent and comprehensive data. *J. Clin. Epidemiol.* **2018**, *96*, 1–11. [CrossRef]
61. McHutchion, L.D.; Pringle, J.M.; Tran, M.-H.N.; Ostevik, A.V.; Constantinescu, G. A survey of public awareness of dysphagia. *Int. J. Speech-Lang. Pathol.* **2021**, *23*, 614–621. [CrossRef]
62. Hróbjartsson, A.; Forfang, E.; Haahr, M.T.; Als-Nielsen, B.; Brorson, S. Blinded trials taken to the test: An analysis of randomised clinical trials that report tests for the success of blinding. *Int. J. Epidemiol.* **2007**, *36*, 654–663. [CrossRef]
63. Kahan, B.C.; Rehal, S.; Cro, S. Risk of selection bias in randomised trials. *Trials* **2015**, *16*, 1–7. [CrossRef]
64. Baijens, L.W.; Clave, P.; Cras, P.; Ekberg, O.; Forster, A.; Kolb, G.F.; Leners, J.C.; Masiero, S.; Mateos-Nozal, J.; Ortego, O.; et al. European Society for Swallowing Disorders—European Union Geriatric Medicine Society white paper: Oropharyngeal dysphagia as a geriatric syndrome. *Clin. Interv. Aging* **2016**, *11*, 1403–1428. [CrossRef]

MDPI
St. Alban-Anlage 66
4052 Basel
Switzerland
Tel. +41 61 683 77 34
Fax +41 61 302 89 18
www.mdpi.com

Journal of Clinical Medicine Editorial Office
E-mail: jcm@mdpi.com
www.mdpi.com/journal/jcm

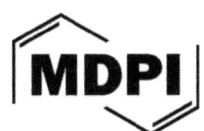

www.ingramcontent.com/pod-product-compliance
Lightning Source LLC
LaVergne TN
LVHW070139100526
838202LV00015B/1853